NEUROFIBROMATOSIS

NEUROFIBROMATOSIS
PHENOTYPE, NATURAL HISTORY, AND PATHOGENESIS

Third Edition

Edited by

J. M. FRIEDMAN, M.D., PH.D.
DAVID H. GUTMANN, M.D.-PH.D.
MIA MACCOLLIN, M.D.
VINCENT M. RICCARDI, M.D.

THE JOHNS HOPKINS UNIVERSITY PRESS

Baltimore and London

This book is dedicated to Elizabeth, Mark, Lindsay, Tony, and all of our other patients, who are our best teachers.

Note: Readers should scrutinize product information sheets for dosage changes or contraindications, particularly for new or infrequently used drugs.

© 1986, 1992, 1999 The Johns Hopkins University Press
All rights reserved. First edition 1986
Printed in the United States of America on acid-free paper
Third edition 1999
9 8 7 6 5 4 3 2 1

The Johns Hopkins University Press
2715 North Charles Street
Baltimore, Maryland 21218-4363
www.press.jhu.edu

Library of Congress Cataloging-in-Publication Data

Neurofibromatosis : phenotype, natural history, and pathogenesis / edited by J.M. Friedman . . . [et al.]. —3rd ed.
    p. cm.
 Includes bibliographical references and index.
 ISBN 0-80 18-6285-X (alk. paper)
 1. Neurofibromatosis.   I. Friedman, J. M. (Jan Marshall), 1947–.
II. Riccardi, Vincent M., 1940–   Neurofibromatosis.
 [DNLM: QZ 380 N4939 1999]
 RC280.N4R525 1999
 616.99'383—dc21
 DNLM/DLC
 for Library of Congress   99-27988
                                                CIP

A catalog record for this book is available from the British Library.

CONTENTS

II. **Neurofibromatosis 2**

FOREWORD

In 1986 Vincent Riccardi and Jan Eichner initiated a monograph on neurofibromatosis. In 1992 Riccardi continued it as a one-author production. It has now reached the perhaps inevitable evolutionary stage of multiple authorship. However, in the classic tradition it remains a collation of extensive personal experience, both in the clinic and in the laboratory, with an exhaustive survey of published records. Now the personal experience is amplified by the multiple authorship.

The first edition established this monograph as a standard source. The second edition appeared soon after the cloning of the genes that are mutant in the two major forms of neurofibromatosis. Only now are we beginning to appreciate the full implications of the basic molecular information—for diagnosis, prognosis, management, and counseling—in addition to understanding the mechanisms by which the mutations (genotype) cause the features of the clinical disorders (phenotype).

Since the last edition, the new genetic information has proved useful in sorting out genetic heterogeneity and phenotypic variability. Careful clinical analysis is even more important now that the possibilities exist for molecular–genetic correlations.

In its previous editions, this book found wide interest and use among health professionals because of the pleiotropic behavior of both the *NF1* and the *NF2* genes, that is, the variety of clinical manifestations. Dermatologists, neurologists, orthopedists, pediatricians, and ophthalmologists are only a few of the medical specialists who care for patients with this group of disorders. Indeed, any physician who is called on to care for such a patient or family should find the book helpful.

Another important group that will welcome this monograph is made up of the families of patients and the patients themselves. An intelligent and well-informed public now expects, and is entitled to, reliable and up-to-date information about the rare disorders that affect selected individuals. A response to that imperative for information is the extensive development of support organizations for individuals with single genetic disorders, with mainly lay leadership. The appendix on resources for patients and their families should prove useful.

This monograph is of general interest to clinical geneticists because it covers a group of disorders that is an important one among the many they treat. The neurofibromatoses illustrate well the three cardinal principles of clinical genetics: pleiotropism and genetic heterogeneity (already referred to) and variability (even within a given family), which we have come to expect of dominantly inherited disorders.

Finally, it can be expected that this monograph will continue to provide useful background to basic scientists who engage in the effort to reveal the remaining fundamental mysteries that surround these rather frequent disorders.

Victor A. McKusick, M.D.
University Professor of Medical Genetics
McKusick-Nathans Institute of Genetic Medicine
Johns Hopkins University School of Medicine

FOREWORD

It has been said that we have learned more about the neurofibromatoses during the past 10 years than during the prior 100. Despite this impressive progress, most physicians around the world are still not very familiar with the diagnosis and management of NF1 and NF2. This can result in a quality of patient care that varies widely and is sometimes substandard—even in developed nations. Those of us involved with patient support groups have heard countless tragic stories from patients and families about nondiagnosis, misdiagnosis, and poor patient care.

This book will make enormous strides toward remedying that situation. The editors have brought together many of the world's leading specialists in neurofibromatosis. Collectively, they represent the major research and clinical areas in NF1 and NF2. These experts give us the current state of knowledge in a clear, detailed, and useful way. Thus, they offer an invaluable reference work for scientists, physicians, and other health care professionals, as well as for people with neurofibromatosis and their families.

Reading the various chapters, it becomes clear that neurofibromatosis is an important research model for cancer and for the development of the nervous system. This growing realization makes an even more compelling case that NF should receive more attention from scientists and medical professionals than it has in the past.

The authors do the reader a valuable service with their candor about the areas where more information is needed. By doing so, they sketch for us the likely road ahead, and they challenge the medical and scientific communities to redouble the energies and resources needed to bring the neurofibromatoses under effective control.

The editors and authors deserve our thanks for such a timely, useful, and well-written volume.

Peter Bellermann
President, The National Neurofibromatosis Foundation, Inc.
Chair, The International Neurofibromatosis Association (Luxembourg)

FOREWORD

The third edition of *Neurofibromatosis: Phenotype, Natural History, and Pathogenesis* continues the tradition of presenting the neurofibromatoses in both clinical and laboratory settings. This updated volume covering both NF1 and NF2 provides a ready reference for the two separate but related genetic disorders. It will promote a better understanding of the neurofibromatoses, which are often confusing to both health professionals and patients.

The addition of new contributors to this edition expands the base of knowledge. It provides health professionals, medical specialists, educators, and social workers with a basic understanding of the various clinical manifestations of the neurofibromatoses. Patients with neurofibromatosis and their families will embrace this latest edition, which contains up-to-date information from some of the best-known clinicians and researchers in the field. These patients, families, and the NF support groups that represent them will be delighted with the efforts of the authors.

I anticipate that the book will be widely used as a reference by patients with newly diagnosed disease, by those experiencing new manifestations, by their families and by NF support groups. Professionals (including NF clinic staff) such as dermatologists, neurologists, neurosurgeons, ophthalmologists, pediatricians, orthopedists, geneticists, educators, and social workers will find this book useful when seeking to understand and explain the issues related to diagnosis, clinical features and complications, and eventually the treatment of patients. The book will be an important one for students during the academic portion of their medical training—an entire volume devoted to neurofibromatosis rather than a few paragraphs of text and a listing in the glossary.

This comprehensive book attempts to reach all of the population involved with issues related to the neurofibromatoses. The past 20 years have provided basic understanding of the many components involved in these complex disorders. Now support groups for the diverse population of patients with NF expect researchers working with these patients to bring this knowledge back to the public in understandable and useful forms. This book is a significant response to this quest for information.

Brenda Duffy
President, Neurofibromatosis, Inc.

PREFACE

Maybe it's a bit of wishful thinking, but, perhaps, the combination of clinical sensitivity, scientific commitment, esthetic and social sensibilities, and modest writing abilities allowed earlier editions of this book to influence how scientific, clinical, and medical-consumer populations currently approach neurofibromatosis (NF)—or, better yet, the neurofibromatoses. The author common to all three editions of this book began his commitment to NF in February 1972. NF-land back then was a lonely place. Actually, the key reasons he dedicated his attention to NF were to derive new information and to organize both old and new information so as to recruit more participants to explore this otherwise poorly charted territory.

Whatever the casual relationships, in the past two decades, the disorders labeled NF and the genes specified as *Nf1* and *Nf2* and their respective gene products, neurofibromin and schwannomin, have created an excitement about the disorder and its pathogenesis in general. This book looks to abet that excitement. The love affair with NF of the book's authors and the other contributors make clear how the neurofibromatoses and other diseases are vanquished: multiple areas of intense focus by researchers and clinicians representing many disciplines.

What do the *Nf1* and *Nf2* genes do? And how do mutations in them cause disease? And, specifically, how do they cause disease in humans? There are only a few clear-cut answers in 2000. But, we're close to major breakthroughs and we trust that we are contributing to that closeness by what we share with you in this book

This book is different from the two previous editions in several ways. Multiple authors and invited contributors from various disciplines will likely enhance the authoritativeness of both the clinical and the scientific sections. NF is no longer simply a "neurocutaneous disorder" or a "neurocristopathy." Rather, echoing the earlier editions, the neurofibromatoses are heterogeneous and involve many different organs and tissues and require analyses from many different disciplines, including clinical, epidemiologic, biochemical, and molecular and in terms of animal models and cell physiology. This fact is obvious in subsequent pages.

This edition combines the Neurofibromatosis Institute Database with the International NF Database under the aegis of Dr. Jan Friedman and the National

NF Foundation. The homogeneity of the former and the size and heterogeneity of the latter make the robust analyses that the reader is likely to find especially informative.

In this edition, there is an increased emphasis on NF2, in both clinical and molecular terms.

There is less speculation and less focus on peripherally related topics (e.g., veterinary neurofibromas and schwannomas). The first edition of this book filled a vacuum. It was, thus, eclectic in nature, with anything possibly related to NF included, primarily to challenge other investigators and clinicians. The second edition was published just as molecular genetic facts began filtering into our knowledge base about NF1 and NF2, and the NIH Consensus Conference had just adopted the nomenclature and precepts outlined in the first edition. Specifically, NF1 and NF2 were not simply phrases coined by or useful to the Baylor NF Program. Now that we all know what NF1 and NF2 are by molecular and broad consensus criteria, the foci of the book have changed.

Relying on clinical data from around the world, we provide our readers the most up-to-date clinical guidance available.

Join us in our elaboration of facts and ideas about the neurofibromatoses as a celebration of both the progress we have made and the potential for the future.

Vincent M. Riccardi, M.D.

ACKNOWLEDGMENTS

The authors wish to achnowledge the love from our families that was vital to our undertaking and completing the work involved in writing this book. Similarly, we wish to thank our many patients with and at-risk for NF1 and NF2. Every one of them taught us something about the neurofibromatoses, and many of them contributed time and, often, samples of themselves to further both clinical and basic research on these fascinating disorders. In keeping with the precedent of the first two editions of the book, the author common to all three editions also wishes to acknowledge the continued support of The Neurofibromatosis Institute, the Salaam wa Saha Fund, the Texas NF Foundation, and Mr. Mark Wagner and his family in Dallas, Texas.

We are very grateful to Dr. Lewis Holmes for his critical reading of this entire book in manuscript and for his valuable suggestions for its improvement. We appreciate Jacek Szudek and Kimberly DeBella's allowing us to include their unpublished analyses of data from the National Neurofibromatosis Foundation International Database. We are grateful to Patricia Birch for her helpful comments on the manuscript and to Nancy North for secretarial assistance. We also appreciate the assistance that Wendy Harris, our editor at the Johns Hopkins University Press, provided in bringing all three editions of this book to fruition.

CONTRIBUTORS

J. M. Friedman, M.D., Ph.D., Professor and Head, Department of Medical Genetics, University of British Columbia, Vancouver, British Columbia, Canada

James G. Gurney, Ph.D., Assistant Professor, Department of Pediatrics, University of Minnesota, Minneapolis, Minnesota

James F. Gusella, Ph.D., Professor, Department of Genetics, Harvard Medical School; and Director, Molecular Neurogenetics Unit, Massachusetts General Hospital, Boston, Massachusetts

David H. Gutmann, M.D.-Ph.D., Associate Professor of Neurology, Pediatrics, and Genetics, Washington University School of Medicine; and Director, Neurofibromatosis Program, St. Louis Children's Hospital, St. Louis, Missouri

Bruce R. Korf, M.D., Ph.D., Associate Chief, Division of Genetics, Children's Hospital and Harvard Medical School, Boston, Massachusetts

Robert Listernick, M.D., Associate Professor, Department of Pediatrics, Northwestern University Medical School; Co-Director, Neurofibromatosis Clinic, Division of General Academic Pediatrics, Children's Memorial Hospital, Chicago, Illinois

Mia MacCollin, M.D., Assistant Professor, Department of Neurology, Harvard Medical School, Boston, Massachusetts

Kathryn North, M.D., B.Sc., Head, Neurogenetics Research Unit, Royal Alexandra Hospital for Children, University of Sydney, New South Wales, Australia

Vincent M. Riccardi, M.D., President, American Medical Consumers, La Crescenta, California

Anat Stemmer-Rachamimov, M.D., Instructor, Department of Pathology, Harvard Medical School, Boston, Massachusetts

David H. Viskochil, M.D., Ph.D., Associate Professor, Department of Pediatrics, University of Utah, Salt Lake City, Utah

NEUROFIBROMATOSIS

1

Historical Background and Introduction

Vincent M. Riccardi, M.D.

HISTORICAL PERSPECTIVES

Neurofibromatosis, or NF, is not a new or recently discovered disease or set of diseases. The most common form, NF1, known worldwide as von Recklinghausen disease for Friedrich von Recklinghausen (Warkany 1981), has been well recognized since 1882 (Crump 1981; von Recklinghausen 1882). The second well-known form, NF2, was characterized in the 1930s and specified as an entity distinct from NF1 in 1981 by Riccardi (Riccardi 1981c). Artistic renderings of presumed NF1 patients have been available as early as the fifteenth century (Madigan and Masello 1988; Zanca 1980). Medical reports of NF1, preceding that of von Recklinghausen, included the eighteenth-century descriptions by Tilesius (1793) and Akenside (1785). Virchow (1857) and Hitchcock (1862) described this disorder in multiple family members, and its genetic nature was documented by Thomson (1900), Adrian (1901), and Prieser and Davenport (1918).

Since the end of the nineteenth century, there have been innumerable case reports and reviews from around the world. By the middle of the twentieth century, reasonably accurate broad surveys were published, most notably those of Borberg (1951) and Crowe, Schull, and Neel (1956). But clinical and investigative programs concentrating on NF as a disorder unto itself were not established until 1978 (Riccardi 1981b). In the meantime, the play, *The Elephant Man,* which dealt with the dual social standards of Victorian England, chronicled the life and travails of Joseph Merrick (Treves 1923). Merrick, often identified erroneously as John Merrick (Karp 1982), actually had the disorder known as *Proteus syndrome* (Cohen 1988), but was mistakenly thought to have NF1 and some of its most serious complications (Montague 1971; Sparks 1980). Although he did not have NF, the wide-scale assumption that he did and his heart-rending plight were nonetheless useful in bringing NF to public attention.

Direct analysis of genetic material, the DNA that constitutes the genes for NF1 and NF2, has allowed us to complement the clinical approach to understanding these diseases. Instead of proceeding from what we know about the disorder to the basic defect, we identify the basic defect at the DNA level and then work toward considering the disease features. Using this approach, we now have highly detailed information about the structure and function of both normal and mutant genes at the NF1 and NF2 loci in humans, mice, fruit flies, and other species.

Five major factors have modified our current approach to understanding the neurofibromatoses in general and NF1 and NF2 in particular:

1. the contributions of *molecular biology;*
2. the development of a number of high-quality, scientifically based *NF referral centers* for combinations of clinical care, clinical investigation, and basic research;
3. the use of *magnetic resonance imaging,* which has allowed both more precise anatomic definition of lesions and the potential for insight into the pathophysiology of at least some of the findings (e.g., the hyperintense T_2-weighted signal foci seen in the brains of the majority of young patients with NF1);
4. *computerized manipulation and dissemination of NF-related data and publications,* which have immensely enhanced our ability to identify and focus on specific features that otherwise might not be appreciated as particularly important; and
5. the identification or creation of a number of *animal models,* both of which have been exploited.

THE NEUROFIBROMATOSES

As we begin to make progress in understanding genotype–phenotype correlations and how the mutant gene actually causes problems, we should be differentiating the immediate consequences of the gene at the clinicopathologic level from secondary manifestations and later complications. Certainly, treatment strategies will be influenced by which stage of progress of the disease is being considered.

- A *primary feature* of NF is a primary clinicopathologic manifestation of the mutant gene (for example, a café-au-lait spot, a neurofibroma, iris Lisch nodules, or dysplastic vertebrae).
- A *secondary feature* is the clinicopathologic consequence of the primary feature's progression over time (for example, the dystrophic kyphoscoliosis that can result from dysplastic vertebrae).
- A *complication* is the clinicopathologic consequence of the secondary feature's progression (for example, spinal cord compression that results from dystrophic kyphoscoliosis). At times, distinguishing between secondary features and complications may not be straightforward. In addition, in some instances it may make sense to consider two or more levels of complication (for example, spinal cord impingement as the primary complication and the resulting paraplegia as a secondary complication, and so on).

- There may be occasion to refer merely to a generic *problem,* which could refer to a primary feature, a secondary feature, a complication, or any combination of them.

ROUTINE EVALUATION OF PATIENTS

The two prior editions of this book described a "routine evaluation protocol" and encouraged its application for the purposes of diagnosing, screening, or evaluating patients with or at risk for any of the neurofibromatoses (Riccardi 1988a, 1988b). That protocol includes:

> personal medical and developmental histories
> family history and pedigree construction
> physical examination, with emphasis on the skin, skeleton, and nervous system
> ophthalmologist's ocular examination
> IQ/psychologic testing
> neuroimaging (CT scan or MRI) of the orbits and brain
> plain radiographs of skull, chest, and spine
> electroencephalogram
> audiogram, brainstem auditory evoked response (BAER), or both.

The object of the evaluation in any given instance is determined by the needs of the situation, which fall into one of three general categories.

1. The diagnosis of NF of unspecified type is being entertained, but the initial three steps of the protocol leave a diagnosis wanting as to whether NF is even present or what the specific type of NF may be. Here, the purpose is to add data that will warrant the diagnosis of NF and, it is to be hoped, specify the type.
2. On general clinical grounds, the diagnosis of a specific type of NF is clear, with no immediate indications of current or potential serious problems. The purpose is to screen for less readily apparent or presymptomatic lesions. While I continue to urge its use in these regards, I also recognize that this approach is not universally accepted.
3. The type of NF diagnosis is clear, with one or more current or potentially serious problems. The issue is to provide a context for proceeding with the further evaluation of the presenting problem. Not infrequently, a patient with NF1 presenting with one type of problem actually has another problem of equal or greater severity that also demands attention.

Of course, every patient with or at risk for NF will be evaluated using the first four approaches, preferably by one or more persons expert in NF: history taking, pedigree construction, comprehensive physical examination, and ocular examination by an ophthalmologist. From a nosologic standpoint, the ocular examination by an ophthalmologist with the necessary aid of a slit-lamp biomicroscope is intended to identify Lisch nodules, optic gliomas, or other ocular complications that would warrant the diagnosis of NF1, or to identify subcapsular cataracts or other ocular findings that would abet the diagnosis of NF2. From a management standpoint, identifying problems, such as a visual deficit, before they become extreme or irreversible is a key impetus. Supplementation of the ocular examination with an electroretinogram or measurement of visual evoked response as a screening tool has been encouraged (Lund and Skovby 1991).

The rationale for neuroimaging studies of the brain and visual pathways is discussed from several vantage points throughout the book, especially in the chapters dealing with the nervous system (Chapter 8) and the eye (Chapter 9). Although there is some controversy over routine screening for optic pathway gliomas in young patients with NF1 (see Chapter 9), I am firm in my commitment to such routine screening. The "wait-and-see" approach is compromised by the fact that if an optic pathway glioma is present, the result is "wait and not see"; that is, permanent loss of vision is at stake.

Plain radiographs of the skull provide excellent means for identifying the presence and extent of sphenoid wing dysplasia and other craniofacial skeletal defects, particularly if the neuroimaging strategy relies on magnetic resonance imaging (MRI), which is relatively poor for bone definition.

Plain radiographs of the spine are useful for screening for the presence of paraspinal neurofibromas, vertebral scalloping or dysplasia, and scoliosis.

Plain radiographs of the chest are equally useful for identifying or documenting the presence of neurofibromas (or other tumors) impinging on the thoracic cavity, particularly at the pulmonary apices and in the mediastinum.

An electroencephalogram (EEG) is justified, perhaps arguably, by the high frequency of EEG abnormalities in NF1, even in the absence of seizures (see Chapter 8). From a practical standpoint in the long-term follow-up of patients with NF1, this is among the most useful of tests. Given the high likelihood of a positive finding, albeit nonspecific, the situation is similar to obtaining an electrocardiogram for someone with an increased risk of a cardiac arrhythmia: it just makes good sense to know as many details as possible about the patient's condition.

While the occurrence of a vestibular schwannoma is very rare in NF1, even if the diagnosis is unequivocally NF1, clarification of auditory abilities is particularly useful for children because of the high frequency of school performance problems. Therefore, I recommend an audiogram, a brainstem audio-evoked response (BAER) study, or both.

Certainly, all school-age children warrant an evaluation of cognitive and learning abilities, for reasons discussed extensively in Chapter 7.

NF HETEROGENEITY

Heterogeneity is critical to understanding NF. Even the most casual observers will appreciate such tremendous variation among patients with NF that they will promptly query whether NF is one disease or, alternatively, a series of clinically similar, but distinct disorders. A related question is whether all instances of café-au-lait spots or neurofibromas, schwannomas, optic gliomas, and so forth, represent NF in some form or another.

Given the increasing availability of analytical methods that focus on the genetic material itself, one might ask, why try to sort out the morass of heterogeneity from the clinical vantage point? Why not wait to employ molecular diagnostic methods and sort out the puzzle pieces that way? The concerns are several. First, we are still at a stage where clinical factors determine strategies and expectations. For example, there must be some clinical context for dealing with a positive molecular test result where a negative one was expected, and, conversely, for dealing with a negative result where a positive result was expected. Moreover, it will be many years before molecular diagnostic techniques can be applied uniformly and intelligently for all who might need them. Finally, for the vast majority of patients with NF1 or NF2, molecular techniques are not required for most areas of decision making. This aspect of ongoing clinical care warrants emphasis: we can still make many cogent decisions about NF1 and NF2 based on sound clinical precepts as reviewed here, combined with a certain degree of direct clinical experience.

The notion of heterogeneity obtains when what appears to be a singular disorder is actually two or more disorders with extensive clinical and/or pathogenetic similarities. "Clinical heterogeneity" indicates that two or more clinically defined disorders mimic each other, leaving it open to question as to whether they have distinct etiologies or merely alternative pathogenetic mechanisms. On the other hand, "genetic heterogeneity" refers to two or more clinically or pathogenetically similar disorders, with at least one of them having a known (and specified) genetic etiology and the other or others having alternative genetic explanations (e.g., allelic mutations or mutations at another gene locus) or a nongenetic etiology (phenocopy).

Without question, the notion of clinical heterogeneity applies to NF. Although all cases of bona fide NF have features or natural history elements in common, there is certainly a very broad spectrum. The geneticist's concept of "variable expressivity" does not account for many of the differences seen along this spectrum. Those features that seem to "breed true" as a distinctive feature within a given family represent yet another aspect of heterogeneity, specifically, genetic heterogeneity. (Some investigators have argued that the ostensibly high frequency of new NF mutations may actually reflect nothing more than the unwitting summation of mutations at multiple loci.)

One type of situation highlights the importance of NF heterogeneity. Pulst and coworkers (1989; Sears et al. 1990) made reference to spinal NF regarding two families with paraspinal neurofibromas as their key feature of NF. In one family, with café-au-lait spots but no Lisch nodules or cutaneous or subcutaneous neurofibromas, linkage to the DNA markers identifying the *NF1* locus was established, suggesting allelism. In the second family there were no café-au-lait spots, cutaneous or subcutaneous neurofibromas, or Lisch nodules. Linkage to chromosome 17 markers was discounted, and the family ultimately showed linkage to chromosome 22 markers about the *NF2* locus.

Watson syndrome (Watson 1967) is considered to be an allelic form of NF1 (Allanson et al. 1990; Hall and Allanson 1991). Patients with Watson syndrome not only have that syndrome's defining primary features of café-au-lait spots and, less frequently, neurofibromas and Lisch nodules, but also variably have pulmonic stenosis and mental retardation (Upadhyaya et al. 1990). Genetic linkage data for both Watson's original families and others indicate a chromosome 17 locus the same as for *NF1* (Upadhyaya et al. 1990). NF and its clinical overlap with Noonan syndrome (Fig. 1-1) are discussed in Chapter 2.

Although a gene mutation is the etiology for NF1 and NF2, the pathogenesis (i.e., the mechanisms by which the mutation leads to or accounts for the individual and combined phenotypic features) remains obscure. In addition, there are multiple genetic considerations at the cellular and molecular levels.

1. Genetic heterogeneity in terms of allelism must be presumed, and the possibility of mutations at other gene loci and phenocopies must not be automatically discounted.
2. There are numerous types of mutations, including a point mutation involving alteration of a single base pair of the gene's DNA, deletions of larger

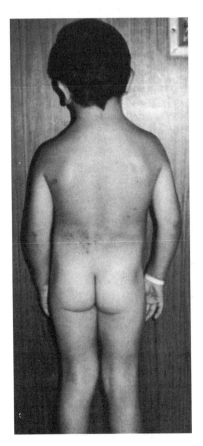

Figure 1-1. Posterior view of a patient with NF1, showing multiple café-au-lait spots, a broad neck, and genu valgum.

numbers of base pairs (Scotti et al. 1987), deletions of the entire gene (Kayes et al. 1990), or rearrangements such as inversions, insertions, and translocations.

3. There is the possibility of modifier genes, linked or unlinked to the *NF1* gene, that influence or limit its expression in one or more tissues. In addition, although not yet proved, it is possible for one or more primary features to have a parent-of-origin effect.

4. Although the *NF1* mutation is dominant by virtue of its segregation pattern from one generation to the next, obviously it is not expressed in gross pathologic terms in all the cells in which it is present (e.g., neurofibromas occur at more or less discrete sites, not continuously throughout the body). At the cellular level the gene may not be dominant in the strict sense but rather may be recessive and thereby require another (i.e., permissive) genetic or epigenetic event for complete or perhaps even partial expression. Such events or phenomena include allelic exclusion or loss of heterozygosity, a second mutation at the original locus or at a second locus, direct cell–cell interaction, and cellular interaction mediated through the local secretion of various compounds.

OTHER FORMS OF NEUROFIBROMATOSIS

One aspect of NF genetic heterogeneity is the proposal, originally published in 1982 by Riccardi (1982a, 1982b), of six other types of NF beyond NF1 and NF2.

CLINICAL OVERLAP OF NF AND NON-NF CONDITIONS

One might be tempted to rely on a molecular diagnosis as the ultimate criterion for whether or not some form of NF is present. For the present, at least from the clinical investigation standpoint, we note that the many instances in which the available molecular markers for *NF1* or *NF2* fail to identify mutations at the respective loci may be used for considering potential additional loci, phenocopies, and so on. One might consider, for example, that DNA homologous to that of the *NF1* gene on the long arm of chromosome 17 is also present on the long arm of chromosome 15, though with no known function or disease associated with it.

Other Specified Disorders

Knudson (1981) emphasized the apparent pathogenetic interrelationship of NF with a number of other conditions, including the multiple endocrine neoplasias (MEN) (Griffiths et al. 1983) and neuroblastoma IV-S (Paul et al. 1991). While the areas of clinical overlap of NF1 with these conditions may be substantial, there is no imperative to subsume either into the NF category, or vice versa. The fact that MEN-1 and MEN-2A have their gene loci on the long arm of chromosome 10 and the long arm of chromosome 11, respectively, neither adds to nor detracts from this approach. Rather, as with the example of Noonan syndrome, the emphasis might best be on exploring the commonalities in the context of the differences. That is, rather than extending the notion of heterogeneity to subsume both in one category, more might be gained by focusing on the differences. The serious student of NF might also wish to consider any one of a large number of other disorders with NF features, especially café-au-lait spots, to be instructive about NF itself (Bhawan et al. 1976).

Other Unspecified Disorders

Over the course of 25 years, I have evaluated 60 or so patients with features that warranted considering the diagnosis of NF (of any type), but for whom an NF diagnosis could not be substantiated. For example, the patient in Figure 1-2 had one area of hyperpigmentation, hemihypertrophy, and mental retardation. These features led her pediatrician to presume some form of NF was present, although we could not confirm that diagnosis. Little, if anything, is gained by subsuming such patients under the rubric of NF on the basis of "heterogeneity." There are limits to the notion of heterogeneity, and in some instances it is more prudent to acknowledge a nonspecific overlap of certain clinical features.

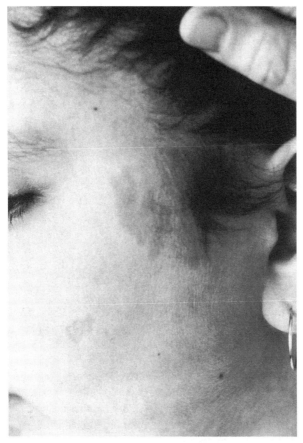

Figure 1-2. The left preauricular region of a patient without NF1, showing her single area of café-au-lait spot–like hyperpigmentation. This finding, in the context of her mental retardation and true hemihypertrophy, led her physician to diagnose NF1 erroneously.

Suggestive Combinations of Clinical Features

More perplexing is the nonspecific, nonsyndromic combination of clinical features. On the one hand, a specific non-NF alternative diagnosis is not readily apparent or compelling; on the other hand, categorically discounting the diagnosis of some form of NF seems arbitrary, respecting our lack of appreciation of the "clinical limits" of this group of diseases.

It is in precisely this context that a totally negative evaluation according to the protocol outlined above portrays its utility. Given totally normal protocol data, what is the point in presuming NF as the diagnosis? On the other hand, the patients described by Wasserteil et al. (1987), including one with only a facial diffuse plexiform neurofibroma, ipsilateral meningiomas, and a contralateral single café-au-lait spot, tax the imagination.

Differential Diagnosis of Isolated Features

When does an isolated café-au-lait spot or another form of hyperpigmentation or an isolated neurofibroma warrant the diagnosis of NF? While NF1 virtually never manifests itself in this way (i.e., solely as one or two café-au-lait spots), clinicians nonetheless often raise the diagnostic possibility of NF in general, and NF1 in particular, on the basis of such minimal findings.

The primary diagnostic charge in such cases is to consider whether any form of NF is present or likely, a task that requires respect for the heterogeneity discussed above. Since some forms of NF are compatible with a single café-au-lait spot, this task may be formidable. It is worth reiterating that not every café-au-lait spot requires the diagnosis of NF.

There are four key items for sorting out the diagnostic possibilities:

1. the specific nature of the lesion or problem itself,
2. the presence and nature of other clinical findings,
3. the age of the patient, and
4. a family history of NF or similar instances of aberrant pigmentation.

For an adult in or beyond the third decade, with no family history of NF, no associated clinical findings on routine evaluation, and a single large café-au-lait spot, one can be fairly certain that the diagnosis of NF1 does not apply (Fig. 1-3). Additional data from a standard protocol evaluation can add conviction to such a nondiagnosis and extend the exclusion to other forms of NF as well. For younger patients, including all children beyond infancy, the same conclusions can be drawn, though some degree of tentativeness (in inverse proportion to the patient's age) may be warranted. For infants, a diagnosis of exclusion should always be reconsidered as the child gets older, although, in the meantime, one can be reasonably optimistic with the family.

For adults, children, and infants with a patch of skin hyperpigmentation that is not typical of a café-au-lait spot, especially in terms of variations in pigment intensity within the patch and an indistinctness of its borders (Fig. 1-4), one can generally be very confident that NF is not the diagnosis, given the absence of

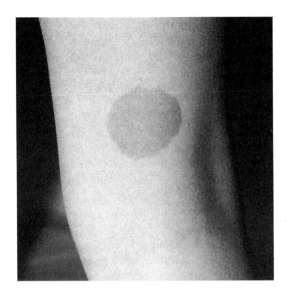

Figure 1-3. The right popliteal fossa of a patient without NF1, showing a discrete area of café-au-lait spot–like hyperpigmentation not associated with any other features of NF.

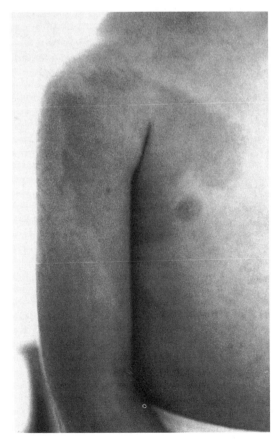

Figure 1-4. The anterior right shoulder and adjacent parts of a patient without NF1, showing contiguous areas of café-au-lait spot–like hyperpigmentation, which led her physician to diagnose NF1 erroneously.

other data pointing toward NF. At times a firm alternative diagnosis, such as a nevus spilus (Fig. 1-5) (Takahashi 1976), can be made. The point here is not that the patchy hyperpigmentation of NF is always in the form of an unequivocal café-au-lait spot, for certainly "atypical" café-au-lait spots do occur in patients with bona fide NF1 (Fig. 1-6). Rather, the point is that it would be very unusual for this to be the only skin pigment disturbance in NF1.

When more than one area of skin hyperpigmentation is present, the situation is more complex and broad generalizations are difficult, meaning that each such patient will have to be evaluated in depth and a conclusion based on the full array of specific details. One group of subjects warrants discussion here. Not infrequently, red-headed children, often of Irish or Welsh parentage, manifest multiple areas of patchy hyperpigmentation that are highly suggestive of NF. In such circumstances, in the absence of other findings, a normal variation of skin pigmentation is the most likely diagnosis. I have seen this problem on a number of occasions, and full evaluations have not substantiated a diagnosis of NF. The point here is not that such patients should be presumed not to have NF, but rather that a much greater flexibility in drawing diagnostic conclusions based solely on skin pigmentation variation is warranted for them.

Solitary neurofibromas of any type (Fig. 1-7) do not automatically warrant the diagnosis of NF and, conversely, such instances require that the clinician be all the more circumspect about excluding the diagnosis of NF in one form or an-

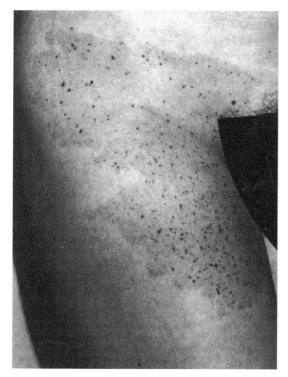

Figure 1-5. The right groin of a patient without NF1, showing a nevus spilus, which led her physician to diagnose NF1 erroneously.

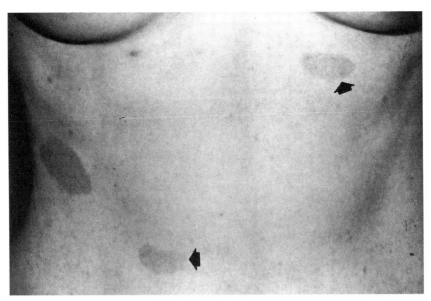

Figure 1-6. The lower chest and abdomen of a patient with NF1, showing café-au-lait spots of varying color intensities and border definitions, the ones at the arrows being very pale and poorly defined.

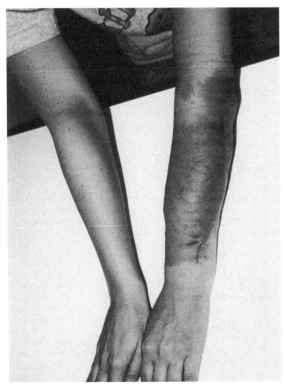

Figure 1-7. Diffuse plexiform neurofibroma of the left forearm of a female patient who had no other features of neurofibromatosis of any type.

other (Riccardi 1984). A full diagnostic evaluation is warranted for all individuals presenting with a solitary neurofibroma. One anatomic location in particular warrants special emphasis: the palm. While palmar neurofibromas do occur in NF1, they are especially frequent among patients with other forms of NF characterized by multiple CNS tumors (e.g., NF2).

Other features of NF beyond skin hyperpigmentation defects and neurofibromas also occur as isolated disorders not automatically warranting the diagnosis of NF, although their presence should prompt an appropriate in-depth evaluation. The features of special concern in this regard include optic gliomas, acoustic neuromas, malignant schwannomas, pheochromocytomas, tibial pseudarthrosis, and kyphoscoliosis (particularly involving the cervical and/or upper thoracic spine).

While it should go without saying that a negative family history for NF does not contradict or preclude a diagnosis of NF, all too often clinicians have made such an error. At least half of all NF1 index cases represent new mutations, and the proportion of new mutations is even higher for NF2. Thus, a negative family history for either disorder in no way detracts from considering this set of diagnoses for any given patient.

NF1 DYSPLASIA AND NEOPLASIA

Dysplasia is aberrant growth, generally in terms of the make-up of the tissue. *Neoplasia* is aberrant growth, generally in terms of one cellular component of the tissue showing "new growth" that outstrips the growth of the remaining, ostensibly normal cellular components. NF1 manifests both types of aberrant growth.

NF1 is highly variable in its expression from one family to another, from one person to another within a family, and from one body segment to another within a given person. It is also progressive, worsening at varying rates over weeks, months, and years, with respect to the types of lesions and their size and/or number. While NF1 manifests itself diffusely throughout the entire body, the specific lesions tend to be more or less discrete, with both apparently random and nonrandom determinants. Specific features (e.g., optic gliomas, kyphoscoliosis) are not more likely to occur if already present in another affected family member. On the whole, then, some aspects of NF1 seem to be intrinsic to the mutation itself (e.g., the presence of café-au-lait spots, neurofibromas, Lisch nodules), some appear to be determined in part by additional specific factors (e.g., trauma, skinfolds), and some appear simply to reflect chance (e.g., the location of café-au-lait spots).

For many years authors have referred to NF1 as a mesodermal defect or, alternatively, a neuroectodermal defect, with utterly no justification for the former other than the fact that structures with components of mesodermal origin are involved. A neuroectodermal defect seems somewhat more plausible since the definitive lesions of NF1 appear to derive from embryonic neural crest cells.

This neurocristopathy approach (Bolande 1974, 1981) has relatively wide acceptance, though a current knowledge of neural crest embryology does not readily account for all of NF1's features, including, for example, learning disabilities, pseudarthroses, pectus excavatum, and short stature. In any case, a primary neural crest defect would not logically require that every NF1 feature has a singular origin in a neural crest defect. The disease is too complex and multifarious for every element of the phenotype to have one simple explanation. As discussed below, I favor the notion that several pathogenetic mechanisms probably come into play in the life of each NF1 patient.

Even if we accept a neurocristopathy pathogenesis of NF in general and NF1 in particular, we still are at a loss as to how to explain thoroughly the different types of neural crest aberrations, including the more or less static café-au-lait spots and the progressively growing neurofibromas and other tumors. Focus on the neural crest merely allows us to target attention; it does not account for all facets of the disorder. Based on the circumstantial evidence given here, I have argued in the past (Riccardi 1979, 1981a) that, while the primary defect involves neural crest derivatives, at least some features of the disease require additional considerations, such as direct interaction between cells of neural crest origin and those of a different type (e.g., mast cells). In addition, one must always keep in mind the distinctions between primary features (e.g., neurofibromas), secondary features (e.g., scoliosis due to massive neurofibroma growth), and tertiary features or complications (e.g., spinal cord compression due to severe scoliosis, in turn due to massive neurofibroma growth).

NF1 IS A PROGRESSIVE DISEASE

The *natural history of disease* is an important biologic concept, as well as a clinically useful medical tool. A systematic accounting of a disease's features and their development and progression allows one to apply deductive logic to identify additional, previously uncharacterized features. It also makes it possible to apply inductive logic to identify basic pathogenetic mechanisms, etiology, or both. The sum of features that might be present at any one time and the temporal relationships (timing of appearance) of these features are central to this concept, thus, the reference to "history." And "natural" refers to what would evolve in the natural course of events without therapeutic intervention.

Numerous investigators have studied the natural history of NF1 and NF2, both to elucidate specific details about these particular diseases and to delineate the features that define or characterize natural history of disease investigations in general. In addition, a clinical genetics perspective has led many to look at natural history specifically in terms of the phenomena referred to as genetic heterogeneity, variable expressivity, and pleiotropism. *Genetic heterogeneity* entails the notion that what appears at first blush to be a singular disorder, in reality comprises multiple disorders deriving from a variety of gene mutations at one or more gene loci. The concept of *variable expressivity* deals with the fact that a given mutation (i.e., within a particular family) may manifest itself in widely disparate ways in terms of the types of lesions and their overall severity. (There are actually two relevant terms and notions here. Variable expressivity is an attribute of the disorder or phenotype. Thus, we say that the disease, NF1, is characterized by variable expressivity. *Variable expression* is an attribute of the mutant gene, and we say that the *NF1* mutation is characterized by variable expression.) Pleiotropism means that the mutation manifests itself in multiple tissues and organ systems.

In any one person NF1 becomes more obvious and more severe with the passage of time. Not only do early-onset lesions tend to become more obvious and more serious, but varied types of new lesions characteristically develop at different times.

The pathogenetic mechanisms underlying the basic nature and progression of NF1 have remained obscure precisely as a function of the three genetic notions of heterogeneity, variability, and pleiotropism. NF1 can be manifest in so many different ways and in so many tissues and organs from one family to another, from one person to another within a given family, and from one body part to another and from one time to another in a given person that a singular schema to account for all of its facets has been wanting. Moreover, almost all NF1 investigations and publications show varying degrees of ascertainment and reporting bias, narrow focus, and a retrospective vantage point. These types of problems are compounded by the large number of patients with NF1, since it is relatively easy to accumulate numerous patients whose collective features, by virtue of chance or investigator bias, suggest associations or causal relationships that actually detract from the timely identification and pursuit of the truly fundamental issues.

The literature on NF1 has also been seriously flawed both by a lack of uniformity in the definition and use of certain terms (e.g., considering an optic glioma sometimes as a hamartoma and sometimes as a neoplasm) and by a frankly incorrect use of other terms (e.g., referring to a neurofibroma as a neuroma).

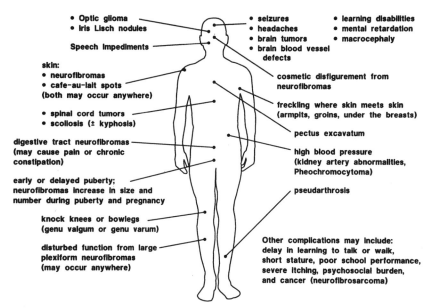

Figure 1-8. Summary of the features of NF1. *Source*: Powell, 1988. Reprinted with permission of S. Karger AG, Basel.

The conceptual and pragmatic limitations notwithstanding, it is still possible to clarify major elements of the natural history of NF1, utilizing data from the older literature and findings from more recent large surveys. There are three approaches to describing the natural history of NF1. The first has to do with delineating each of the features of NF1 as such and distinguishing primary features (e.g., café-au-lait spots, neurofibromas, optic gliomas), secondary features (seizures, learning disabilities, scoliosis, or malignancy), and complications (neurologic and respiratory compromise from severe kyphoscoliosis or leg amputation from congenital tibial pseudarthrosis). The second approach has to do with timing: the age of onset and worsening of the various clinical problems and pathologic aberrations. The third approach has to do with characterizing the nature and progression of all features of NF1 for each of the body's organ systems and tissues. Figure 1-8 summarizes the array of problems of all types—primary features, secondary features and complications—that characterize NF1 as a whole.

OVERALL MORBIDITY AND MORTALITY

Accurate estimates of overall severity of NF1 are now available from a variety of sources (Samuelsson and Akesson 1989; Huson et al. 1989a, 1989b; Samuelsson and Riccardi 1989a, 1989b; Samuelsson and Samuelsson 1989). Even so, almost all available data are derived from horizontal, cross-sectional studies. Detailed longitudinal studies are not available. Mulvihill et al. (1990) and Sorensen et al. (1986a, 1986b), however, provided data dealing with long-term follow-up of the NF1 cohort identified by Borberg (1951). Data from the work reported here combined with those of Mulvihill (1986) and Sorensen et al. (1986a, 1986b) confirm that NF1 is progressive, unpredictable, and associated with an excess of untimely deaths related to the disorder itself. On the other hand, death among patients with NF1 is often from other causes, whether as totally independent co-morbidities or accidents.

NF1 severity is determined by many factors, age being paramount among them. The next section describes a method of grading the clinical severity of NF. Table 1-1 demonstrates that the likelihood of reaching NF1 severity grade 3 is at least 50% by the age of 15 years. The likelihood of reaching NF1 severity grade 4 is at least 10% by age 15 and 25% by age 30. In addition, minimal (grade 1) or mild (grade 2) NF1 in the childhood years in no way precludes an ultimate development of moderate (grade 3) or severe (grade 4) problems (Reynolds and Pineda 1988).

NF1 is a serious disease with a clear-cut compromise of health and life expectancy. Whether these considerations can be translated into a quantitative characterization of NF1 mortality at this time is problematic. First, the necessary data just are not available. Second, the course of NF1 is so variable that, in a very important sense, an "average decrease" in life expectancy is a fiction of sorts that limits its utility in advising individual patients and families. Third is the issue of ascertainment bias discussed elsewhere. Do the apparent risks that

Table 1-1. Probability of patients with NF1 reaching severity
grade 3 or 4, as a function of age

Age (yr)	Grade 3 (%)	Grade 4 (%)
5	24	6
10	36	8
15	51	11
20	59	15
25	60	19
30	79	25
40	92	30
60	—	49

derive from identified index cases and their affected family members apply to all persons bearing the NF1 mutation, including those not yet brought to medical attention? On the one hand, we could argue that the generalizations derived from one set of index cases obtain for subsequent index cases ascertained in the same way. On the other hand, we would also argue that the data derived from a comprehensive NF program probably are directly applicable to all patients with NF1.

SEVERITY OF NF1: A DETAILED ANALYSIS

A key element of evaluating patients with NF1 is to determine whether they have average, greater, or lesser severity compared with the total population of subjects with NF1. To address this issue, I considered severity as described below. In addition to the current level of severity, I also considered the number of years spent in each of four possible levels of severity and the reasons for being included in the two most serious levels of severity.

SEVERITY GRADES

The severity grade refers to the severity level of the NF (whether NF1 or other types of NF), based on the results of the evaluation protocol described above.

- *Grade 1,* or *minimal NF,* means the presence of few NF features, with no compromise of health or well-being. Perhaps it is most accurate to say that, except for café-au-lait spots and iris Lisch nodules, grade 1 is defined by the absence of features, while grades 2 to 4 are predicated on the presence of specific features and an ordered level of compromise.
- *Grade 2,* or *mild NF,* reflects the presence of enough stigmata to make the disease obvious and a source of concern, but without significant compromise of health. For example, the patient may exhibit facial café-au-lait spots or a modest number of cutaneous or deep neurofibromas.
- *Grade 3,* or *moderate NF,* is assigned when the features of NF are associated with unequivocal compromise of health and well-being, but the com-

promise can be reasonably well managed, is not intractable, or will not invariably lead to a shortened life span. Because there are many features of NF that can lead to this level of clinical problems, the category of severity grade 3 is necessarily broad, spanning a relatively large age range.

- *Grade 4, or severe NF,* indicates the presence of serious compromise that is intractable, is managed or treated only with difficulty, or, at least statistically, is associated with a shortened life span. Mental retardation, drug-resistant seizures, brain tumors, and malignant tumors contribute to this category of complications.

Table 2-1 in Chapter 2 lists the clinical features used to determine severity grade in NF1. At times, it simply is not possible to decide about the level of severity. In such instances, rather than arbitrarily assigning a severity grade, the feature is merely noted as being present. There are two reasons for not being able to decide the level of severity. First, the distinction between any two severity grades seems to be indeterminate. For example, the presence of learning disabilities or school performance problems may be an unequivocal fact, but whether either warrants a grade 3 or a grade 4 assignment may not be so clear. Second, there may be one or more additional confounding factors, such as a serious hearing deficit, making quantification of the learning disabilities difficult.

SEVERITY PROFILES

Although useful for a wide variety of overview and comparative studies, the approach that uses static severity grades has some serious intrinsic limitations. In particular, age is not accounted for. And since NF severity is a function of age, merely itemizing severity grade scores and/or comparing them among and between groups of patients may be misleading in connection with respective groups or natural history of the disease in general.

Thus, we have *severity profiles* (Riccardi 1981b, 1981c) that designate the number of years spent in each of the four severity grades for each patient. For example, a severity profile 03-10-07-08 designates that the patient is in his twenty-eighth year (3+10+7+8) and that he has spent 8 years in grade 1, 7 years in grade 2, 10 years in grade 3, and 3 years in grade 4. Such severity profiles have two primary benefits for students of NF natural history. First, by comparing severity profiles among large numbers of NF patients, it quickly becomes apparent that the progression to higher severity grades on a year-by-year basis is highly individual, that is, highly variable in a way that is not quite so obvious in narrative descriptions. Second, by not overshadowing the patient's prior milder course with a restricted focus on his or her more serious current problems, the earlier, milder states are given a more realistic perspective. They emphasize that a less serious course early on does not in any way preclude more serious problems eventually. But severity profiles are relatively cumbersome to use for large-scale comparisons and on their own they do not allow for useful prognostications or determinations of a priori risks.

The data contained in these profiles can be used in another helpful way: for construction of life-table risk estimates (Chase et al. 1983). Given that there is no regressing to a lower severity grade once a higher one has been attained, the number of years that have elapsed up to the point of entering grade 2, 3, or 4 is indicated by the sum of years spent in the preceding grade or grades. In the example used above, the patient entered grade 3 at age 15 and grade 4 at age 25. Then, if entrance into severity grade 3 is taken as equivalent to "death" (the standard end point for life-table calculations), a life table indicating the percentage of survivors (i.e., those who did not reach grade 3) as a function of age can be portrayed. More useful, however, are the reciprocal data depicting the percentage likelihood of reaching grade 3 as a function of age. Figure 1-9 displays a probability curve for reaching grade 3 for 238 NF1 Clinical Research Program study subjects. A similar approach can be used to determine the percentage probability curve for the age-related attainment of severity grade 4. Figure 1-10 displays this curve for the 238 study subjects. Note the differences in the shapes of these two curves.

The life-table method for estimating age-related probabilities is far superior to merely calculating percentage frequencies for each age, since the significance of over- or under-representation of various ages is minimized. In addition, it now becomes possible to compare subgroups of the study population in terms of not only their respective frequencies of specific features and average severity grade

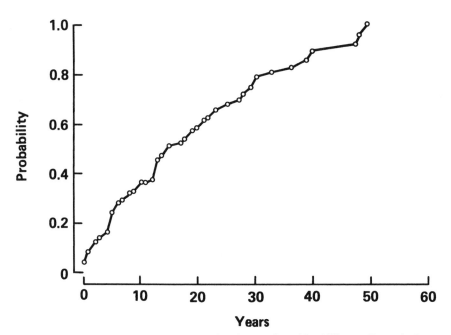

Figure 1-9. Probability curve depicting the chance of reaching NF1 severity grade 3 as a function of age, for both sexes combined.

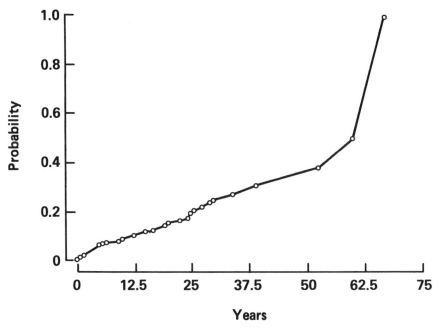

Figure 1-10. Probability curve depicting the chance of reaching NF1 severity grade 4 as a function of age, for both sexes combined.

scores, but also their respective life-table curves. That is, do any two subgroups have the same age-related likelihoods of reaching grade 3 or 4? Thus, this type of comparison should be especially instructive concerning the similarities or dissimilarities of various subgroups relevant to questions of natural history. For example, Figure 1-11 depicts the likelihood curves of reaching grade 3 for original and nonoriginal cases. Not only do they appear to be similar visually, a Gehan Generalized Wilcoxon Test of life-table curves indicates they are not different ($p > .30$). Figure 1-12 depicts the probability curves for NF1 males and females reaching grade 3 as a function of age. A statistical analysis indicates these curves show differences that are not significant ($p = .099$). Figure 1-13, dealing with a comparison of males and females attaining severity grade 4, depicts curves that are not different from each other ($p = .179$). Other data not shown have been derived to effect the following comparisons: original versus nonoriginal cases for grade 4 (no difference, $p > .30$); mother affected versus father affected for grade 3 (no difference, $p > .30$) and for grade 4 (no difference, $p > .30$); index cases versus nonindex cases for grade 3 (slight difference, $p = .04$) and for grade 4 (no difference, $p = .42$); probands versus affected cases for grade 3 (no difference, $p = .133$) and for grade 4 (no difference, $p = .91$); sporadic cases versus probands for grade 3 (no difference, $p = .19$) and for grade 4 (no difference, $p = .11$); and sporadic cases versus affected cases for grade 3 (difference significant, $p = .02$) and for grade 4 (no difference, $p = .30$).

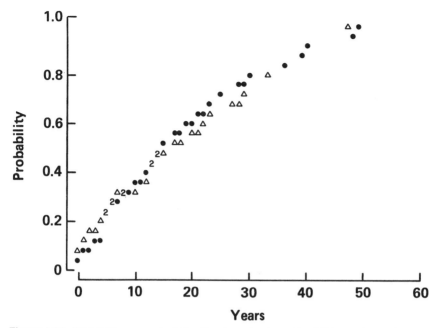

Figure 1-11. Probability curves depicting the chances of reaching NF1 severity grade 3 as a function of age, for both sexes combined, for original cases (solid circles) and nonoriginal cases (open triangles).

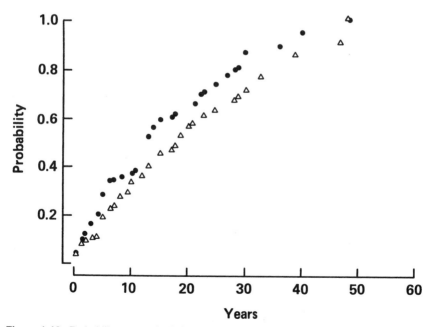

Figure 1-12. Probability curves depicting the chances of reaching NF1 severity grade 3 as a function of age, for males (solid circles) and females (open triangles).

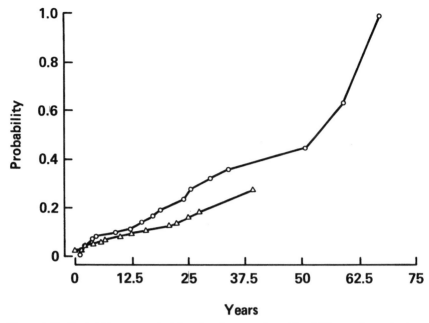

Figure 1-13. Probability curves depicting the chances of reaching NF1 severity grade 4 as a function of age, for males (circles) and for females (triangles).

Therefore, if we use life-table data (probability curves) for severity grades 3 and 4 to compare various subgroups at all ages, we note the following: no significant differences between any groups in terms of life-table data for grade 4, but some differences in life-table data for grade 3, primarily index cases versus affected cases and sporadic cases versus affected cases (with the latter difference presumably accounting for the former, since probands were not different from affected cases). With respect to grade 3, if we further divide the original subgroups (i.e., probands, affected cases, and so on) into patients less than 20 years old and those 20 and older, some rather surprising results are noted (data not shown). First, there are very highly significant differences between the two age groupings within each of the primary groups, with the younger patients showing an earlier attainment of grade 3. Second, for the patients younger than 20 years there are no significant differences between any of the primary groups (including index versus affected cases and sporadic cases versus affected cases). And third, for the patients at 20 years and older, there is persistence of the differences between index cases and affected cases and between sporadic cases and affected cases.

Specifically, then, the only significant differences among these comparisons are for older patients. It is not at all clear why this is so. The data would suggest, however, that extrapolating overall severity (including a priori risks) from only young patients would skew expectations toward earlier onset and from only older (> 20 years) patients would skew expectations toward later onset. These data indicate that distinctiveness based on index code and origin of the mutation are not cogent arguments on their own against treating Clinical Research Program patients with NF1 as a reasonable approximation of a representative sample of NF1 in the general population. That is, the basis for inclusion of patients in such a study population and the timing of attainment of severity grade 3 are the consequences of a wide variety of factors, including those reflecting the biology of the disease, social factors, and methodologic factors such as methods of ascertainment and semantics of terminology used to categorize various patients.

REFERENCES

Adrian C. 1901. Uber Neurofibromatose und ihre Komplikationen. *Beitr Klin Chir* 31:1–98.

Akenside M. 1785. Observations on cancers. (First reported case of NF-1). *Med Trans Coll Physicians Lond* 1:64–92.

Allanson JE, Watson GH, Partington M, Upadhyaya M, Harper P, and Huson SM. 1990. Watson syndrome: is it a subtype of neurofibromatosis? *Proc Greenwood Genet Ctr* 9:63–64.

Bhawan J, Purtilo DT, Riordan JA, Saxena VK, and Edelstein L. 1976. Giant and "granular melanosomes" in leopard syndrome: an ultrastructural study. *Cutan Pathol* 3:207–16.

Bolande RP. 1974. The neurocristopathies: a unifying concept of disease arising in neural crest maldevelopment. *Hum Pathol* 5:409–29.

———. 1981. Neurofibromatosis: The quintessential neurocristopathy: pathogenetic concepts and relationships. *Adv Neurol* 29:67–75.

Borberg A. 1951. Clinical and genetic investigations into tuberous sclerosis and Recklinghausen's neurofibromatosis. *Acta Psychiatr Neurol Scand* 71:1–239.

Chase GA, Folstein MF, Breitner JCS, Beaty TH, and Self SG. 1983. The use of life tables and survival analysis in testing genetic hypotheses, with an application to Alzheimer's disease. *Am J Epidemiol* 117:590–7.

Cohen MM Jr. 1988. Understanding Proteus syndrome, unmasking the elephant man, and stemming elephant fever. *Neurofibromatosis* 1:260–80.

Crowe FW, Schull WJ, and Neel JV. 1956. *A Clinical, Pathological, and Genetic Study of Multiple Neurofibromatosis.* Springfield, Ill.: Charles C Thomas, pp. 1–181.

Crump T. 1981. Translation of case reports in Uber die multiplen fibrome der haut und ihre beziehung zu multiplen neuromen by F. V. Recklinghausen. *Adv Neurol* 29:259–75.

Griffiths DFR, Williams GT, and Williams ED. 1983. Multiple endocrine neoplasia associated with von Recklinghausen's disease. *BMJ* 287:1341–3.

Hall JG and Allanson JE. 1991. Neurofibromatosis 1: Predicting the relation of gene structure to gene function. *Am J Med Genet* 38:135.

Hitchcock A. 1862. Some remarks on neuroma, with a brief account of three cases of anomalous cutaneous tumours in one family. *Am J Med Sci* 43:320–8.

Huson SM, Compston DAS, Clark P, and Harper PS. 1989a. A genetic study of von Recklinghausen neurofibromatosis in south east Wales. I. Prevalence, fitness, mutation rate, and effect of parental transmission. *J Med Genet* 26:704–11.

Huson SM, Compston DAS, and Harper PS. 1989b. A genetic study of von Recklinghausen neurofibromatosis in south east Wales. II. Guidelines for genetic counselling. *J Med Genet* 26:712–21.

Karp LE. 1982. More on the elephant man. *Am J Med Genet* 13:355.

Kayes LM, Riccardi VM, and Stephens K. 1990. Evidence for a microdeletion in a patient with Neurofibromatosis 1 and mental retardation. *Am J Hum Genet* 47:A223. (abstract)

Knudson AG Jr. 1981. A geneticist's view of neurofibromatosis. *Adv Neurol* 29:237–42.

Lund AM and Skovby F. 1991. Optic gliomas in children with neurofibromatosis type 1. *Eur J Pediatr* 150:835–8.

Madigan P and Masello MJ. 1988. Report of a neurofibromatosis-like case: Monstrorum Historia, 1642. *Neurofibromatosis* 2:53–6.

Montague A. 1971. *The Elephant Man: A Study of Human Dignity.* London: Dutton.

Mulvihill JJ. 1986. Neurofibromatosis: a genetic epidemiologist's point of view. *Ann NY Acad Sci* 486:38–44.

Mulvihill JJ, Parry DM, Sherman JL, Pikus A, Kaiser-Kupfer MI, and Eldridge R. 1990. Neurofibromatosis 1 (Recklinghausen disease) and neurofibromatosis 2 (bilateral acoustic neurofibromatosis): an update. *Ann Intern Med* 113:39–52.

Paul SR, Tarbell NJ, Korf B, Kretschmar CS, Lavally B, and Grier HE. 1991. Stage IV neuroblastoma in infants: long-term survival. *Cancer* 67:1493–7.

Powell PP. 1988. Schematic presentation of von Recklinghausen neurofibromatosis (NF-1): an aid for patient and family. *Neurofibromatosis* 1:164–5.

Prieser SA and Davenport CB. 1918. Multiple neurofibromatosis (von Recklinghausen disease) and its inheritance. *Am J Med Sci* 156:507–41.

Pulst SM, Riccardi VM, Ren M, Barker DF, Fain PR, and Korenberg JR. 1989. Spinal neurofibromatosis is linked to the neurofibromatosis 1 region on chromosome 17. *Am J Hum Genet* 45:A158. (abstract)

Reynolds RL and Pineda CA. 1988. Neurofibromatosis: review and report. *J Am Dent Assoc* 117:735–7.

Riccardi VM. 1979. Cell–cell interaction as an epigenetic determinant in the expression of mutant neural crest cells. *Birth Defects* 15(B):89–98.

———. 1981a. Cutaneous manifestations of neurofibromatosis cellular interaction, pigmentation, and mast cells. *Birth Defects* 17(2):129–45.

———. 1981b. Neurofibromatosis: an overview and new directions in clinical investigations. *Adv Neurol* 29:1–9.

———. 1981c. Von Recklinghausen neurofibromatosis. *N Engl J Med* 305:1617–27.

———. 1982a. Neurofibromatosis: clinical heterogeneity. *Curr Probl Cancer* 7(2):1–34.

———. 1982b. The multiple forms of neurofibromatosis. *Pediatr Rev* 3:292–8.

———. 1984. Neurofibromatosis heterogeneity. *J Am Acad Dermatol* 10:518–9.

———. 1988a. Guidelines for organizing a comprehensive neurofibromatosis program. *Neurofibromatosis* 1:105–19.

———. 1988b. Routine cranial neuroimaging of patients with or at risk for neurofibromatosis. *Neurofibromatosis* 1:65–8.

Samuelsson B and Akesson HO. 1989. Neurofibromatosis in Gothenburg, Sweden. IV. Genetic analyses. *Neurofibromatosis* 2:107–15.

Samuelsson B and Riccardi VM. 1989a. Neurofibromatosis in Gothenburg, Sweden. II. Intellectual compromise. *Neurofibromatosis* 2:78–83.

———. 1989b. Neurofibromatosis in Gothenburg, Sweden. III. Psychiatric and social aspects. *Neurofibromatosis* 2:84–106.

Samuelsson B and Samuelsson S. 1989. Neurofibromatosis in Gothenburg, Sweden. I. Background, study design and epidemiology. *Neurofibromatosis* 2:6–22.

Scotti G, Fillizolo F, Scialfa G, and Tampieri D. 1987. Repeated subarachnoid hemorrhages from a cervical meningioma. *J Neurosurg* 66:779–81.

Sears TA, Riccardi VM, Fain P, Barker D, Korenberg JR, and Pulst SM. 1990. Non-allelic heterogeneity of familial spinal neurofibromatosis. *Am J Hum Genet* 47:A77. (abstract)

Sorensen SA, Mulvihill JJ, and Nielsen A. 1986a. Nation-wide follow-up of Recklinghausen neurofibromatosis: Survival and malignant neoplasms. *N Engl J Med* 314:1010–5.

————. 1986b. On the natural history of von Recklinghausen neurofibromatosis. *Ann NY Acad Sci* 486:30–7.

Sparks C. 1980. *The Elephant Man.* New York: Ballantine Books.

Takahashi M. 1976. Studies on café-au-lait spots in neurofibromatosis and pigmented macules of nevus spilus. *Tohoku J Exp Med* 118:255–73.

Thomson A. 1900. *On Neuroma and Neurofibromatosis.* Edinburgh: Turnbull & Spears, pp. 1–123.

Tilesius WG. 1793. *Historia Pathologica Singularis Cutis Turpitudinis.* Leipzig: S.L. Crusius, pp. 1–11.

Treves F. 1923. *The Elephant Man and Other Reminiscences.* London: Cossell.

Upadhyaya M, Sarfarazi M, Huson S, et al. 1990. Linkage of Watson's syndrome to chromosome 17 markers. *J Med Genet* 27:209. (abstract)

Virchow R. 1857. Uber eniem Fall von vielfachen Neuromen (Faser-Kern-geschwultsen) mit ausgezeichneter localer Recidivfahikeit. *Virchows Arch [A]* 12:144.

von Recklinghausen F. 1882. *Uber die Multiplen Fibrome der Haut und ihre Beziehung zu Multiplen Neuromen.* Berlin: August Hirschwald, pp. 1–138.

Warkany J. 1981. Friedrich Daniel von Recklinghausen and his times. *Adv Neurol* 29:251–7.

Wasserteil V, Bruce S, and Riccardi VM. 1987. Non-von Recklinghausen's neurofibromatosis presenting as hemifacial neurofibromas and contralateral café-au-lait spots. *J Am Acad Dermatol* 16:1090–6.

Watson GH. 1967. Pulmonary stenosis, café-au-lait spots, and dull intelligence. *Arch Dis Child* 42:1145–6.

Zanca A. 1980. Antique illustrations of neurofibromatosis. *Int J Dermatol* 19:55–8.

I

Neurofibromatosis 1

2

Clinical and Epidemiological Features

J. M. Friedman, M.D., Ph.D., and Vincent M. Riccardi, M.D.

Neurofibromatosis type 1 (NF1) is one of the most frequent human genetic diseases, with a prevalence of two to three cases per 10,000 population. Café-au-lait macules, neurofibromas, intertriginous freckling, and Lisch nodules develop in most affected patients. Other important clinical manifestations of NF1 include learning disabilities, optic gliomas, increased risk of certain malignancies, and characteristic osseous lesions such as dysplastic scoliosis. The frequency of many of these features depends on age. The average life expectancy of patients with NF1 is reduced by at least 10 to 15 years. Malignancy is the most common cause of death among patients with NF1.

Two especially striking aspects of the natural history of NF1 are its extreme variability and its progressive nature. The expression of NF1 is highly variable from one family to another, from one person to another within a family, and from one part of the body to another within an individual. Although NF1 is generally progressive throughout life, various lesions may appear and worsen at different times and at different rates.

A few clinical subtypes of NF1 have been recognized that appear to "run true" in families. Watson syndrome and the severe phenotype associated with deletions of the entire *NF1* gene are two examples. Other conditions, such as the NF1–Noonan syndrome, exhibit a more complex relationship to NF1, both clinically and genetically.

This chapter provides an overview of the NF1 phenotype as a whole, including its natural history and variability. Detailed discussion of the diagnosis and management of various clinical problems that affect patients is deferred to subsequent chapters. We begin by considering the epidemiology of the disease.

EPIDEMIOLOGY

PREVALENCE

Crowe and his associates (1956) estimated the frequency of patients with neurofibromatosis using data from hospital admissions and state institutions for the mentally retarded. These investigators concluded that the prevalence was 3.0 to

4.0 per 10,000 (between 1/3300 and 1/2500). They considered this to be a conservative estimate.

Most other studies have produced somewhat lower estimates of NF1 prevalence. Littler and Morton (1990) used the population-based Danish study of Borberg (1951) to estimate a prevalence of 2.7 per 10,000 (1/3704) for NF1. Sergeyev (1975) calculated the prevalence to be 1.3 per 10,000 (1/7800) in a sample of 16-year-old Russian males. Samuelsson and Axelsson (1981) and Samuelsson and Samuelsson (1989) estimated a prevalence of 2.2 per 10,000 (1/4600) in Sweden. Fuller et al. (1989) calculated the prevalence of NF1 to be 4.6 per 10,000 (1/2190) in New Zealand. Huson et al. (1988, 1989a) estimated the minimal prevalence of NF1 to be 2.0 per 10,000 (1/4950) in southeast Wales. Adjusting for underascertainment of younger patients, Huson et al. (1989a) calculated the prevalence to be 2.4 per 10,000 (1/4150). Clementi et al. (1990) found an overall NF1 prevalence of 1.5 per 10,000 (1/6711) in northeastern Italy. Poyhonen et al. (1997b) identified 197 NF1 patients in a population of 732,000 in northern Finland, a prevalence of 2.7 per 10,000 (1/3716).

Clementi et al. (1990) observed a higher prevalence among the population under 9 years of age (2.3 per 10,000 or 1/4292). Huson et al. (1988, 1989a) also found a higher prevalence of NF1 among younger patients. The observed frequency of NF1 among people under 20 years old was 2.5 per 10,000 (1/4000) in the Welsh study. Correcting for underascertainment, Huson et al. (1989a) estimated the incidence at birth of *NF1* mutation carriers to be 3.9 per 10,000 (1/2558). The finding of a lower prevalence of NF1 among individuals in their 60s and 70s than earlier in adulthood may result from earlier death among NF1 patients (Huson et al. 1988; Fuller et al. 1989; Samuelsson and Samuelsson 1989). However, it is not clear that this effect is severe enough to explain the magnitude of the observed difference in NF1 prevalence between children and adults. Underascertainment of adult patients may also contribute to the higher observed frequency of NF1 among children (Clementi et al. 1990).

Of these studies, only Poyhonen et al. (1997b) used the full NIH Diagnostic Criteria to identify patients with NF1 (National Institutes of Health Consensus Development Conference 1988; Gutmann et al. 1997). A few patients who did not have NF1 may have been counted as affected in some of the earlier studies, and this would produce an overestimate of disease prevalence. It is more likely, however, that some patients with NF1 were missed because mildly affected individuals do not come to medical attention (Clementi et al. 1990; Huson et al. 1989a).

ETHNIC VARIATION

Patients and families with NF1 have been reported from throughout the world (Cnossen et al. 1998; Friedman and Birch 1997b; Huson et al. 1988; Niimura 1990; North 1993; Poyhonen et al. 1997b; Riccardi 1992; Wong 1994), and there is no population in which NF1 is known not to occur. The prevalence of NF1 has only been measured in Caucasian and Japanese populations (see previous section), but the frequency does not appear to differ greatly among the groups that have been investigated.

No systematic study has been reported of ethnic variation in NF1 disease manifestations. Most serious complications occur with similar frequencies in different ethnic groups (Cnossen et al. 1988; Friedman and Birch 1997b; Huson et al. 1989b; Niimura 1990; Riccardi 1992; Wong 1994). One exception may be carcinoid tumors, which may occur more often in black than in white patients with NF1 (Burke et al. 1990). Optic glioma appears to be less common among black patients with NF1 than among whites, but gliomas are less common among black patients than among white patients in the general population (Bunin 1987; Fan and Pezeshkpour 1992).

NF DATABASES

Several electronic databases have been established to encourage neurofibromatosis research. Those discussed in this section contain information that is available on request to qualified investigators.

NNFF International Database

The NNFF International Database contains extensive demographic, clinical, and genetic data on more than 3000 patients with NF1, including about 400 multiplex families, from 26 participating centers in North America, Europe, Japan, and Australia. The database is maintained by Dr. J.M. Friedman and Patricia Birch at the University of British Columbia to facilitate comprehensive clinical and genetic analysis of neurofibromatosis (Friedman et al. 1993). All information is recorded using a standard format and consistent definitions of clinical features.

The greatest strength of the NNFF International Database is its large size. The limitations include the fact that most contributors are NF clinics at major medical centers, which probably produces an ascertainment bias. Data quality is somewhat variable because it depends entirely on voluntary contributions from clinicians throughout the world. The NNFF International Database is sponsored by the (U.S.) National Neurofibromatosis Foundation.

Neurofibromatosis Institute Database

This database contains information on the large series of NF patients that Dr. V.M. Riccardi has evaluated personally. The NF Institute Database includes standard clinical information on more than 1100 patients with NF1. Longitudinal data are available over several years on about one third of these patients. These data were described in detail in earlier editions of this book (Riccardi and Eichner 1986; Riccardi 1992).

The information in the NF Institute Database is particularly valuable because of its consistency. An enormous amount of information is available on each patient; in many instances this includes results of laboratory and radiological studies as well as very detailed clinical descriptions. One limitation is that most of these data were collected before the NIH diagnostic criteria were established, and some variables were recorded in a format that does not permit direct assessment of these criteria.

NF1 Genetic Analysis Consortium Database

The *NF1* Genetic Analysis Consortium is directed by Dr. Bruce Korf of Harvard University and includes investigators at some 50 centers who are identifying mutations in patients with NF1. The database currently contains complete standardized mutation descriptions for about 250 patients with NF1 (*NF1* Genetic Analysis Consortium Database, 1997). Brief clinical descriptions are recorded on all of these patients, and full information is available on about 25% of them, who also have been reported to the NNFF International Database.

CLINICAL OVERVIEW OF NF1

PHYSICAL FEATURES

Neurofibromas

A neurofibroma is a benign tumor arising from small or large nerves. Neurofibromas can occur anywhere in the body outside of the substance of the brain or spinal cord proper. A neurofibroma is comprised largely of Schwann cells and fibroblasts but also contains numerous perineurial cells, endothelial cells, pericytes, and mast cells and a small number of nerve cells (Lott and Richardson 1981). Occasionally melanin-containing cells, usually pigmented Schwann cells, are also present (Diaz-Flores et al. 1978). Even less frequently there may be a "glandular" organization of tumor components (DeSchryver and Santa Cruz 1984). The natural history and pathogenesis of neurofibromas is discussed in detail in Chapter 6.

Neurofibromas, whether they occur as part of NF1 or as solitary tumors in patients who do not have NF1 (Harkin and Reed 1969), are similar in terms of their histology and biological behavior. From a clinical perspective, there are four types of neurofibromas:

1. discrete cutaneous neurofibromas of the dermis or epidermis;
2. discrete subcutaneous neurofibromas that lie deeper in the skin;
3. deep nodular neurofibromas; and
4. diffuse plexiform neurofibromas.

Cutaneous neurofibromas may be sessile (Figs. 2-1, 2-2, and 2-3) or, at a later stage, pedunculated (Figs. 2-3 and 2-4). Cutaneous neurofibromas can be defined clinically because they move with the skin when it is moved. Sessile neurofibromas, particularly in their early stages, often have a reddish, bluish, or violaceous hue. They are fleshy and soft to the touch and rarely cause pain. Subcutaneous neurofibromas can be distinguished from cutaneous tumors clinically because the skin can be moved over subcutaneous lesions. They usually have a spherical or ovoid shape, are firm or rubbery, and may be painful or tender (Fig. 2-5).

Deep nodular neurofibromas are often called *nodular plexiform neurofibromas*. They resemble discrete cutaneous and subcutaneous lesions but involve major or minor nerves in tissues or organs beneath the dermis. Deep nodular neurofibromas

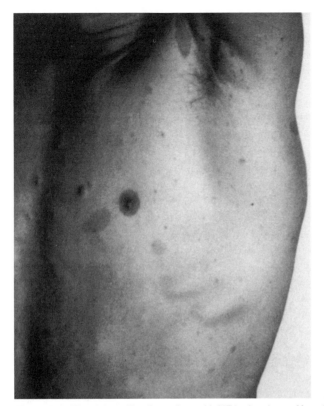

Figure 2-1. The right axilla of a patient with NF1, showing café-au-lait spots, sessile cutaneous neurofibromas, and pectus excavatum typical of NF1.

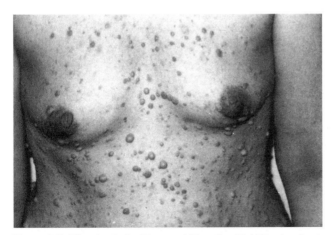

Figure 2-2. The chest of a 38-year-old female with NF1, showing large numbers of sessile cutaneous neurofibromas with prominent involvement of the nipples and areolae.

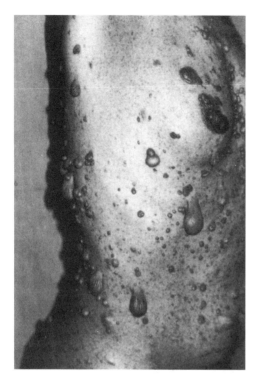

Figure 2-3. The right lateral trunk of a patient with NF1, showing large numbers of sessile and pedunculated cutaneous neurofibromas of various sizes.

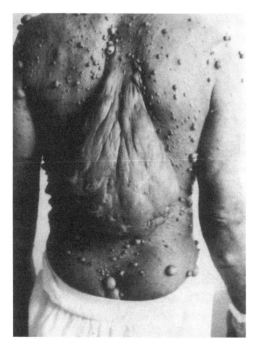

Figure 2-4. The back of a patient with NF1, showing myriad sessile cutaneous neurofibromas and a huge pedunculated neurofibroma. Note the presence of several neurofibromas at the top of the gluteal crease.

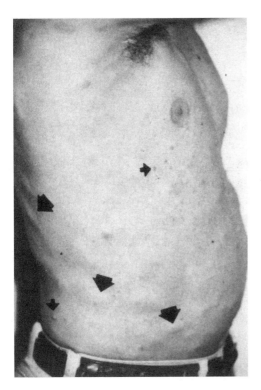

Figure 2-5. Side view of patient with NF1, showing large numbers of subcutaneous (large arrows) and cutaneous (small arrows) neurofibromas.

vary greatly in size and may extend the entire length of a nerve. They often do not come to clinical attention until later in life and are sometimes painful.

Diffuse plexiform neurofibromas are made up of an extensive interdigitating network of tissue, primarily of the types that also characterize discrete neurofibromas. Plexiform neurofibromas may include elements equivalent to schwannomas (Woodruff et al. 1983) or discrete neurofibromas or both in combination. Diffuse plexiform neurofibromas have numerous fingerlike fronds that insinuate themselves extensively into adjacent normal tissues, making total surgical removal impossible unless normal tissue is sacrificed as well. Plexiform neurofibromas may occur superficially, with extensive involvement of the skin and subcutaneous tissues (Figs. 2-6 and 2-7). Diffuse plexiform neurofibromas may also involve deep tissues, including those of the craniofacial region, paraspinal structures, mediastinum, retroperitoneum, and viscera, especially the gastrointestinal tract.

When a diffuse plexiform neurofibroma affects the skin, overlying hyperpigmentation or hypertrichosis or both often occur. The appearance differs from that of a café-au-lait spot in that the skin immediately over a plexiform neurofibroma is often thickened, redundant, or raised, and the dermal hairs are typically thick, coarse, and darkly pigmented. Skin involvement with a plexiform neurofibroma may be absent, relatively limited (Fig. 2-8), or very extensive (Fig. 2-9). The as-

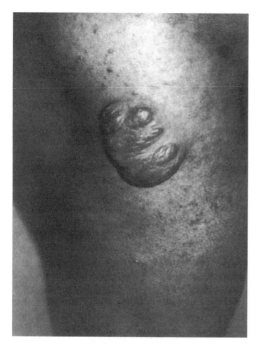

Figure 2-6. A large, diffuse plexiform neurofibroma involving the thigh in a patient with NF1.

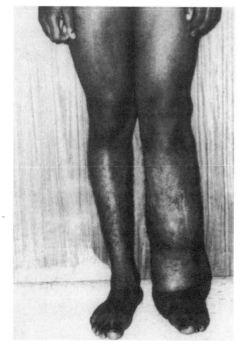

Figure 2-7. Elephantiasis like limb hypertrophy resulting from a diffuse plexiform neurofibroma in a patient with NF1.

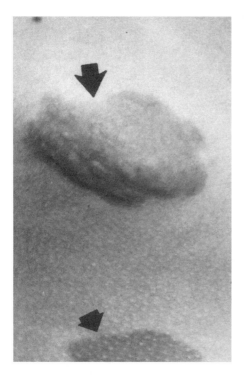

Figure 2-8. The right lower posterior trunk of a patient with NF1, showing an area of hyperpigmentation associated with an underlying diffuse plexiform neurofibroma (large arrow) and an adjacent café-au-lait spot (small arrow).

sociated skin involvement may be the earliest sign of an extensive deep plexiform lesion, either immediately subjacent or at some distance. When the skin over the body's midline is involved, extension into and around the spinal cord is usually present (Fig. 2-10).

Neurofibromas may arise from small nerve radicals, larger nerve branches, individual major nerves (both within and distal to the cervical, brachial, lumbar or sacral plexuses), or dorsal nerve roots in the paraspinal region. Diffuse plexiform neurofibromas affect much more than just the nerve, and the entire region (e.g., a limb) may appear to be dysplastic.

Deep nodular neurofibromas and diffuse plexiform neurofibromas occasionally give rise to malignant peripheral nerve sheath tumors. Malignant peripheral nerve sheath tumors do not appear to arise from discrete cutaneous or subcutaneous neurofibromas. The development and nature of these malignancies are discussed in Chapter 6.

Other Cardinal Features

Café-au-lait Spots. The prototypical café-au-lait spot is 10 to 30 mm in diameter, ovoid in shape, and uniform in color, with the intensity depending on background cutaneous pigmentation (Fig. 2-11). The borders are characteristically sharp and well defined but are sometimes ragged. Variations in color or the

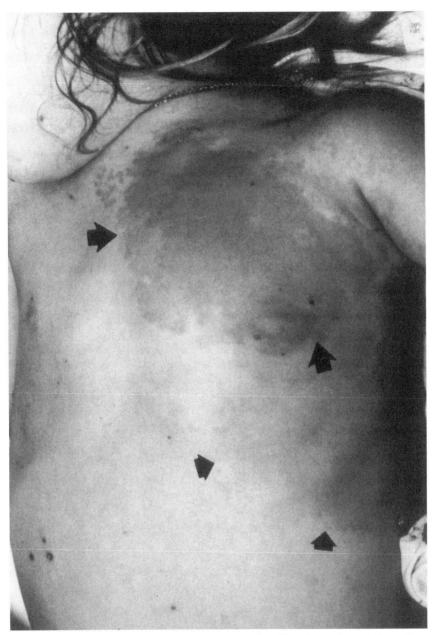

Figure 2-9. The left chest of a patient with NF1, showing diffuse hyperpigmentation adjacent to (small arrows) and overlying (large arrows) a diffuse plexiform neurofibroma with extensive intrathoracic, mediastinal, and retroperitoneal involvement.

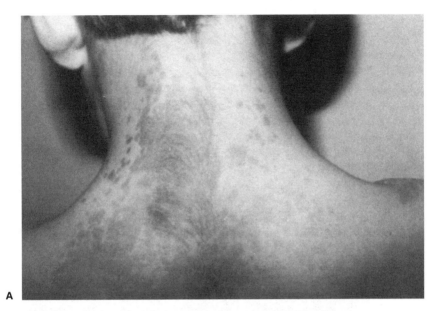

A

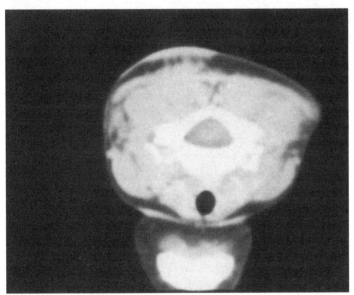

B

Figure 2-10. (A) Hypertrichosis and hyperpigmentation overlying a diffuse plexiform neurofibroma of the posterior neck of a patient with NF1. (B) Cervical CT scan of the same patient, showing a diffuse plexiform neurofibroma underlying the cutaneous hyperpigmentation and hypertrichosis.

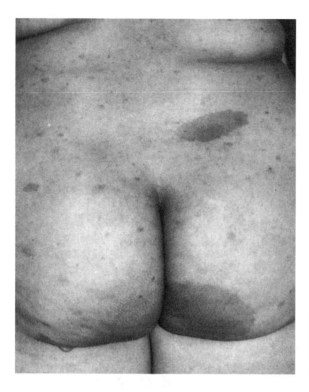

Figure 2-11. The lower back and buttocks of a patient with NF1, showing variation in the size of café-au-lait spots.

smoothness of the borders generally are not thought to be useful in differentiating NF1 from other conditions with multiple café-au-lait spots (Riccardi 1981a, 1982a), although some controversy exists about this (Fois et al. 1993). Café-au-lait spots may be very large, covering much of a body part on one side (Fig. 2-12). Large lesions of the buttocks or trunk are common. Café-au-lait spots may also be smaller than 10 mm in diameter, although differentiation from freckling becomes problematic with decreasing size.

Café-au-lait spots may occur anywhere on the body in patients with NF1 except in the scalp, eyebrows, palms, or soles. Pigment variation in typical café-au-lait spots may be of three types in NF1: (1) two-tone café-au-lait spots, suggesting a café-au-lait spot within a café-au-lait spot (Fig. 2-13); (2) an acquired decrease in pigmentation in scars involving a café-au-lait spot (Fig. 2-14); and (3) increased coloration proportionate to changes in the surrounding skin as a result of sun tanning (Fig. 2-15).

Atypical café-au-lait spots may also be seen in patients with NF1, with variations in the color of the macule, indistinct borders, and odd shapes (Figs. 2-16 and 2-17). Coincidental hyperpigmentation may be superimposed on café-au-lait spots (e.g., by coincident common pigmented nevi). Conversely, a café-au-lait spot overlying a "mongolian spot" may influence the melanin distribution in the mongolian spot (Fig. 2-18). The café-au-lait spot obscures the mongolian spot, and a 2- to 4-mm concentric halo may be produced around the café-au-lait spot.

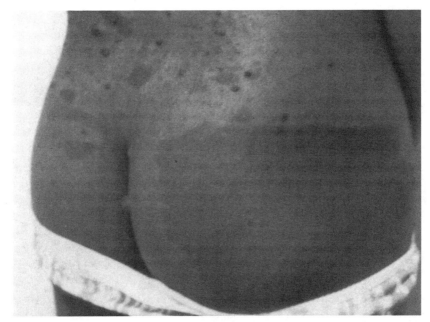

Figure 2-12. A large café-au-lait spot over the buttock of a patient with NF1. Note that the café-au-lait spot is proportionally darker on this patient with black skin than on the patient with white skin shown in Figure 2-11.

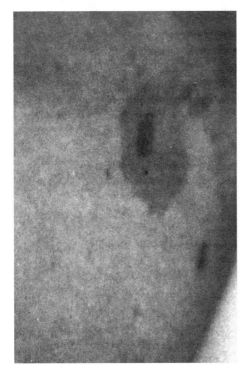

Figure 2-13. Close-up of the skin of an NF1 patient, showing a two-toned café-au-lait spot.

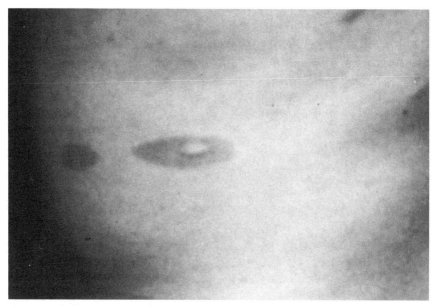

Figure 2-14. The right flank of a patient with NF1, showing normal pigmentation in the scar of a biopsy site in a café-au-lait spot.

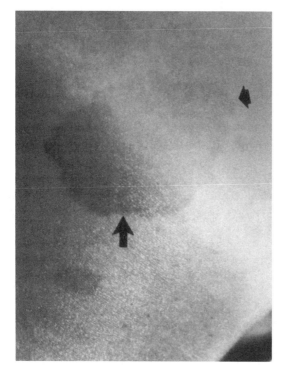

Figure 2-15. The left lateral buttock of a patient with NF1, showing a large café-au-lait spot, part of which has been exposed to the sun (large arrow) and part of which has not (small arrow).

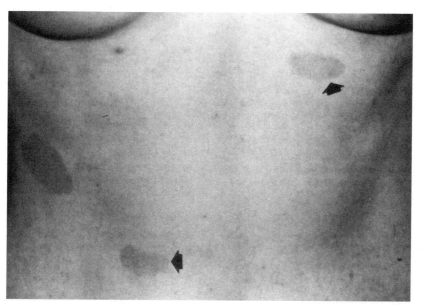

Figure 2-16. The lower chest and abdomen of a patient with NF1, showing café-au-lait spots of varying color intensities and border definitions. The café-au-lait spots at the arrows are very pale and poorly defined in comparison to the typical café-au-lait spot on the right flank.

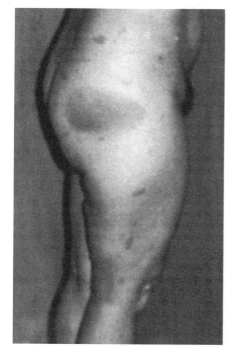

Figure 2-17. Side view of an NF1 patient, showing a large café-au-lait spot with atypically indistinct borders.

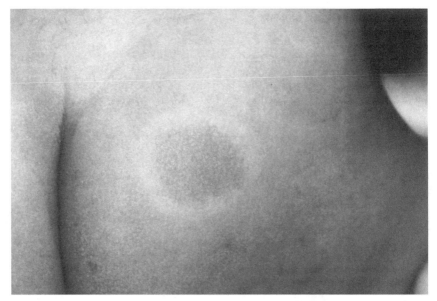

Figure 2-18. The buttock skin of a patient with NF1, showing the "halo" phenomenon that may occur with superimposition of a café-au-lait spot on a mongolian spot.

Beyond this halo, the bluish coloration of the mongolian spot resumes (Ahn et al. 1998; Bocian & Walker 1987).

Café-au-lait spots are characterized histologically by the presence of giant melanosomes (melanin macroglobules) within melanocytes (Fig. 2-19) (Benedict et al. 1968; Martuza et al. 1985; Riccardi and Eichner 1986). The aberrant cellular organelles in café-au-lait spots are not unique to patients with NF1 (Benedict et al. 1968; Bhawan et al. 1976; Konrad et al. 1974; Martuza et al. 1985) and vary in number in individuals with different levels of background pigmentation of the skin. Giant melanosomes are seen in café-au-lait spots of both children and adults with NF1, but the frequency is higher in adults (Riccardi and Eichner 1986). Giant melanosomes are occasionally seen in the unaffected skin of adults with NF1 and, less frequently, in the normal skin of adults without NF1. The presence of giant melanocytes in skin biopsy specimens of café-au-lait spots is, therefore, of little or no use in the diagnosis of NF1.

Axillary and Other Intertriginous Freckling. Although freckles in patients with NF1 usually appear similar to café-au-lait spots in color, freckles are smaller, usually 1 to 3 mm in diameter, and typically occur in clusters. Axillary freckling may be apparent in patients with NF1 at birth but more often appears later in childhood (see Fig. 3-4). Freckling elsewhere develops in childhood or later in life.

Freckling in some patients with NF1 may occur diffusely over the trunk and proximal extremities but in other patients is limited to intertriginous regions or sites of skin apposition, especially in the axillae (Fig. 2-20), inguinal regions,

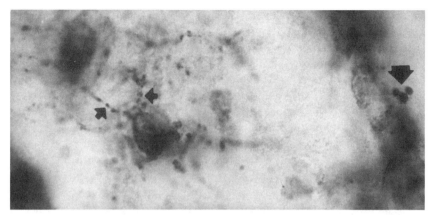

Figure 2-19. Giant melanosomes (large arrow) in a split-thickness skin biopsy specimen from a patient with NF1. Normal-sized melanosomes (small arrows) are also seen in the dendritic processes of a melanocyte (original magnification ×1000).

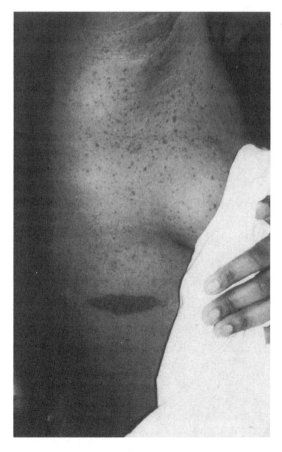

Figure 2-20. The right axilla of a patient with NF1, showing true axillary freckling and a large café-au-lait spot.

upper eyelids, and base of the neck. Two other commonly affected regions are the apposing skin surfaces below the breasts in women (Fig. 2-21) and in skinfolds associated with obesity (Figs. 2-22 and 2-23).

The location of freckles in patients with NF1 suggests that physical factors promote expression of the *NF1* mutation to produce freckling without sun exposure. Such factors might be increased temperature, absence of light, excess moisture, salinity, or some other component of skin secretions. The occasional appearance of freckling at sites where tight clothing, such as a brassiere, rubs against the skin or where itching and scratching are intense (Fig. 2-24) suggests that friction is sometimes important. This may also provide at least a partial explanation for the common occurrence of freckling at the base of the neck, where collars rub.

Lisch Nodules. Iris Lisch nodules are a nearly unique and very frequent feature of NF1 (Lewis and Riccardi 1981; Lisch 1937; Lubs et al. 1991; Riccardi 1981a). Lisch nodules are pigmented hamartomas, (Fig. 2-25 and 2-26) that must be distinguished from iris nevi, which are frequently seen in normal individuals. Lisch nodules are almost always bilateral and present in roughly equal numbers in both irises. The only clearly established exception to this rule is in young children, when only one or two Lisch nodules may be apparent (Huson et al. 1987). However many are present, Lisch nodules are not associated with visual compromise or other ocular manifestations of NF1.

Careful slit-lamp biomicroscopic examination by an experienced ophthalmologist is necessary to determine the presence or absence of Lisch nodules when

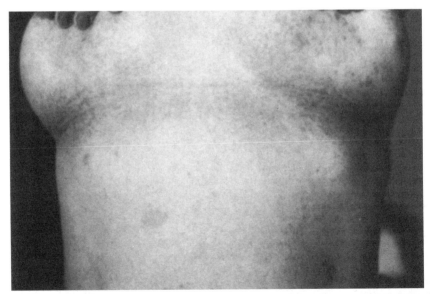

Figure 2-21. The lower chest of a woman with NF1, showing extensive acquired freckling where the breasts (here held up) appose the chest wall.

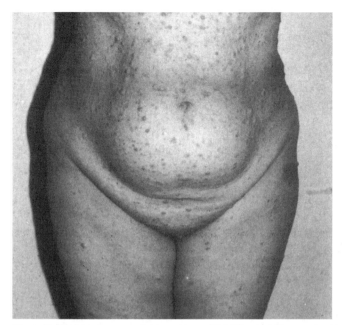

Figure 2-22. The lower trunk of a patient with NF1, showing acquired freckling at skinfold sites, especially on the abdomen.

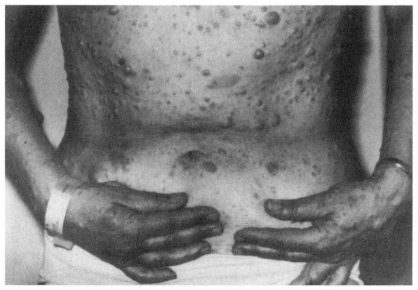

Figure 2-23. The abdomen of a patient with NF1, showing acquired freckling on apposing surfaces of an abdominal skin fold.

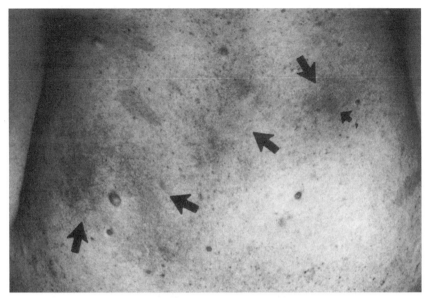

Figure 2-24. Close-up view of the back of a patient with NF1, showing diffuse hyperpigmentation (small arrow) and clusters of freckles (large arrows) in areas of intense itching and scratching.

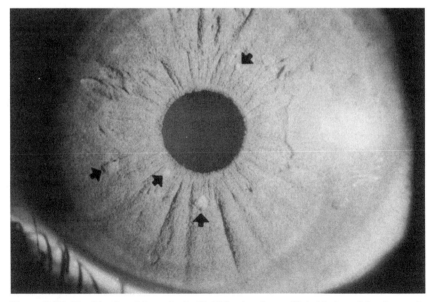

Figure 2-25. The iris of a white patient with NF1, showing multiple Lisch nodules (arrows). *Source:* Photograph courtesy of R.A. Lewis, M.D.

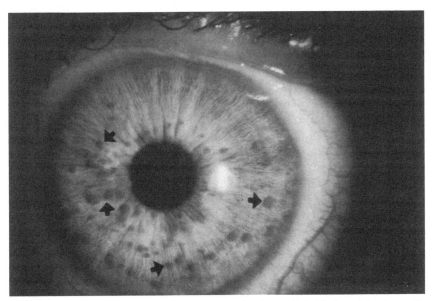

Figure 2-26. The iris of a black patient with NF1, showing multiple Lisch nodules (arrows). *Source:* Photograph courtesy of R.A. Lewis, M.D.

only a few are present and/or the patient is very young. Lisch nodules are seen with the slit lamp to be three-dimensional translucent masses punctuated by melanin-containing cells, usually imparting a gray-tan hue. On a blue, hazel, or very light brown iris, Lisch nodules stand out as being darker (see Fig. 2-25). They can usually be seen easily with an ordinary hand-held ophthalmoscope and their elevated nature demonstrated by shadowing with oblique illumination. On brown or dark brown irises, Lisch nodules appear lighter than the background and look flatter because the translucent prominence is less obvious (see Fig. 2-26). Lisch nodules develop as a function of age (Huson et al. 1987; Lewis and Riccardi 1981; Mautner et al. 1988; Riccardi 1981a; Zehavi et al. 1986). They are uncommon in small children but occur in most patients with NF1 who are over 10 years of age (see Fig. 3-3).

Pathologically, Lisch nodules are characterized as melanocytic hamartomas (Perry and Font 1982). Factors contributing to the origin and growth of these masses are unknown (Rubenstein et al. 1990), but it is interesting to note that Lisch nodules develop in iris tissue that is of neural crest origin.

Optic Gliomas. Gliomas in patients with NF1 may involve any portion of the optic pathway, from the optic nerve at its connection with the globe to the optic radiations in the occipital lobes of the brain. Although optic pathway gliomas occur in about 15% of patients with NF1 (see Chapter 9), these tumors usually remain asymptomatic throughout life. The benign biologic behavior of most optic pathway gliomas in NF1 differs from that of histologically similar tumors in patients who do not have neurofibromatosis. Optic pathway gliomas are discussed in detail in Chapter 9.

Distinctive Osseous Lesions. Dysplastic scoliosis with vertebral scalloping and tibial pseudarthrosis are among the most serious and characteristic clinical manifestations of NF1. Dysplastic scoliosis can produce spinal cord compression with consequent acute or chronic neurologic complications. Although scoliosis occurs in at least 10% of all patients with NF1, the severe dysplastic form is much less frequent.

Tibial and other long bone bowing and thinning are congenital dysplastic lesions that occur in a small percentage of patients with NF1. Pathologic fractures and pseudarthrosis are common complications of this osseous dysplasia, which is usually very difficult to treat effectively. Both vertebral and long bone dysplasia are discussed in Chapter 11.

ABNORMALITIES OF FUNCTION

The most frequent abnormalities of function in NF1 involve the central nervous system. They are described in detail in Chapters 7 to 9. Learning disabilities affect 30 to 65% of patients, but frank mental retardation is uncommon (see Chapter 7). Visual deficits associated with optic gliomas are the most common sensory abnormality (see Chapter 9). Other sensory or motor deficits may result from central nervous system tumors or from neurofibromas involving or impinging on spinal nerve roots or major peripheral nerves. These complications can be very serious or even life threatening; fortunately, they are uncommon. Complications of the skeletal abnormalities that characterize NF1 can also have serious functional consequences. Scoliosis, especially the dysplastic form (see Chapter 11), can produce pulmonary restriction and other major functional handicaps, even if neurologic involvement does not occur. Tibial pseudoarthrosis may lead to amputation (see Chapter 11).

The occurrence of plexiform neurofibromas within or adjacent to vital organs can cause obstruction (e.g., to the gastrointestinal tract, renal excretory system, or birth canal) (Brown et al. 1997; Kimmelman 1979). Neurofibromas may also produce local erosion with consequent bleeding into the gastrointestinal, urinary, or respiratory tract, within the abdominal, pleural, or retroperitoneal space, or into soft tissues (Du Toit 1987; Frank et al. 1981; Jeng et al. 1988; Melin et al. 1994; Tung et al. 1997; Waxman et al. 1986). Most deep nodular and plexiform neurofibromas are asymptomatic, however (Tonsgard et al. 1998).

Local hypertrophy is sometimes associated with the presence of a plexiform neurofibroma, especially of the limb or face. Such lesions can impair function and cause substantial disfigurement (Figs. 2-27 and 2-28). Discrete cutaneous and subcutaneous neurofibromas are often of cosmetic significance and occasionally can seriously impair a patient's ability to function normally in society.

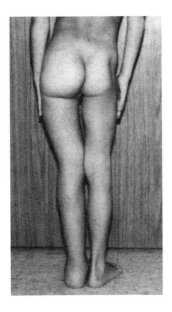

Figure 2-27. The posterior lower limbs of a patient with NF1, showing a diffuse plexiform neurofibroma with segmental hypertrophy extending from the left upper buttock to the sole of the foot.

THE OVERALL PHENOTYPE IN PATIENTS WITH NF1

Body Habitus

Patients with NF1 are usually shorter than average and have larger than average head circumferences. The weight of most patients with NF1 is similar to that of unaffected people of the same age and sex, but serious obesity is less common among older children and adults with NF1. Growth in people with NF1 is discussed in detail in Chapter 11.

"Typical Facies"

Some clinicians consider the facial appearance of patients with NF1 to be distinctive (Kaplan and Rosenblatt 1985; Norman 1972; Pivnick et al. 1997; Westerhof et al. 1984)). Figure 2-29 shows a patient who exhibits the characteristic facial features, including a broad-based nose and apparent ocular hypertelorism. Although patients with NF1 often do have a characteristic facial appearance, it is not clear that this is sufficiently distinctive to be of clinical importance (Pivnick et al. 1997).

The typical pigmentary abnormalities, macrocephaly, and superimposed consequences of facial neurofibromas, including asymmetry and local tumor prominences, may immediately suggest a diagnosis of NF1 to an experienced clinician. Individuals with NF1 who have a truly distinctive facial appearance often just share the facial characteristics of other family members. While aberrations of the facial skeleton (e.g., sphenoid wing dysplasia) certainly do occur among patients

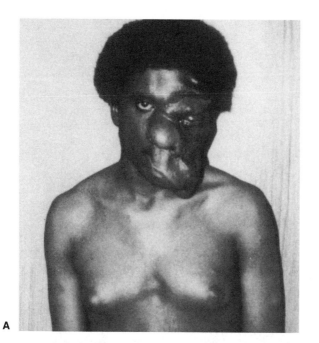

A

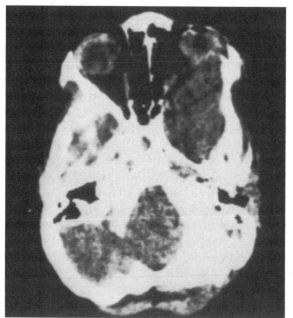

B

Figure 2-28. (A) Severe facial disfigurement and functional impairment from a diffuse plexiform neurofibroma in a man with NF1. The patient also has gynecomastia. (B) Cranial CT scan of the same patient, showing intraorbital and intracranial extension of the diffuse facial plexiform neurofibroma.

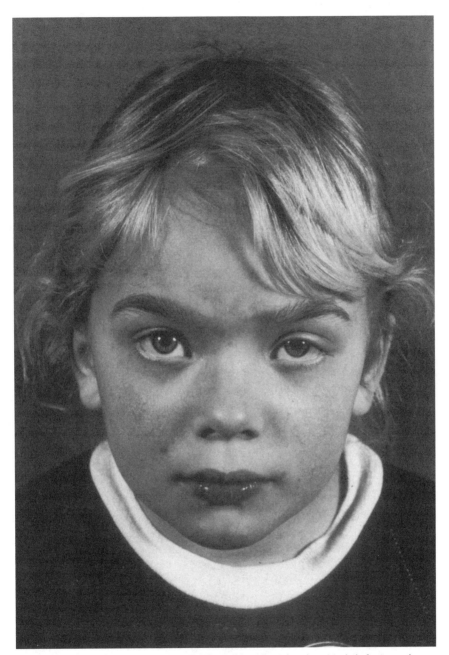

Figure 2-29. The face of a patient with NF1, said to show the characteristic features, including telecanthus. *Source:* Courtesy of Westerhof et al. 1984. Reprinted with permission.

with NF1, the spectrum of changes is so great that no single set of facial characteristics defines patients with NF1 as a group.

Aging

A prematurely aged appearance of the face is often, but not always, seen in middle-aged adults with NF1. This "older" appearance probably results from a combination of ruddy pigmented coloration and laxity of the skin. Skin laxity occurs in adults with NF1 whether or not facial cutaneous neurofibromas are present in large numbers. This observation suggests that the *NF1* mutation may affect the integrity of connective tissues. This same process may sometimes produce joint laxity, especially of the fingers and wrists, and an unusual and distinctive softness and smoothness of the skin in the fourth or fifth decades of life. Occasional reports of coincidental NF1 and Ehlers–Danlos syndrome (De Angelis and Cirillo 1968; Goodman et al. 1962; Taylor et al. 1984; Turkington and Grode 1964) may represent extreme manifestations of this phenomenon. Mutation analysis has not been reported in such patients for either the *NF1* locus or loci associated with Ehlers–Danlos syndrome.

NATURAL HISTORY

In any affected person, NF1 becomes more obvious and more severe with the passage of time. Moreover, lesions of different kinds characteristically develop at different times of life (Friedman and Birch 1997b; Goldberg et al. 1996; Huson et al. 1989b; Reynolds and Pineda 1988). Little is known about the factors that contribute to disease progression, and disease activity at one point in life does not necessarily predict severity later (Riccardi 1992; Zöller et al. 1995). From a clinical perspective, the natural history of NF1 is obscured by variable expressivity of the disease and the pleiotropy of *NF1* mutations. Allelic heterogeneity (i.e., the effects of different specific mutations of the *NF1* locus) may have some influence on the phenotype as well.

Variable *expressivity* means that a mutation may produce widely disparate types of lesions and very different overall disease severity in affected individuals. NF1 exhibits extremely variable expressivity, even within a single family. A related but distinct concept is pleiotropy. *Pleiotropy* means that a mutation can involve many different tissues or organs in an affected individual. *NF1* mutations are also extremely pleiotropic. At one time this was attributed to the fact that NF1 can involve many different tissues of neural crest origin (Bolande 1974, 1981), but tissues that are not derived from the embryonic neural crest, such as the bones and blood, may also be affected.

Genetic heterogeneity is the existence of more than one genotype that can produce a clinically similar or identical phenotype. The term is usually employed to mean *locus heterogeneity* (i.e., the occurrence of a particular disease as the result of mutations at more than one genetic locus). Before NF1 and NF2 were distinguished as separate clinical entities, genetic heterogeneity clearly existed within the "neurofibromatoses." This confounded many clinical descriptions of neurofibromatosis. The establishment of generally accepted diagnostic criteria for NF1 and NF2 (Gutmann et al. 1997; National Institutes of Health Consensus Development Conference 1988) has now improved this situation substantially. There is no evidence for locus heterogeneity within NF1 itself (Barker et al. 1987; Mathew et al. 1989; Riccardi 1993; Seizinger et al. 1987).

MORBIDITY AND MORTALITY

Overall Function and Adaptation

Estimates of the overall severity of NF1 are available from a variety of sources (Huson et al. 1989a, 1989b; Riccardi 1992; Samuelsson and Samuelsson 1989), but most available data are derived from cross-sectional studies. Longitudinal follow-up of three groups of patients has provided important additional information on the natural history of NF1. Borberg (1951) described a nationwide cohort of Danish patients with neurofibromatosis who have now been followed for more than 50 years (Sørensen et al. 1986a, 1986b). More recently, Zöller and associates (1995, 1997a, 1997b) described a 12-year medical and psychiatric follow-up of a population-based series of Swedish patients with NF1 who were originally assembled by Samuelsson and Samuelsson (1989). Riccardi (1992) reported experience with serial evaluations of a larger, clinic-based group of patients with NF1 in the previous edition of this book. All of these studies demonstrate that NF1 is a progressive, although unpredictable, disease associated with a variety of clinical manifestations and complications. NF1 can remain quite mild in some patients, but life expectancy is reduced overall.

Severity Scales

The severity of NF1 is determined by many factors, of which age is the most important. Nevertheless, it is obvious from simple clinical observation that some patients have more severe disease manifestations than others of the same age. Some patients have debilitating or even fatal disease early in life, while others live to an advanced age with only mild manifestations. To provide an assessment of overall disease severity, some clinicians employ graded scales based on the clinical features of NF1 present in a particular patient at a given time in his or her life. One such scale is given in Table 2-1 (Riccardi 1992). Other authors (Carey et al. 1979; Samuelsson and Samuelsson 1989) have proposed alternative systems to assess the severity of NF1, but none of these scales has been generally adopted. Although severity scales provide a relatively easy way to describe the current clinical state of a patient, their general usefulness is limited because they do not predict the future course of the disease.

Mortality and Causes of Death

Most NF1-related deaths occur in childhood or middle adulthood. Death in childhood usually results from an intracranial tumor or, less frequently, from a malignant peripheral nerve sheath tumor, leukemia, or embryonal tumor. The progressive growth of a diffuse plexiform neurofibroma involving the cervical region or upper mediastinum may also cause death in a child with NF1.

Table 2-1. The NF1 severity grading system described by Riccardi (1992)

Feature	Severity Grade			
	1	2	3	4
ANATOMIC/STRUCTURAL				
Pigmentation				
Café-au-lait spots	+	+	+	0
Axillary freckling	+	+	0	0
Other freckling	+	+	0	0
Hyperpigmentation overlying plexiform neurofibroma	+	+	+	0
Other hyperpigmentation	+	+	+	0
Hypopigmentation	+	+	+	0
Neurofibromas				
Skin				
Cutaneous	+	+	+	+
Subcutaneous	+	+	+	+
Deep	E	+	+	+
Diffuse				
Orbital/periorbital	E	E	+	+
Other craniofacial	E	E	+	+
Chest	E	+	+	+
Paraspinal/cervical	E	E	+	+
Paraspinal/thoracic	E	E	+	+
Paraspinal/lumbosacral	E	E	+	+
Abdomino-retroperitoneal	E	E	+	+
Limb	E	E	+	+
Visceral	E	+	+	+
Schwannoma/non–central nervous system	+	+	+	+
Central nervous system tumors				
Glioma/orbit	E	E	+	+
Other orbit tumor	E	E	+	+
Glioma/chiasm	E	E	+	+
Glioma/other	E	E	+	+
Schwannoma/brain	E	E	+	+
Meningioma/brain	E	E	+	+
Other brain tumor	E	E	+	+
Spinal cord tumor	E	E	+	+
Pheochromocytoma	E	E	+	+
Carcinoid	E	E	+	+
Other benign tumor	E	+	+	+
Malignancy	E	E	E	+
Ocular				
Lisch nodules	+	0	0	0
Corneal nerves	+	0	0	0
Choroidal hamartomas	+	0	0	0
Congenital glaucoma, etc.	E	+	+	+
Ptosis	E	+	+	0
Cataract	E	+	+	+
Skeletal	E	+	+	0
Short stature	+	0	0	0
Macrocephaly	+	0	0	0
Craniofacial dysplasia	E	+	+	+

Table 2-1. *Continued*

	Severity Grade			
Feature	1	2	3	4
Spine				
Vertebral dysplasia	E	+	+	+
Scoliosis/kyphoscoliosis	E	+	+	+
Lumbar scalloping	+	0	0	0
Pseudarthrosis				
Tibial	E	E	+	+
Other	E	E	+	+
Genu valgum/varum	E	+	+	0
Pectus excavatum	+	+	+	0
Other skeletal	E	+	+	+
Colon ganglioneuromatosis	E	+	+	0
Xanthogranulomas	+	+	0	0
Vascular				
Angiomas	E	+	+	+
Renal	E	E	+	+
Cerebral	E	E	+	+
Other vascular	E	+	+	+
Cerebrospinal fluid spaces				
Ventricle dilation	E	E	+	0
Hydrocephalus	E	E	+	+
Other cerebrospinal fluid	E	+	+	+
Excessive dental caries	E	+	+	0
EEG abnormality	E	+	+	0
Other anatomic/structural	E	+	+	+
FUNCTIONAL				
Death	E	E	E	+
Whole person	E	E	+	+
Cosmesis disfigurement	E	+	+	+
Hypertrophic impairment	E	E	+	+
Neurologic				
Weakness/paralysis	E	E	+	+
Incoordination	E	+	+	+
Pain	E	+	+	+
Seizures	E	E	+	+
Other neurologic	E	+	+	+
Strabismus	E	+	+	0
Visual impairment	E	E	+	+
Hearing impairment	E	+	+	+
Speech impediment	E	+	+	0
Intellectual				
Developmental delay	E	+	+	+
Learning disability	E	+	+	+
School performance problems	E	+	+	+
Mental retardation	E	E	E	+
Psychologic				
Psychosocial burden	E	+	+	+
Psychiatric disturbance	E	E	+	+

(cont.)

Table 2-1. *Continued*

	Severity Grade			
Feature	1	2	3	4
Headache	E	+	+	0
Puberty disturbance	E	E	+	+
Pruritus	E	+	+	+
Constipation	E	+	+	0
Gastrointestinal hemorrhage	E	E	+	+
Hypertension	E	E	+	+
Surgery	E	+	+	+
Other functional	E	+	+	+

Note: The table lists clinical features used to determine each severity grade. For a detailed explanation of the severity scales, see Chapter 1. *Key:* + = the feature is consistent with the severity grade designated; if more than one severity grade is designated, this feature has graded levels of severity; if only one severity grade is designated, then the feature is merely of diagnostic utility (grade 1) or it requires the highest severity grade (4). E = the feature excludes the designated severity grade. 0 = the feature is not a criterion for the designated severity grade.

NF1-related death in early or middle adulthood usually results from a malignant peripheral nerve sheath tumor or sarcoma of another tissue. Other problems that can lead to early death in patients with NF1 include acute hydrocephalus, severe seizures, gastrointestinal hemorrhage, intracranial hemorrhage related to NF1 vasculopathy, progressive spinal cord encroachment by plexiform neurofibromas or unstable dysplastic scoliosis, and complications of hypertension caused by arterial dysplasia or pheochromocytoma. All of these conditions are discussed in subsequent chapters of this book.

Two population-based long-term follow-up studies provide the best available mortality data on adult patients with NF1. Sørensen and associates (1986b) estimated survival over 39 years for 76 probands with NF1 and 79 of their affected relatives identified through Danish hospital admission records (Borberg 1951). Survival was significantly reduced among the patients with NF1 in comparison with the general population. The effect was more marked in the probands than in their relatives, but the reduction was also significant for affected relatives, so ascertainment bias is unlikely to be the only explanation. The most common causes of death—cancer, myocardial infarction, cerebrovascular accidents, and pneumonia—were similar to those in the general population. Central nervous system tumors, especially gliomas, and second primary neoplasms appeared to be unusually frequent among patients with NF1.

The series reported by Zöller et al. (1995) includes information on 70 patients with NF1 from Göteborg, Sweden, whose average age was 43.6±15.4 years at the time of ascertainment. Over the next 12 years, 22 of these patients died, whereas 5.1 deaths would have been expected in the general population. The mean age at death for the patients with NF1 was 61.6 years. The average life expectancy for the Swedish population from which the patients were drawn was 75 years. Malignancy, the most common cause of death, occurred in 17 (24%) of the 70 patients reported by Zöller et al. (1995, 1997b). Hypertension was significantly associated with mortality—10 of 12 patients with NF1 who had high blood pressure died during the period of observation. Cardiovascular disease, hemorrhage, or embolism caused the death of 7 individuals, but this may have been unrelated to the NF1 in some or all of these cases.

PROGRESSION OF THE DISEASE THROUGHOUT LIFE

Neurofibromas

Neurofibromas may develop at any time in the life of persons with NF1. The occurrence of neurofibromas provides a vivid illustration of how the disease can vary with age. The occasional finding of an aberrant hair whorl over the spine when there are underlying paraspinal neurofibromas (Fig. 2-30) indicates that these tumors are sometimes present during fetal development. This clinical finding, which is often called the "Riccardi sign" (Flannery and Howell 1987), is important because of the frequent association of dysplastic scoliosis as well. The aberrant hair whorl is thought to reflect alteration of hair patterning by an abnormality of the shape or organization of underlying tissues before 16 weeks of fetal development (Jones 1997).

Further evidence for the in utero occurrence of neurofibromas is provided by their occasional presence in newborns with NF1. Congenital neurofibromas are characteristically (perhaps exclusively) of the diffuse plexiform type. Diffuse

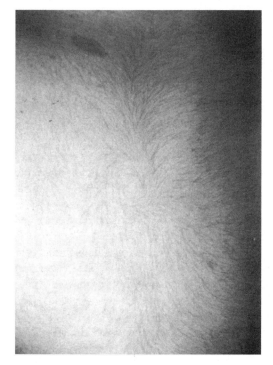

Figure 2-30. Close-up of the back of a patient with NF1, showing a midline hair whorl overlying paravertebral neurofibromas and associated vertebral dysplasia (Riccardi sign).

plexiform neurofibromas are virtually all congenital, even if they do not become apparent until later in life. Consequently, some infants with NF1 present with a diffuse plexiform neurofibroma (or with an area of cutaneous hyperpigmentation that overlies an associated plexiform neurofibroma) before any other signs of NF1 are apparent. While congenital diffuse plexiform neurofibromas may be quiescent in infancy, more often they exhibit active growth during this time.

The two body areas most likely to be involved with a congenital diffuse plexiform neurofibroma are the craniofacial region and the neck and superior mediastinal region. Craniofacial involvement is usually in one of two distinctive patterns: (1) involvement of the second division of the trigeminal nerve, in which the orbit and periorbital regions are primarily affected, or (2) involvement of the third division of the trigeminal nerve, in which the buccal, oropharyngeal, and retro pharyngeal regions are primarily affected. Each of these patterns occurs in at least 5% of patients with NF1. Sphenoid wing dysplasia is often seen in association with an orbital or periorbital diffuse plexiform neurofibroma but may also occur in the absence of such a tumor. The cervical/pharyngeal/mediastinal congenital diffuse plexiform neurofibromas warrant special attention because their aggressive growth in infancy and childhood can lead to severe compromise or death (Apter et al. 1975). Congenital diffuse plexiform neurofibromas occurring elsewhere in the body, particularly in the perineum or limbs, may also be troublesome early in life. Diffuse plexiform neurofibromas may also progress during adolescence.

It is unusual for discrete cutaneous or subcutaneous neurofibromas or deep nodular neurofibromas to become apparent during infancy or early childhood. These tumors more often appear in later childhood or during adolescence (Friedman and Birch 1997b; Huson 1994; Huson et al. 1988). The onset of puberty is often associated with a substantial increase in the number and size of discrete neurofibromas, but dermal neurofibromas do not begin to develop until the late second or third decade of life in some patients with NF1.

During early adulthood, the skin of the trunk tends to become peppered with relatively large numbers of discrete neurofibromas. This occurs as the more or less sequential development of tumors ranging in size from 3 to 12 mm over a number of years. There is typically marked variation in growth from one neurofibroma to another. A second, less common, pattern is characterized by the rapid development of innumerable dermal neurofibromas over a period of months. This is sometimes called "eruptive neurofibromatosis" (Fitzpatrick et al. 1983).

A sudden increase in the number and size of cutaneous neurofibromas often occurs during pregnancy (Dugoff and Sujansky 1996). As pregnancy progresses, cutaneous neurofibromas tend to appear engorged—larger, turgid, and mildly inflamed. Growth in size of diffuse plexiform neurofibromas may also occur during pregnancy. In both instances, some regression in size often occurs within weeks of parturition, and reversion to the pre-pregnancy state is common.

The middle and late adulthood of most patients with NF1 are characterized by a progressive but highly variable increase in the number and size of neurofibromas throughout the body. Late adulthood is a relatively quiescent period in terms of neurofibroma development compared with earlier in life. It is unusual for an elderly person with NF1 to have serious new problems related to neurofibromas, but additional complications from long-standing tumors may occur.

Other Disease Manifestations

The purpose of this section is to outline briefly the timing of onset of other features of NF1. The object is to provide an overview of the temporal course of the disease with respect to age. Detailed discussion of the nature and evolution of these problems can be found in other parts of this book.

Infancy. Café-au-lait spots may be present at birth and usually increase in number during infancy. New café-au-lait spots rarely appear after the first few years of life (see Fig. 3-2). Long-bone bowing, which may lead to pseudarthrosis, is a congenital lesion, although it may not be obvious at birth. Optic glioma and seizures are among the more common serious manifestations of NF1 that may become apparent in the first year of life. Congenital glaucoma and deafness are less frequent but may also present in infancy.

Childhood. Learning disabilities usually become apparent when children with NF1 begin school. Delayed gross motor development or difficulties with speech may be seen in younger children, and mental retardation, although much less frequent, often presents earlier. Visual impairment resulting from optic gliomas usually develops within the first six years of life. Symptoms of brain tumors may also become evident in childhood. Leukemia, although more common in children with NF1 than in other children, is a rare complication of NF1.

Dystrophic scoliosis usually presents during middle childhood and may do so with rapid progression of the curve or with neurological impairment, especially if there are associated paraspinal neurofibromas. Dystrophic scoliosis does not usually develop before about 6 years of age, and most patients with NF1 who are affected with dystrophic scoliosis have unremarkable spines clinically in early childhood. Dystrophic scoliosis is unlikely to occur if it is not apparent by the end of the first decade of life.

Short stature and macrocephaly are often diagnosed in patients with NF1 during childhood. Precocious puberty may occur, especially in children with optic chiasm gliomas. Hypertension is occasionally seen in children with NF1. When high blood pressure does develop in this age group, a demonstrable cause such as renal artery stenosis or aortic coarctation can often be found.

Adolescence. Worsening of preexisting problems (e.g., scoliosis) often occurs during adolescence. Cosmetic disfigurement or learning disabilities may produce serious psychologic consequences in teenagers with NF1. Malignant peripheral nerve sheath tumors begin to develop at this time, but fortunately, they are uncommon in adolescents.

Adulthood. The most frequent problem among young adults with NF1 is an increase in the number and size of neurofibromas, with both cosmetic disfigurement and functional compromise (e.g., pain, paralysis, gastrointestinal hemorrhage, or renovascular hypertension) as a consequence. Malignant peripheral nerve sheath tumors most often occur in the third decade of life but may develop earlier or later (Poyhonen et al. 1997b; Zöller et al. 1997b). If pseudarthrosis, dystrophic scoliosis, optic glioma, diffuse plexiform neurofibromas, or other characteristics of early childhood have not developed, they will not do so when patients with NF1 are adults.

VARIABILITY

Although NF1 is progressive over the course of an affected individual's life, the rate of progression and the occurrence of serious disease manifestations and complications vary greatly from patient to patient. Affected members of a single family, all of whom have the same mutation of the *NF1* locus, may have very different disease manifestations. There are several possible sources of the extreme variability that characterizes NF1:

Allelic heterogeneity has a limited role in determining clinical variability. Allelic effects are probably responsible for the severe phenotype seen with deletions of the entire *NF1* gene (Kayes et al. 1992, 1994; Leppig et al. 1996, 1997; Riva et al. 1996; Tonsgard et al. 1997; Upadhyaya et al. 1998; Valero et al. 1997; Wu et al. 1995, 1997b) and for the intrafamilial consistency seen with Watson syndrome (Allanson et al. 1991; Upadhyaya et al. 1992) and some instances of familial café-au-lait syndrome (Abeliovich et al. 1995). A few other possible examples are discussed under "Clinical Subtypes" below, but strong allele–phenotype correlations in NF1 are exceptional.

Three other genes are known to be embedded within an intron of the *NF1* locus, and involvement of one or more of these genes might affect the NF1 phenotype (Habib et al. 1998; Viskochil et al. 1991). However, direct evidence for an effect of these genes on the clinical manifestations of NF1 is lacking.

Polymorphic variations in the normal allele could affect expression of the mutant allele. There is currently no evidence to support this conjecture in NF1.

Loci with partial homology to the *NF1* gene have been found on several chromosomes (Gasparini et al. 1993; Legius et al. 1992; Purandare et al. 1995; Ritchie et al. 1998). Although many of these loci are simply pseudogenes, some are transcribed and might influence *NF1* expression.

Epistasis is the effect of genes at other loci or, more generally, of the "genetic background." Evidence for the action of modifying genes is provided by a study of concordance for various clinical features of NF1 among affected relatives (Easton et al. 1993). The higher frequency of tumors observed among women with NF1 than among affected men (Samuelsson and Axelsson 1981; Sørensen et al. 1986b) may also be due to epistasis.

The *NF1* transcript is subject to posttranscriptional control of various kinds. Alternative splicing produces isoforms that exhibit differential expression during development and in different tissues (Danglot et al. 1995; Geist and Gutmann 1996; Gutmann 1998; Skuse and Cappione 1997). Stability, transport, and editing of the *NF1* mRNA transcript are often altered in cells from affected patients (Hoffmeyer et al. 1994, 1995; Metheny et al. 1995). In some patients with *NF1* nonsense mutations, the mutant exon may be spliced out during mRNA processing, preventing premature termination of the neurofibromin that is produced (Hoffmeyer et al. 1998). These processes could affect neurofibromin activity in affected tissues and play a role in clinical variability.

Somatic mosaicism has been demonstrated in a family in which the disease was milder in the parent, who had an *NF1* mutation in only a portion of cells, than in the child, who had the mutation in all cells (Tonsgard et al. 1997). Somatic mosaicism for an *NF1* mutation may contribute to the phenotypic variability in this family, but it is not yet clear how important this phenomenon is in general (Rasmussen et al. 1998; Zlotogora 1993).

Epigenetic effects such as imprinting may contribute to the clinical variability of NF1, although there is little evidence to support this possibility. In one series, children who inherited NF1 from their mothers appeared to be more severely affected than children who inherited the disease from their fathers (Hall 1981; Miller and Hall 1978), but this finding has not been confirmed in subsequent larger studies (Huson et al. 1989a; Riccardi and Wald 1987).

Nongenetic factors such as environmental exposures, diet, or trauma may be responsible for some of the variability in NF1. By far the most important nongenetic factor that affects the phenotype of NF1 is age. Local tissue injury may also play a role in development of neurofibromas (Riccardi 1992).

Chance probably accounts for much of the clinical variability in NF1 (Riccardi 1993). Evidence of acquired mutations of the normal *NF1* allele in peripheral neurofibromas of patients with NF1 (Colman et al. 1995; Sawada et al. 1996) suggests that random "second hit" somatic mutations may be important in the development of at least some of the characteristic benign tumors that give neurofibromatosis its name.

CLINICAL SUBTYPES

Segmental NF1

The term *segmental NF* has been used in various ways by different authors, and some reported cases probably are just mild manifestations of generalized NF1. The strictest and most useful definition of segmental NF1 is that put forward by Riccardi (1982b, 1984): café-au-lait spots (and/or freckling) and accompanying neurofibroma(s) restricted to a single side of the body, with no crossing of the midline. Defined in this way, segmental NF1 can be considered a more or less specific subtype of NF1 (Miller and Sparkes 1977; Riccardi 1984; Saul and Stevenson 1984; Viskochil and Carey 1994).

The significance of not crossing the midline relates to the observation that café-au-lait spots in the usual form of NF1 show no limitation of distribution with respect to the midline (Riccardi 1981b). Café-au-lait spots occur randomly over the trunk in patients with generalized NF1, and some lesions may actually straddle the midline. The respect that neurofibromas, café-au-lait spots, and freckling show for the midline in segmental NF1 suggests that a distinctive embryologic and/or genetic mechanism operates in such patients. The responsible mechanism is thought to be postzygotic somatic mutation of the *NF1* gene (Crowe et al. 1956; Miller and Sparkes 1977; Riccardi 1982b). Although somatic mosaicism for an *NF1* mutation has not yet been demonstrated in any patient with segmental NF1, one observation that supports this interpretation is the fact that segmental NF1 is never inherited (Miller and Sparkes 1977; Riccardi 1992; Viskochil and Carey 1994). One would expect the parents of a child with segmental NF1 to be unaffected if both transmitted a normal *NF1* allele to the conceptus and the pathogenic mutation arose later in embryogenesis.

Patients with segmental NF1 may have children with generalized NF1 (Boltshauser et al. 1989; Moss and Green 1994; Rubenstein et al. 1983). This would be expected if segmental NF1 is caused by a postzygotic *NF1* mutation that can sometimes involve the germ cells as well as somatic tissues. A child who inherits NF1 from a parent with segmental disease would be expected to carry the pathogenic *NF1* mutation in all the cells of his or her body.

Interpreting segmental NF1 as a manifestation of somatic mosaicism implies that all cells containing the *NF1* mutation in an individual are clonally related (i.e., all should be linear descendants of the embryonic cell that sustained the mutation). Embryonic development in mammals is generally not characterized by progressive restriction of developmental potential in clonally related cells that are restricted to particular circumscribed regions. Extensive mixing of cells with various clonal histories is generally the rule in mammalian embryonic development. One of the few developmental boundaries that does exist in mammals is the midline, and it is established very early in embryogenesis (Wolpert et al. 1998).

For somatic mosicaism to affect a region of the body large enough to be recognized as segmental NF1, the mutation must have occurred very early in embryogenesis, but after the midline was established as a developmental boundary. The earlier in embryogenesis a mutation occurs, the more likely it is that the cells that carry it will be distributed widely throughout the body. Therefore, it would not be surprising to find mosaicism for the *NF1* mutation in many different tissues of such patients. This may explain the occurrence of the *NF1* mutation in germline as well as somatic cells in some patients with typical segmental NF1 (Viskochil and Carey 1994), the finding of iris Lisch nodules in patients with otherwise typical segmental NF1 (Moss and Green 1994; Weleber and Zonana 1983), and the occurrence of somewhat localized forms of NF1 in patients who do not meet Riccardi's strict definition of segmental NF1 (Roth et al. 1987; Viskochil and Carey 1994).

The limited "window" of embryogenesis during which a postzygotic *NF1* mutation would be expected to produce the phenotype of segmental NF1 probably accounts for the fact that all patients reported to date with mosaicism for an *NF1* mutation have exhibited generalized, rather than segmental, disease (Ainsworth et al. 1997; Colman et al. 1996; Rasmussen et al. 1998; Tonsgard et al. 1997; Wu et al. 1997a). Segmental NF1 may occur when the mutation arises a little later in development. Instances in which the mutation occurs still later are probably not recognized as neurofibromatosis clinically but might present with an apparently isolated lesion, such as a malignant nerve sheath tumor, in which inactivation of the *NF1* gene may be pathogenically important (Legius et al. 1993; Lothe et al. 1995).

Large-Deletion Phenotype

A more or less distinct phenotype has been described in patients who have deletions of the entire *NF1* locus (Kayes et al. 1992, 1994; Leppig et al. 1996, 1997; Riva et al. 1996; Tonsgard et al. 1997; Valero et al. 1997; Upadhyaya et al. 1998; Wu et al. 1995, 1997b). The features of reported patients include an unusually large number of discrete dermal neurofibromas early in life, developmental delay or mental retardation, and dysmorphic but not entirely characteristic facies.

It is unclear how consistently this phenotype is actually associated with deletion of the entire *NF1* locus. Families have been reported in which large deletions of the *NF1* locus segregate not only with NF1 but also with associated features of this phenotype (Leppig et al. 1997; Wu et al. 1997b). On the other hand, many patients with NF1 who have similar features do not have large deletions (Tonsgard et al. 1997; Wu et al. 1995), and large *NF1* deletions have been observed in patients without this unusual phenotype (Rasmussen et al. 1998).

Watson Syndrome

Pulmonic stenosis, multiple café-au-lait spots, and dull intelligence are the cardinal features of Watson syndrome (Allanson et al. 1991; Watson 1967). Affected patients may also have other manifestations of NF1, including axillary freckling, Lisch nodules, multiple neurofibromas, short stature, macrocephaly, and characteristic "unidentified bright objects" (UBOs) on MRI scan of the brain (Allanson et al. 1991; Leão and Robeiro da Silva 1995; Watson 1967).

Watson syndrome is transmitted as an autosomal dominant trait with less phenotypic variability than is usually seen in NF1. Studies have demonstrated linkage of Watson syndrome to the *NF1* locus (Allanson et al. 1991), and an 80-kb deletion of the *NF1* gene has been reported in one patient with Watson syndrome (Upadhyaya et al. 1992). Thus, Watson syndrome appears to be an allelic variant of NF1.

Familial Café-au-Lait Spots

Café-au-lait spots without other characteristic features of NF1 can be transmitted as an autosomal dominant trait (Arnsmeier et al. 1994; Charrow et al. 1993; Riccardi 1980, 1982b; Whitehouse 1966). In most families that have been studied, this trait is not linked to the *NF1* locus (Brunner et al. 1993; Charrow et al. 1993), although linkage to *NF1* appears likely in one large kindred (Abeliovich et al. 1995). The phenotype is consistent in affected members of this family: all have multiple café-au-lait spots and none has any other features of NF1.

Other Possible Subtypes of NF1

Small numbers of patients with NF1 have been reported with phenotypes defined by unusual combinations of features or apparent familial consistency. Further clinical, genetic, and molecular studies of such patients are necessary to determine if these phenotypes represent discrete NF1 subtypes.

Carcinoid of the Duodenum, Pheochromocytoma, and NF1. Pheochromocytomas are neoplasms that can cause severe and sometimes fatal hypertension. They arise in the adrenal medulla or various other organs associated with the sympathetic nervous system. Although they are an uncommon complication of NF1, pheochromocytomas are much more common in patients with NF1 than in others. Pheochromocytomas develop from neural crest–derived chromaffin cells. Although most pheochromocytomas in patients with NF1 are benign, the tumors usually show loss of heterozygosity for DNA markers in the region of the *NF1* locus (Gutmann et al. 1994; Xu et al. 1992). Loss of heterozygosity for DNA markers in the region of the *NF1* gene is not found in most pheochromocytomas in patients who do not have NF1. Pheochromocytomas are discussed in detail in Chapter 12.

Carcinoid tumors are neoplasms that contain a variety of peptide hormones. Most carcinoids develop in the wall of the gastrointestinal tract, but they may also occur in other sites. Carcinoids are usually slow-growing, and they often remain asymptomatic for years. Like pheochromocytomas, carcinoid tumors are more frequent in patients with NF1 than in others, and multiple primary carcinoid tumors may develop in patients with NF1 (Burke et al. 1990; Dawson et al. 1984; Hough et al. 1983). Carcinoid tumors in patients with NF1 almost always arise in or near the ampulla of Vater and contain somatostatin (see discussion in Chapter 12). Although carcinoids of the small intestine usually exhibit chromaffin staining, they do not appear to be of neural crest origin. The carcinoid tumors that arise in patients with NF1 have an unusual histopathological appearance (Burke et al. 1989, 1990; Dayal et al. 1986; Griffiths et al. 1987) and are more often malignant than one would expect in general.

Patients with NF1 who have a pheochromocytoma have a remarkably high frequency of a coincidental carcinoid tumor, and vice versa (Cantor et al. 1982; Griffiths et al. 1983, 1987; Wheeler et al. 1986). Griffiths et al. (1987) found pheochromocytomas in 6 (22%) of 27 patients with NF1 with duodenal carcinoid tumors, a frequency more than 20 times higher than that expected for patients with NF1 in general. This observation suggests that patients with NF1 who have pheochromocytoma and duodenal carcinoid may represent a distinct subset.

Familial Spinal NF. Familial spinal NF is a genetically heterogeneous condition, but at least some instances appear to result from mutations of the *NF1* gene (Ars et al. 1998; Poyhonen et al. 1997a; Pulst et al. 1991). As expected, familial spinal NF may be transmitted as an autosomal dominant trait. Affected patients may have typical cutaneous manifestations of NF1, although these are generally not severe (Ars et al. 1998; Poyhonen et al. 1997a). What is unusual is the occurrence of neurofibromas of multiple spinal nerve roots. These tumors are often asymptomatic, but they may cause serious neurologic deficits (Ars et al. 1998; Poyhonen et al. 1997a; Pulst et al. 1991).

NF1 with Familial Malignant Peripheral Nerve Sheath Tumors. Malignant peripheral nerve sheath tumors (MPNSTs) are an uncommon but very serious and often fatal complication of NF1 (see Chapter 6). Several families have been reported in which an MPNST has developed in more than one relative with NF1 (Dales et al. 1983; Meis et al. 1992; Shearer et al. 1994; Poyhonen et al. 1997b). Although this could be no more than a reporting bias, the familial occurrence of MPNST does appear to be unusually frequent. The nature of the inherited *NF1* mutation has not yet been described in any of these families.

Gastrointestinal NF. A few patients have been described who have multiple intestinal neurofibromas without other typical features of NF1 (Heimann et al. 1988; Verhest et al. 1988; Shekitka and Sobin 1994). The condition is transmitted as an autosomal dominant trait, although penetrance, at least for the intestinal manifestations, is incomplete. It is not clear whether or not mutations of *NF1* locus are involved in the pathogenesis of gastrointestinal NF.

Late Onset NF. A few patients have been reported who have multiple discrete dermal neurofibromas but no café-au-lait spots or iris Lisch nodules (Riccardi 1982a, 1982b, 1983). These patients also lack most of the other typical features of NF1. The neurofibromas, which may not appear until the third decade of life or later, may be cutaneous, subcutaneous, or both, and may be relatively localized or diffusely distributed.

The nature of this condition and its relationship (if any) to NF1 is obscure. None of the reported cases has been familial, and mutations of the *NF1* locus have not been demonstrated in any of these patients. A possible association between late-onset NF and systemic lupus erythematosus (Bitnun and Bassan 1975; Carr and Howe 1989; Riccardi 1983) suggests that this condition might be an autoimmune phenocopy of NF1 (Riccardi 1992). Other possibilities include somatic mosaicism for an *NF1* mutation, a mutation of a different gene, or the uncommon chance occurrence of several sporadic neurofibromas in an individual who does not have NF1.

NF–Noonan Syndrome. Noonan syndrome is characterized by short stature, typical facial appearance (Figure 2-31), broad or webbed neck, an unusual sternal deformity, cryptorchidism, and congenital heart disease (Allanson 1987; Noonan

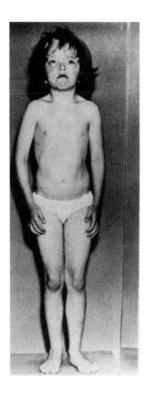

Figure 2-31. A five-year-old girl with NF1-Noonan syndrome. She has multiple café-au-lait spots, axillary freckling, and neurofibromas over her abdomen and buttocks. Her appearance is also typical of Noonan syndrome, with down-slanting palpebral fissures, malar hypoplasia, ptosis, a broad neck, and pectus excavatum. Source: Allanson et al. 1984. Photograph provided by Dr. Judith Allanson and reprinted with permission.

1994; Sharland et al. 1992a). Noonan syndrome is etiologically heterogeneous. Linkage to the long arm of chromosome 12 has been demonstrated in one large family with dominantly inherited Noonan syndrome (Brady et al. 1997; Jamieson et al. 1994). Other families with Noonan syndrome do not show linkage to chromosome 12q (Jamieson et al. 1994), but linkage to the *NF1* locus on chromosome 17 is unlikely in most families studied (Bahuau et al. 1996; Edman Ahlbom et al. 1995; Flintoff et al. 1993; Sharland et al. 1992b).

Most patients with Noonan syndrome do not have NF1 (Sharland et al. 1992a). Nevertheless, the facial, skeletal, and cardiac features of Noonan syndrome occur much more frequently than expected among patients with NF1 (Allanson et al. 1985; Carey 1998; Colley et al. 1996; Mendez 1985; Meschede et al. 1993; North 1993; Opitz and Weaver 1985; Quattrin et al. 1987; Stern et al. 1992; Tassabehji et al. 1993). The concurrence of NF1 and Noonan syndrome has been reported both in sporadic cases and in multiple members of some families (Colley et al. 1996; Quattrin et al. 1987; Stern et al. 1992; Tassabehji et al. 1993). In the familial instances, the Noonan phenotype may not be observed in all relatives who have NF1 (Colley et al. 1996; Stern et al. 1992). In some families with NF–Noonan syndrome, relatives have been found who have Noonan syndrome without features of NF1 (Buehning and Curry 1995; Bahuau et al. 1996, 1998; Colley et al. 1996). In one such family, the NF1 phenotype was determined by a mutation of the *NF1* locus but the Noonan phenotype segregated independently (Bahuau et al. 1996, 1998). It seems likely that two different autosomal dominant mutations are responsible for the NF1 and Noonan phenotypes in these families, but proof of this interpretation will require molecular demonstration of both mutations.

Deletions of the entire *NF1* locus have been found in three unrelated families with NF–Noonan syndrome (Colley et al. 1996; Kayes et al. 1994). An unusual in-frame 42-base tandem duplication of the *NF1* locus was observed in one other family with NF–Noonan syndrome (Tassabehji et al. 1993). Linkage of the NF1 phenotype to the *NF1* locus was demonstrated in another family in which some members also have features of Noonan syndrome (Stern et al. 1992). The most reasonable interpretation of these findings is that a mutation of the *NF1* locus can (but does not necessarily) produce a concurrent Noonan syndrome phenotype in some families.

Familial NF1 with Overgrowth. NF1 and a generalized overgrowth syndrome have been observed in a mother and son who both have a deletion of the entire *NF1* locus (van Asperen et al. 1998). In addition to excessive postnatal growth, both patients have facial and other features similar to those seen in the Weaver syndrome, (Ardinger et al. 1986; Cohen 1989) and the child has an advanced skeletal age. However, some of these features (e.g., developmental delay, macrocephaly, and hypertelorism) overlap with those of NF1, and it is uncertain whether a clinical diagnosis of Weaver syndrome is appropriate. No molecular diagnostic test for Weaver syndrome is currently available, and the cause of the overgrowth in this family is unknown.

Encephalocraniocutaneous Lipomatosis. Encephalocraniocutaneous lipomatosis is a rare sporadic syndrome characterized by unilateral craniofacial alopecia and lipomas with ipsilateral porencephaly and cerebral atrophy (Ciatti et al. 1998; Grimalt et al. 1993). Other features include ocular lesions, macrocephaly, severe psychomotor retardation, and seizures.

Encephalocraniocutaneous lipomatosis shares very few clinical features with NF1. It is, therefore, somewhat surprising that Legius et al. (1995) found a de novo nonsense mutation in the *NF1* gene in a 2-year-old patient with typical features of encephalocraniocutaneous lipomatosis. This child had more than five café-au-lait spots and foci of increased T_2-weighted signal intensity on cranial MRI scan but did not meet the NIH diagnostic criteria for NF1. Molecular studies showed no evidence of mosaicism for the mutation.

Although it is possible that this child has NF1 as a result of a new mutation and coincidental encephalocraniocutaneous lipomatosis of some other cause, the concurrence of these two events is striking. This particular *NF1* mutation was not found in one other patient with encephalocraniocutaneous lipomatosis who was studied (Legius et al. 1995), but thorough molecular evaluation of the *NF1* locus in other patients with this condition has not yet been reported.

Associations of Clinical Features

It is usually asserted that every affected individual with NF1 is at risk for all the myriad complications of the disease because no particular feature or specific mutant allele has consistently been found to predict the occurrence of any complication. The failure to find associations between various features in patients with NF1 may be the result of the infrequency of most important complications and the inadequate size of most patient series that have been studied.

Some investigations have suggested that associations do exist between particular features of NF1 in individual patients. For example, an association between the presence of juvenile xanthogranulomata and development of juvenile chronic myelogenous leukemia in patients with NF1 has been proposed (Morier et al. 1990; Zvulunov et al. 1995). However, juvenile chronic myelogenous leukemia is very rare among children with NF1, so finding juvenile xanthogranulomas does not warrant an extensive search for malignancy (Gutmann et al. 1996). Zvulunov and associates (1998) also suggested an association between the occurrence of macrocephaly and more severe manifestations of NF1, although this has not been seen in other, larger studies (Riccardi 1992; see following paragraphs). An association between UBOs on brain MRI and neurocognitive deficit was also found in some studies but not others (North et al. 1997; see Chapter 7).

Analysis of the occurrence of 10 selected features among 1479 NF1 probands from the NNFF International Database is shown in Table 2-2. The chance probabilities of the observed associations between each pair of traits within individual NF1 probands is given in the upper portion of each cell in the table. The lower portion of each cell shows a similar analysis using comparable variables in 1022 probands from the NF Institute Database. Combined odds ratios for both databases are shown in Table 2-3.

Nineteen of 45 possible associations in the NNFF International Database are statistically significant at $p < .05$ and have odds ratios with 95% confidence intervals that do not include 1.0. In the NF Institute data, 10 of 28 possible associations are statistically significant. There is a remarkable concordance between the findings in the NNFF International Database and the independent NF Institute Database. The associations are either both statistically significant or both not significant in 24 of 28 comparisons. The probability of observing this degree of concordance by chance is very small.

Each observed association requires careful analysis. Many of them probably reflect the fact that most features of NF1 increase in frequency with age. However, some associations may represent variable manifestations of a common underlying pathogenic abnormality. This may explain the association between the occurrence of café-au-lait spots and intertriginous freckling, for example. Other associations may provide insights into the pathogenesis of NF1. One example may be the strong association observed between the occurrence of optic glioma and other neoplasms (excluding neurofibromas). This association appears to reflect an unusually high frequency of other central nervous system gliomas among NF1 patients with optic gliomas (Table 2-4; Kuenzle et al. 1994; Bilaniuk et al. 1997; Friedman and Birch 1997a). Patients with NF1 with optic glioma do

Table 2-2. Associations between the occurrence of ten traits among 1479 individual NF1 probands from the NNFF International Database (top number in each cell) and among 1022 probands from the NF Institute Database (bottom number in each cell)

	Intertriginous Freckling	Discrete Neurofibroma	Plexiform Neurofibroma	Xantho-granuloma	Lisch Nodules	Scoliosis	Pseud-arthrosis	Optic Glioma	Other Malignancy
Café-au-lait spots	<.001	.007	NS	NS	NS	NS	NS	NS	NS
Intertriginous freckling		<.001 <.001	.034 .001	.031 NS	<.001 <.001	.004 .019	NS NS	NS NS	NS
Discrete neurofibroma			<.001 <.001	<.001 NS	<.001 <.001	.001 <.001	NS NS	NS NS	<.001
Plexiform neurofibroma				.019 NS	<.001 <.001	<.001 <.001	NS NS	NS NS	NS
Xanthogranuloma					.011 NS	NS NS	NS NS	NS NS	NS
Lisch nodules						<.001 <.001	NS NS	NS NS	.039
Scoliosis						<.001	NS NS	NS NS	NS
Pseudarthrosis								NS NS	NS
Optic glioma									.001

Note: The number given in each cell is the probability (*p* value) that both traits would occur together with the frequency observed on the basis of chance alone. Probabilities were calculated using a two-tailed Fisher's exact test. NS = not significant. *Source:* This analysis was performed by Jacek Szudek and is used with his permission.

Table 2-3. Combined odds ratios and 95% confidence intervals for the association data of Table 2-2

	Intertriginous Freckling	Discrete Neurofibroma	Plexiform Neurofibroma	Xantho-granuloma	Lisch Nodules	Scoliosis	Pseud-arthrosis	Optic Glioma	Other Malignancy
Café-au-lait spots	2.7 (1.8–4.1)	.61 (.41–.89)	.82 (.54–1.2)	1.8 (.45–1.6)	.87 (.54–1.4)	.71 (.46–1.1)	1.5 (.38–1.3)	1.2 (.46–3.3)	.62 (.31–1.4)
Intertriginous freckling		3.0 (2.3–3.7)	1.7 (1.3–2.2)	.52 (.28–.95)	2.9 (2.1–3.9)	1.7 (1.3–2.4)	.56 (.32–1.0)	1.4 (.85–2.2)	2.0 (1.0–3.8)
Discrete neurofibroma			3.1 (2.5–3.8)	.39 (.22–.69)	4.2 (3.4–5.3)	2.3 (1.8–2.3)	.60 (.36–.99)	.91 (.67–1.2)	2.9 (1.8–4.6)
Plexiform neurofibroma				.64 (.31–1.3)	2.0 (1.6–2.6)	2.2 (1.8–2.7)	1.0 (.60–1.8)	.97 (.70–1.3)	1.5 (.94–2.3)
Xanthogranuloma					.39 (.20–3.7)	.43 (.18–1.0)	1.5 (.34–6.4)	1.4 (.51–3.6)	1.5 (.53–4.3)
Lisch nodules						2.7 (2.0–3.7)	.77 (.39–1.5)	1.0 (.68–1.5)	2.0 (1.1–3.7)
Scoliosis							1.7 (.96–3.0)	.97 (.67–1.4)	1.9 (1.3–3.0)
Pseudarthrosis								.78 (.31–1.9)	1.2 (.36–3.9)
Optic glioma									2.3 (1.3–4.1)

Note: Calculations were made using the method of Einarson et al. (1988). *Source:* This analysis was performed by Jacek Szudek and is used with his permission.

Table 2-4. Association between the occurrence of optic glioma and other CNS tumors but not non-CNS malignancies in 684 individuals with NF1 who had cranial imaging studies

Optic Glioma	Other CNS Tumor		Non-CNS Malignancy	
	Present	Absent	Present	Absent
Present	17	137	4	150
Absent	8	522	20	510
	$X^2 = 28.1$		$X^2 = 0.2$	
	$p < .000001$		$p = .65$	
	Odds ratio = 8.1		Odds ratio = 0.7	
	(95% CI = 3.2–22.1)		(95% CI = 0.2–2.1)	

Note: Probabilities were calculated using Fisher's exact test.
Source: Data from Friedman and Birch (1997a).

not have malignant tumors outside of the central nervous system more often than expected. The association between the occurrence of optic and other central nervous system gliomas does not result from observation bias, radiation treatment for optic glioma, or age (Friedman and Birch 1997a).

The associations found among various clinical features suggest that there are fundamental pathophysiological similarities among certain manifestations of NF1 but not others. Observation of these associations is also compatible with the hypothesis that some patients with NF1 are at greater risk than others for the development of particular disease complications. For example, the associations between occurrence of clinical features may reflect genetic factors. Familial tendencies do exist for some of these features developing, such as café-au-lait spots, Lisch nodules, and other malignancy (Table 2-5).

Table 2-5. Associations between the occurrence of the 10 traits in Table 2-2 in both affected members of 249 NF1 parent–child pairs

Feature in Parents and Children	Fisher's Exact Test Probability	Odds Ratio with 95% Confidence Interval
Café-au-lait spots	.007	5.0 (1.4–19.2)
Intertriginous freckling	NS	1.6 (0.7–3.6)
Discrete neurofibroma	NS	1.5 (0.7–3.3)
Plexiform neurofibroma	.029	3.1 (1.1–8.6)
Xanthogranuloma	NS	–
Lisch nodules	.0002	6.4 (2.3–18)
Scoliosis	NS	1.8 (0.8–3.8)
Pseudarthrosis	NS	–
Optic glioma	NS	–
Other malignancy	.0062	18 (2.0–140)

Note: The *p* value listed is the probability that the trait would occur in both family members on the basis of chance alone. Probabilities were calculated using a two-tailed Fisher's exact test. NS = not significant. *Source:* This analysis was performed by Jacek Szudek and is used with his permission.

PATHOGENIC INSIGHTS PROVIDED BY THE CLINICAL MANIFESTATIONS OF NF1

NF1 features either pose limitations on any pathogenic schema (i.e., they must be accounted for directly and immediately) or, of and by themselves, suggest particular pathogenic mechanisms. The box lists "pathogenic pearls" in NF1 that are especially useful in these ways.

This compilation of observations has several recurrent themes:

1. Multiple tissues and cell types contribute to the primary lesions of NF1.
2. Although the body as a whole is diffusely involved, the lesions themselves are patchy or localized.
3. There appears to be a role for a variety of local factors and influences, ranging from cellular interactions and hormones to mechanical forces. The presence of the mutant *NF1* gene does not itself explain the nature, degree, and timing of all disease manifestations.

REFERENCES

Abeliovich D, Gelman-Kohan Z, Silverstein S, Lerer I, Chemke J, Merlin S, and Zlotogora J. 1995. Familial café au lait spots: a variant of neurofibromatosis type 1. *J Med Genet* 32:985–6.

Ahn JS, Kim SD, Hwang JH, Youn SW, Kim KH, and Park KC. 1998. Halo-like disappearance of mongolian spot combined with café au lait spot. *Pediatr Dermatol* 15:70–1.

Ainsworth PJ, Chakraborty PK, and Weksberg R. 1997. Example of somatic mosaicism in a series of de novo neurofibromatosis type 1 cases due to a maternally derived deletion. *Hum Mutat* 9:452–7.

Allanson JE. 1987. Noonan syndrome. *J Med Genet* 24:9–13.

Allanson JE, Hall JG, and Van Allen MI. 1985. Noonan phenotype associated with neurofibromatosis. *Am J Med Genet* 21:457–62.

Allanson JE, Upadhyaya M, Watson GH, Partington M, MacKenzie A, Lahey D, MacLeod H, Sarfarazi M, Broadhead W, Harper PS, and Huson SM. 1991. Watson syndrome: is it a subtype of type 1 neurofibromatosis? *J Med Genet* 28:752–6.

Apter N, Chemke J, Hurwitz N, and Levin S. 1975. Neonatal neurofibromatosis: unusual manifestations with malignant clinical course. *Clin Genet* 7:388–93.

Ardinger HH, Hanson JW, Harrod MJ, Cohen MM Jr, Tibbles JA, Welch JP, Young-Wee T, Sommer A, Goldberg R, Shpritzen RJ, et al. 1986. Further delineation of Weaver syndrome. *J Pediatr* 108:228–35.

Arnsmeier SL, Riccardi VM, and Paller AS. 1994. Familial multiple café au lait spots. *Arch Dermatol* 130:1425–6.

Ars E, Kruyer H, Gaona A, Casquero P, Rosell J, Volpini V, Serra E, Lázaro C, and Estavill X. 1998. A clinical variant of neurofibromatosis type 1: familial spinal neurofibromatosis with a frameshift mutation in the *NF1* gene. *Am J Hum Genet* 62:834–41.

Bahuau M, Flintoff W, Assouline B, Lyonnet S, Le Merrer M, Prieur M, Guilloud-Bataille M, Feingold N, Munnich A, Vidaud M, and Vidaud D. 1996. Exclusion of allelism of Noonan syndrome and neurofibromatosis type 1 in a large family with Noonan-syndrome-neurofibromatosis association. *Amer J Med Genet* 66:347–55.

Bahuau M, Houdayer C, Assouline B, Blanchet-Bardon C, Le Merrer M, Lyonnet S, Giraud S, Récan D, Lakhdar H, Vidaud M, and Vidaud D. 1998. Novel recurrent non-

PATHOGENIC PEARLS

—Mental retardation, learning disabilities, developmental delay, speech defects, general incoordination, macrocephaly, and seizures must be accounted for, yet no universal explanation is even vaguely apparent. The same is true for short stature, pectus excavatum, and genu varum/valgum.

—Identical twins with NF1 are generally discordant in their café-au-lait spots and neurofibroma distribution and overall NF1 phenotype including severity grades, although Crawford and Buckler (1983), Cartwright (1982), and Pascual-Castroviejo et al. (1988) reported monozygous twin sets concordant for optic gliomas. For at least some of the features, their presence and specific qualities are not intrinsically determined by the mutant gene itself but rather appear more to reflect extrinsic influences, including random ones (Riccardi et al. 1979; Bauer et al. 1988). It is of some interest that all but one of the reported twin sets have been female.

—The concordance of the borders of the hyperpigmentation overlying a diffuse plexiform neurofibroma with the borders of the tumor itself suggests there must be some factor or factors to mediate this symmetry.

—The increase in the number and size of neurofibromas during puberty and pregnancy and the proclivity for neurofibroma development in the sexually mature female areola suggest an important direct or, more likely, indirect influence of one or more sex hormones.

—The occasional presence of cutaneous hypopigmented macules in NF1 suggests that the mutant gene can influence the behavior of skin melanocytes in more than one way or that a single intracellular defect can have quite opposite effects.

—The development of normal levels of pigmentation in a punch biopsy scar in the center of a café-au-lait spot suggests that the hyperpigmentation of the café-au-lait spot does not represent a fixed, permanent feature of the café-au-lait spot melanocytes (which presumably provide the melanocytes in the scarred region) and further, that local factors acting over very small distances may determine melanocyte expression of the NF1 mutation. The halo phenomenon around café-au-lait spots superimposed on a mongolian spot also suggests an interaction between café-au-lait spot melanocytes and the surrounding skin and/or the inability of melanosomes to leak from café-au-lait spot melanocytes. The presence of two-tone café-au-lait spots suggests that the hyperpigmentation is not merely an all-or-nothing phenomenon but one with degrees of severity.

—The development of freckling in areas of skin apposition and where clothing rubs against the skin suggests that local factors, very likely friction and/or elevated temperature, influence the expression of the NF1 mutation in melanocytes.

—Café-au-lait spots are not seen in the scalp or eyebrows, the only congenitally hairy skin areas, suggesting that hair follicles from these regions (or other aspects of embryologic skin development) obviate the expression of the NF1 mutation in the melanocytes there. Otherwise, except for an apparent paucity of café-au-lait spots on the face and glans penis, NF1 café-au-lait spots are distributed randomly over the body (Riccardi 1981b).

—Discrete cutaneous neurofibromas appear to occur to some degree in all areas of the body, though they tend to be heaviest on the trunk (front and back equally) and are apparently lightest over the shins. Local trauma may contribute to the origin of at least some cutaneous neurofibromas. A neurofibroma on the forearm developed in a young woman who had forcefully closed a car door on her forearm at that site. Several days later she noted intense itching in that region, and about 10 days later a neurofibroma appeared there de novo, progressing over several months' time to the size of a small grape. Throughout its growth and for some time thereafter, local itching was present and was often intense. Other patients have related similar anecdotes. In particular, patients may note that the neurofibroma-associated itching may be precipitated or aggravated by increased body heat, including that caused by exertion.

—Juvenile xanthogranulomas occur in the skin of a small percentage of young NF1 patients. Their relationship to the NF1 mutation is totally obscure.

—The parents of children with diffuse cutaneous plexiform neurofibromas often comment spontaneously on the child's frequent, if not incessant, scratching at the tumor site. The scratching is especially notable when the tumor appears to be increasing in size. As noted previously (Riccardi 1981b, 1992) itching associated with growing or large numbers of neurofibromas is not infrequent among patients with NF1, both children and adults. This observation led Riccardi to postulate that mast cells in the neurofibromas may be the cause of the itching and even of tumor growth.

—The variety of benign tumors, most of nervous system origin, is quite remarkable for NF1. Any pathogenetic schema for NF1 would have to account for this variety, whether or not a common neural crest origin is presumed. One type of tumor not ordinarily associated with NF1 is the lipoma and its variants. Lipomas may occur as part of NF1 (Sinha et al. 1973; Laptev 1978). In addition, when present in large numbers suggesting multiple subcutaneous neurofibromas, multiple lipomatosis may be incorrectly presumed to represent NF1. Lipomatous tumors may also more legitimately overlap with NF, as indicated in the report of familial angiolipomatosis by Goodman and Baskin (1989), in the report of Bamforth et al. (1989), and in consideration of the overlap of the neurofibromatoses with other disorders (Budka 1974; Saul and Stevenson 1986). Finally, neurofibrosarcomas in NF1 not infrequently have elements of liposarcoma (Riccardi and Elder 1986) or liposarcoma may be the entirety of the malignancy (Baker and Greenspan 1981; Baker et al. 1982; Vivot et al. 1986).

—The involvement of blood vessels, ranging from aortic coarctation to capillary angiomas, as a primary feature of NF1 bears specific emphasis. In general, this aspect of NF1 has not received its full due in discussions of this sort, presumably because its significance has not been fully appreciated and its relationship to other features of the disease is so obscure.

—The potentially adverse influence of NF1 in a mother on the severity of NF1 in her offspring (Miller and Hall 1978; Hall 1981) is mentioned here only to dismiss it. No such adverse effect of maternal NF1 has been documented (Riccardi and Wald 1987). Other than perhaps mechanical trauma, there are no known environmental influences on the evolution or severity of NF1. This includes birth control pills, other commonly used prescription and nonprescription drugs, and dietary intake.

sense mutation causing neurofibromatosis type 1 (NF1) in a family segregating both NF1 and Noonan syndrome. *Am J Med Genet* 75:265–72.

Baker ND and Greenspan A. 1981. Pleomorphic liposarcoma, grade IV, of the soft tissue, arising in generalized plexiform neurofibromatosis. *Skeletal Radiol* 7:150–3.

Baker ND, Tchang FK, and Greenspan A. 1982. Liposarcoma complicating neurofibromatosis: report of two cases. *Bull Hosp Joint Dis Orthop Inst* 42:172–86.

Bamforth JSG, Riccardi VM, Thiesen P, et al. 1989. Encephalocraniocutaneous lipomatosis: report of two cases and review of the literature. *Neurofibromatosis* 2:166–73.

Barker D, Wright E, Nguyen K, Cannon L, Fain P, Goldgar D, Bishop DT, et al. 1987. Gene for von Recklinghausen neurofibromatosis is in the pericentromeric region of chromosome 17. *Science* 236:1100–2.

Benedict PH, Szabó G, Fitzpatrick TB, and Sinesi SJ. 1968. Melanotic macules in Albright's syndrome and in neurofibromatosis. *JAMA* 205:618–26.

Bhawan J, Purtilo DT, Riordan JA, Saxena VK, and Edelstein L. 1976. Giant and "granular melanosomes" in LEOPARD syndrome: an ultrastructural study. *J Cutan Pathol* 3:207–16.

Bilaniuk LT, Molloy PT, Zimmerman RA, Phillips PC, Vaughan SN, Liu GT, Sutton LN, and Needle M. 1997. Neurofibromatosis type 1: brain stem tumours. *Neuroradiology* 39:642–53.

Bitnun S and Bassan H. 1975. Neurofibromatosis and systemic lupus erythematosus. *N Engl J Med* 292:429–30.

Bocian M and Walker AP. 1987. Halo phenomenon in neurofibromatosis: the influence of café-au-lait spots on mongolian spots. *Proc Greenwood Genet Ctr* 6:160.

Bolande RP. 1974. The neurocristopathies: a unifying concept of disease arising in neural crest development. *Hum Pathol* 5:409–29.

―――. 1981. Neurofibromatosis—the quintessential neurocristopathy: pathogenic concepts and relationships. *Adv Neurol* 29:67–75.

Boltshauser E, Stocker H, and Mächler M. 1989. Neurofibromatosis type 1 in a child of a parent with segmental neurofibromatosis (NF-5). *Neurofibromatosis* 2:244–5.

Borberg A. 1951. Clinical and genetic investigations into tuberous sclerosis and Recklinghausen's neurofibromatosis: contributions to elucidation of interrelationship and eugenics of the syndromes. *Acta Psychiatr Neurol Scand Suppl* 71:1–239.

Brady AF, Jamieson CR, van der Burgt I, Crosby A, van Reen M, Kremer H, Mariman E, Patton MA, and Jeffery S. 1997. Further delineation of the critical region for Noonan syndrome on the long arm of chromosome 12. *Eur J Hum Genet* 5:336–7.

Brown JA, Levy JB, and Kramer SA. 1997. Genitourinary neurofibromatosis mimicking posterior urethral valves. *Urology* 49:960–2.

Brunner HG, Hulsebos T, Steijlen PM, der Kinderen DJ, van den Steen A, and Hamel BCJ. 1993. Exclusion of the neurofibromatosis 1 locus in a family with inherited café-au-lait spots. *Am J Med Genet* 46:472–4.

Budka H. 1974. Intracranial lipomatous hamartomas (intracranial "lipomas"): a study of 13 cases including combinations with medulloblastoma, colloid and epidermal cysts, angiomatosis and other malformations. *Acta Neuropathol* 28:205–22.

Buehning L and Curry CJ. 1995. Neurofibromatosis-Noonan syndrome. *Pediatr Dermatol* 12:267–71.

Bunin G. 1987. Racial patterns of childhood brain cancer by histologic type. *J Natl Cancer Inst* 78:875–80.

Burke AP, Federspiel BH, Sobin LH, Shekitka KM, and Helwig EB. 1989. Carcinoids of the duodenum: a histologic and immunochemical study of 65 tumors. *Am J Surg Pathol* 13:828–37.

Burke AP, Sobin LH, Shekitka KM, Federspiel BH, and Helwig EB. 1990. Somatostatin-producing duodenal carcinoid in patients with von Recklinghausen's neurofibromatosis: a predilection for black patients. *Cancer* 65:1591–5.

Cantor AM, Rigby CC, Beck PR, and Mangion D. 1982. Neurofibromatosis, phaeochromocytoma, and somatostatinoma. *BMJ* 285:1618–9.

Carey JC. 1998. Neurofibromatosis-Noonan syndrome. *Am J Med Genet* 75:263–4.

Carey JC, Laub JM, and Hall BD. 1979. Penetrance and variability in neurofibromatosis: a genetic study of 60 families. *Birth Defects Orig Artic Ser* 15(5B):271–81.

Carr ME and Howe CWS. 1989. Lupus anticoagulant and neuroectodermal antigens in a patient with neurofibromatosis. *South Med J* 82:921–3.

Cartwright SC. 1982. Concordant optic glioma in a pair of monozygotic twins with neurofibromatosis. *Clin Pediatr* 21:236–8.

Charrow J, Listernick R, and Ward K. 1993. Autosomal dominant multiple café-au-lait spots and neurofibromatosis-1: evidence of non-linkage. *Am J Med Genet* 45:606–8.

Ciatti S, Del Monaco M, Hyde P, and Bernstein EF. 1998. Encephalocraniocutaneous lipomatosis: a rare neurocutaneous syndrome. *J Am Acad Dermatol* 38:102–4.

Clementi M, Barbujani G, Turolla L, and Tenconi R. 1990. Neurofibromatosis-1: a maximum likelihood estimation of mutation rate. *Hum Genet* 84:116–8.

Cnossen MH, de Goede-Bolder A, van den Broek KM, Waasdorp CME, Oranje AP, Stroink H, Simonsz HJ, van den Ouweland AMW, Halley DJJ, and Niermeijer MF. 1998. A prospective 10 year follow up study of patients with neurofibromatosis type 1. *Arch Dis Child* 78:408–12.

Cohen MM Jr. 1989. A comprehensive and critical assessment of overgrowth and overgrowth syndromes. *Adv Hum Genet* 18:181–303, 373–6.

Colley A, Donnai D, and Evans DGR. 1996. Neurofibromatosis/Noonan phenotype: a variable feature of type 1 neurofibromatosis. *Clin Genet* 49:59–64.

Colman SD, Williams CA, and Wallace MR. 1995. Benign neurofibromas in type 1 neurofibromatosis (NF1) show somatic deletion of the NF1 gene. *Nat Genet* 11:90–2.

Colman SD, Rasmussen SA, Ho VT, Abernathy CR, and Wallace MR. 1996. Somatic mosaicism in a patient with neurofibromatosis type 1. *Am J Hum Genet* 58:484–90.

Crawford MJ and Buckler JMH. 1983. Optic glomata affecting twins with neurofibromatosis. *Dev Med Child Neurol* 25:370–3.

Crowe FW, Schull WJ, and Neel JV. 1956. *A Clinical, Pathological, and Genetic Study of Multiple Neurofibromatosis. Springfield, Ill.: Charles C Thomas.*

Dales RL, McEver VW, Quispe G, and Davies RS. 1983. Update on biologic behavior and surgical implications of neurofibromatosis and neurofibrosarcoma. *Surg Gynecol Obstet* 156:636–40.

Danglot G, Regnier V, Fauvet D, Vassal G, Kujas M, and Bernheim A. 1995. Neurofibromatosis 1 (NF1) mRNAs expressed in the central nervous system are differentially spliced in the 5′ part of the gene. *Hum Mol Genet* 4:915–20.

Dawson BV, Kazama R, and Paplanus SH. 1984. Association of carcinoid with neurofibromatosis. *South Med J* 77:511–3.

Dayal Y, Tallberg KA, Nunnemacher G, DeLellis RA, and Wolfe HJ. 1986. Duodenal carcinoids in patients with and without neurofibromatosis: a comparative study. *Am J Surg Pathol* 10:348–57.

De Angelis P and Crillo C. 1968. [A case of von Recklinghausen's neurofibromatosis associated with Ehlers-Danlos syndrome.] *Pediatria (Napoli)* 76:134–49.

DeSchryver K and Santa Cruz DJ. 1984. So-called glandular schwannoma: ependymal differentiation in a case. *Ultrastruct Pathol* 6:167–75.

Diaz-Flores L, Sanchez G, Garcia Del Moral R, Aneiros J, and Varela H. 1978. Cells with intermediate characteristics between teloglial, melanic, and nerve sheath cells: melanogliocyte. *Morfologia Norm Patol* 2:253–71.

Dugoff L and Sujansky E. 1996. Neurofibromatosis type 1 and pregnancy. *Am J Med Genet* 66:7–10.

Du Toit DF. 1987. Gastric haemorrhage in a patient with neurofibromatosis. *S Afr Med J* 71:730–1.

Easton DF, Ponder MA, Huson SM, and Ponder BAJ. 1993. An analysis of variation in expression of neurofibromatosis (NF) type I (NFI): evidence for modifying genes. *Am J Hum Genet* 53:305–13.

Edman Ahlbom B, Dahl N, Zetterqvist P, and Annerén G. 1995. Noonan syndrome with café-au-lait spots and multiple lentigines syndrome are not linked to the neurofibromatosis type 1 locus. *Clin Genet* 48:85–9.

Einarson TR, Leeder JS, and Koren G. 1988. A method for meta-analysis of epidemiological studies. *Drug Intell Clin Pharm* 22:813–24.

Fan KJ and Pezeshkpour GH. 1992. Ethnic distribution of primary central nervous system tumors in Washington, D.C., 1971–1985. *J Natl Med Assoc* 84:858–63.

Fitzpatrick ME, McDermott M, May D, Hofeldt FD. 1983. Eruptive neurofibromatosis associated with anorexia nervosa. Arch Dermatol 119:1019–21.

Flannery DB and Howell CG. 1987. Confirmation of the Riccardi sign. *Proc Greenwood Genet Ctr* 6:161.

Flintoff WF, Bahuau M, Lyonnet S, Gilgenkrantz S, Lacombe D, Marçon F, Levilliers J, Kachaner J, Munnich A, and Le Merrer M. 1993. No evidence for linkage to the type 1 or type 2 neurofibromatosis loci in Noonan syndrome families. *Am J Med Genet* 46:700–5.

Fois A, Calistri L, Balestri P, Vivarelli R, Bartalini G, Mancini L, Berardi A, and Vanni M. 1993. Relationship between café-au-lait spots as the only symptom and peripheral neurofibromatosis (NF1): a follow-up study. *Eur J Pediatr* 152:500–4.

Frank DJ, Majid N, and England D. 1981. Massive gastrointestinal bleeding in a patient with von Recklinghausen's disease: case report. *Milit Med* 146:438–9.

Friedman JM and Birch P. 1997a. An association between optic glioma and other tumours of the central nervous system in neurofibromatosis type 1. *Neuropediatrics* 28:131–2.

———. 1997b. Type 1 neurofibromatosis: a descriptive analysis of the disorder in 1,728 patients. *Am J Med Genet* 70:138–43.

Friedman JM, Greene C, Birch P, and the NNFF International Database Participants. 1993. National Neurofibromatosis Foundation International Database. *Am J Med Genet* 45:88–91.

Fuller LC, Cox B, and Gardner RJM. 1989. Prevalence of von Recklinghausen neurofibromatosis in Dunedin, New Zealand. *Neurofibromatosis* 2:278–83.

Gasparini P, Grifa A, Origone P, Coviello D, Antonacci R, and Rocchi M. 1993. Detection of a neurofibromatosis type I (NF1) homologous sequence by PCR: implications for the diagnosis and screening of genetic diseases. *Mol Cell Probes* 7:415–8.

Geist RT and Gutmann DH. 1996. Expression of a developmentally-regulated neuron-specific isoform of the neurofibromatosis 1 (NF1) gene. *Neurosci Lett* 211:85–8.

Goldberg Y, Dibbern K, Klein J, Riccardi VM, and Graham JM. 1996. Neurofibromatosis type 1: an update and review for the primary pediatrician. *Clin Pediatr (Phila)* 35:545–61.

Goodman JC and Baskin DS. 1989. Autosomal dominant familial angiolipomatosis clinically mimicking neurofibromatosis. *Neurofibromatosis* 2:326–31.

Goodman RM, Levitsky JM, and Friedman IA. 1962. The Ehlers-Danlos syndrome and multiple neurofibromatosis in a kindred of mixed derivation, with special emphasis on hemostasis in the Ehlers-Danlos syndrome. *Am J Med* 32:976–83.

Griffiths DFR, Williams GT, and Williams ED. 1983. Multiple endocrine neoplasia associated with von Recklinghausen's disease. *BMJ* 287:1341–3.

———. 1987. Duodenal carcinoid tumours, phaeochromocytoma and neurofibromatosis: islet cell tumour, phaeochromocytoma and the von Hippel-Lindau complex: two distinctive neuroendocrine syndromes. *Q J Med* 64:769–82.

Grimalt R, Ermacora E, Mistura L, Russo G, Tadini GL, Triulzi F, Cavicchini S, Rondanini GF, and Caputo R. 1993. Encephalocraniocutaneous lipomatosis: case report and review of the literature. *Pediatr Dermatol* 10:164–8.

Gutmann DH. 1998. Recent insights into neurofibromatosis type 1: clear genetic progress. *Arch Neurol* 55:778–80.

Gutmann DH, Aylsworth A, Carey JC, Korf B, Marks J, Pyeritz RE, Rubenstein A, and Viskochil D. 1997. The diagnostic evaluation and multidisciplinary management of neurofibromatosis 1 and neurofibromatosis 2. *JAMA* 278:51–7.

Gutmann DH, Cole JL, Stone WJ, Ponder BA, and Collins FS. 1994. Loss of neurofibromin in adrenal gland tumors from patients with neurofibromatosis type 1. *Genes Chromosomes Cancer* 10:55–8.

Gutmann DH, Gurney JG, and Shannon KM. 1996. Juvenile xanthogranuloma, neurofibromatosis 1, and juvenile chronic myeloid leukemia. *Arch Dermatol* 132:1390–1.

Habib AA, Gulcher JR, Högnason T, Zheng L, and Stefánsson K. 1998. The OMgp gene, a second growth suppressor within the NF1 gene. *Oncogene* 16:1525–31.

Hall JG. 1981. Possible maternal and hormonal factors in neurofibromatosis. *Adv Neurol* 29:125–31.

Harkin JC and Reed RJ. 1969. Tumors of the peripheral nervous system. In: *Atlas of Tumor Pathology.* Second series. Washington, DC: Armed Forces Institute of Pathology, pp. 67–100.

Heimann R, Verhest A, Verschraegen J, Grosjean W, Draps JP, and Hecht F. 1988. Hereditary intestinal neurofibromatosis. I. A distinctive genetic disease. *Neurofibromatosis* 1:26–32.

Hoffmeyer S, Assum G, Griesser J, Kaufmann D, Nürnberg P, and Krone W. 1995. On unequal allelic expression of the neurofibromin gene in neurofibromatosis type 1. *Hum Molec Genet* 4:1267–72.

Hoffmeyer S, Assum G, Kaufmann D, and Krone W. 1994. Unequal expression of *NF1* alleles. *Nat Genet* 6:331.

Hough DR, Chan A, and Davidson H. 1983. Von Recklinghausen's disease associated with gastrointestinal carcinoid tumors. *Cancer* 51:2206–8.

Huson SM. 1994. Neurofibromatosis 1: a clinical and genetic overview. In: Huson SM and Hughes RAC, eds. *The Neurofibromatoses: A Pathogenic and Clinical Overview.* Chapman and Hall Medical, London, pp 160–203.

Huson SM, Compston DAS, Clark P, and Harper PS. 1989a. A genetic study of von Recklinghausen neurofibromatosis in southeast Wales. I. Prevalence, fitness, mutation rate, and effect of parental transmission on severity. *J Med Genet* 26:704–11.

Huson SM, Compston DAS, and Harper PS. 1989b. A genetic study of von Recklinghausen neurofibromatosis in south east Wales: II. Guidelines for genetic counselling. *J Med Genet* 26:712–21.

Huson SM, Harper PS, and Compston DAS. 1988. Von Recklinghausen neurofibromatosis: a clinical and population study in South-East Wales. *Brain* 111:1355–81.

Huson S, Jones D, and Beck L. 1987. Ophthalmic manifestations of neurofibromatosis. *Br J Ophthalmol* 71:235–8.

Jamieson CR, van der Burgt I, Brady AF, van Reen M, Elsawi MM, Hol F, Jeffery S, Patton MA, and Mariman E. 1994. Mapping a gene for Noonan syndrome to the long arm of chromosome 12. *Nat Genet* 8:357–60.

Jeng K-S, Yang K-C, Ching H-J, and Shih C-C. 1988. An unusual cause of gastrointestinal hemorrhage—intestinal neurofibromatosis. *J Clin Gastroenterol* 10:585–7.

Jones KL. 1997. *Smith's Recognizable Patterns of Human Malformation,* 5th ed. Philadelphia: W.B. Saunders, pp. 740–6.

Kaplan P and Rosenblatt B. 1985. A distinctive facial appearance in neurofibromatosis von Recklinghausen. *Am J Med Genet* 21:463–70.

Kayes LM, Riccardi VM, Burke W, Bennett RL, and Stephens K. 1992. Large de novo DNA deletion in a patient with sporadic neurofibromatosis 1, mental retardation, and dysmorphism. *J Med Genet* 29:686–90.

Kayes LM, Burke W, Riccardi VM, Bennett R, Ehrlich P, Rubenstein A, and Stephens K. 1994. Deletions spanning the neurofibromatosis 1 gene: identification and phenotype of five patients. *Am J Hum Genet* 54:424–36.

Kimmelman CP. 1979. Otolaryngologic aspects of neurofibromatosis. *Arch Otololaryngol* 105:732–6.

Konrad K, Wolff K, Hönigsmann H. 1974. The giant melanosome: a model of deranged melansome morphogenesis. *J Ultrstruct Res* 48:102–23.

Kuenzle C, Weissert M, Roulet E, Bode H, Schefer S, Huisman T, Landau K, and Boltshauser E. 1994. Follow-up of optic pathway gliomas in children with neurofibromatosis type 1. *Neuropediatrics* 25:295–300.

Laptev VV. 1978. [Lipoma of the small intestinal mesentery in a patient with neurofibromatosis]. *Khirurgiia* 11:134–5.

Leão M and Ribeiro da Silva ML. 1995. Evidence of central nervous system involvement in Watson syndrome. *Pediatr Neurol* 12:252–4.

Legius E, Marchuk DA, Hall BK, Andersen LB, Wallace MR, Collins FS, and Glover TW. 1992. *NF-1* related locus on chromosome 15. *Genomics* 13:1316–8.

Legius E, Marchuk DA, Collins FS, and Glover TW. 1993. Somatic deletion of neurofibromatosis type 1 gene in a neurofibrosarcoma supports a tumour suppressor gene hypothesis. *Nat Genet* 3:122–6.

Legius E, Wu R, Eyssen M, Marynen P, Fryns JP, and Cassiman JJ. 1995. Encephalocraniocutaneous lipomatosis with a mutation in the NF1 gene. *J Med Genet* 32:316–9.

Leppig KA, Kaplan P, Viskochil D, Weaver M, Ortenberg J, and Stephens K. 1997. Familial neurofibromatosis 1 microdeletions: cosegregation with distinct facial phenotype and early onset of cutaneous neurofibromata. *Am J Med Genet* 73:197–204.

Leppig KA, Viskochil D, Neil S, Rubenstein A, Johnson VP, Zhu XL, Brothman AR, and Stephens K. 1996. The detection of contiguous gene deletions at the neurofibromatosis 1 locus with fluorescence in situ hybridization. *Cytogenet Cell Genet* 72:95–8.

Lewis RA and Riccardi VM. 1981. Von Recklinghausen neurofibromatosis: incidence of iris hamartomata. *Ophthalmology* 88:348–54.

Lisch K. 1937. Ueber Beteilgung der Augen, insbesondere das vorkommen von Irisnötchen bei der Neurofibromatose (Recklinghausen). *Z Augenheilkd* 93:137–43.

Littler M and Morton NE. 1990. Segregation analysis of peripheral neurofibromatosis (NF1). *J Med Genet* 27:307–10.

Lothe RA, Slettan A, Saeter G, Brøgger A, Brresen A-L, and Nesland JM. 1995. Alterations at chromosome 17 loci in peripheral nerve sheath tumors. *J Neuropathol Exp Neurol* 54:65–73.

Lott IT and Richardson EP. 1981. Neuropathological findings and the biology of neurofibromatosis. *Adv Neurol* 29:23–32.

Lubs M-LE, Bauer MS, Formas ME, and Djokic B. 1991. Lisch nodules in neurofibromatosis type 1. *N Engl J Med* 324:1264–6.

Martuza RL, Phillippe I, Fitzpatrick TB, Zwaan J, Seki Y, and Lederman J. 1985. Melanin macroglobules as a cellular marker of neurofibromatosis: a quantitative study. *J Invest Dermatol* 85:347–50.

Mathew CGP, Thorpe K, Easton DF, Chin KS, Jadayel D, Ponder M, Moore G, et al. 1989. Linkage analysis of chromosome 17 markers in British and South African families with neurofibromatosis type I. *Am J Hum Genet* 44:38–40.

Mautner VF, Umnus-Schnelle S, Koppen J, and Heise U. 1988. [Diagnosis of Recklinghausen's neurofibromatosis]. *Dtsch Med Wochenschr* 113:1149–1151.

Meis JM, Enzinger FM, Martz KL, and Neal JA. 1992. Malignant peripheral nerve sheath tumors (malignant schwannomas) in children. *Am J Surg Pathol* 16:694–707.

Melin MM, Grotz RL, and Nivatvongs S. 1994. Gastrointestinal hemorrhage complicating systemic neurofibromatosis. *Am J Gastroenterol* 89:1888–90.

Mendez HMM. 1985. The neurofibromatosis-Noonan syndrome. *Am J Med Genet* 21:471–6.

Meschede D, Froster UG, Gullotta F, and Nieschlag E. 1993. Reproductive failure in a patient with neurofibromatosis-Noonan syndrome. *Am J Med Genet* 47:346–51.

Metheny LJ, Cappione AJ, and Skuse GR. 1995. Genetic and epigenetic mechanisms in the pathogenesis of neurofibromatosis type 1. *J Neuropathol Exp Neurol* 54: 753–60.

Miller M and Hall JG. 1978. Possible maternal effect on severity of neurofibromatosis. *Lancet* 2:1071–3.

Morier P, Mérot Y, Paccaud D, Beck D, and Frenk E. 1990. Juvenile chronic granulocytic leukemia, juvenile xanthogranulomas, and neurofibromatosis: case report and review of the literature. *J Am Acad Dermatol* 22:962–5.

Moss C and Green SH. 1994. What is segmental neurofibromatosis? *Brit J Dermatol* 130:106–10.

National Institutes of Health Consensus Development Conference. 1988. Neurofibromatosis: conference statement. *Arch Neurol* 45:575–8.

NF1 Genetic Analysis Consortium Database. 1997. <http://www.clam.com/nf/nf1gene/nf1gene.home.html>.

Niimura M. 1990. Neurofibromatosis in Japan. In: Ishibashi Y and Hori Y (eds.). *Tuberous Sclerosis and Neurofibromatosis: Epidemiology, Pathophysiology, Biology, and Management.* Amsterdam: Elsevier, pp. 23–31.

Noonan J. 1994. Noonan syndrome: an update and review for the primary pediatrician. *Clin Pediatr (Phila)* 33:548–55.

Norman ME. 1972. Neurofibromatosis in a family. *Am J Dis Child* 123:159–60.

North K. 1993. Neurofibromatosis type 1: review of the first 200 patients in an Australian clinic. *J Child Neurol* 8:395–402.

North KN, Riccardi V, Samango-Sprouse C, Ferner R, Moore B, Legius E, Ratner N, and Denckla MB. 1997. Cognitive function and academic performance in neurofibromatosis 1: consensus statement from the NF1 Cognitive Disorders Task Force. *Neurology* 48:1121–7.

Opitz JM and Weaver DD. 1985. The neurofibromatosis-Noonan syndrome. *Am J Med Genet* 21:477–90.

Pascual-Castroviejo I, Verdu A, Roman M, et al. 1988. Optic glioma with progressive occlusion of the aqueduct of Sylvius in monozygotic twins with neurofibromatosis. *Brain Dev* 10:24–9.

Perry HD and Font RL. 1982. Iris nodules in von Recklinghausen's neurofibromatosis: electron microscopic confirmation of their melanocytic origin. *Arch Ophthalmol* 100:1635–40.

Pivnick EK, Schaefer GB, Lin AE, Park VM, Tolley EA, Lawrence MD, and Huson SM. 1997. Delineation of a common facial appearance in neurofibromatosis type 1 (NF1). *Am J Hum Genet* 61:A110.

Poyhonen M, Leisti E-L, Kytölö S, and Leisti J. 1997a. Hereditary spinal neurofibromatosis: a rare form of NF1? *J Med Genet* 34:184–7.

Poyhonen M, Niemela S, and Herva R. 1997b. Risk of malignancy and death in neurofibromatosis. *Arch Pathol Lab Med* 121:139–43.

Pulst SM, Riccardi VM, Fain P, and Korenberg JR. 1991. Familial spinal neurofibromatosis: clinical and DNA linkage analysis. *Neurology* 41:1923–7.

Purandare SM, Breidenbach HH, Li Y, Zhu XL, Sawada S, Neil SM, Brothman A, White R, Cawthon R, and Viskochil D. 1995. Identification of neurofibromatosis 1 (*NF1*) homologous loci by direct sequencing, fluorescence *in situ* hybridization, and PCR amplification of somatic cell hybrids. *Genomics* 30:476–85.

Quattrin T, McPherson E, and Putnam E. 1987. Vertical transmission of the neurofibromatosis/Noonan syndrome. *Am J Med Genet* 26:645–9.

Rasmussen SA, Colman SD, Ho VT, Abernathy CR, Arn PH, Weiss L, Schwartz C, Saul RA, and Wallace MR. 1998. Constitutional and mosaic large NF1 gene deletions in neurofibromatosis type 1. *J Med Genet* 35:468–71.

Reynolds RL and Pineda CA. 1988. Neurofibromatosis: review and report of case. *J Am Dent Assoc* 117:735–7.

Riccardi VM. 1980. Pathophysiology of neurofibromatosis. IV. Dermatologic insights into heterogeneity and pathogenesis. *J Am Acad Dermatol* 3:157–66.

———. 1981a. Von Recklinghausen neurofibromatosis. *N Engl J Med* 305:1617–27.

———. 1981b. Cutaneous manifestation of neurofibromatosis: cellular interaction, pigmentation, and mast cells. *Birth Defects Orig Artic Ser* 27(2):129–45.

———. 1982a. The multiple forms of neurofibromatosis. *Pediatr Rev* 3:292–8.

———. 1982b. Neurofibromatosis: clinical heterogeneity. *Curr Probl Cancer* 7(2):1–34.

———. 1983. Neurofibromatosis in a patient with systemic lupus erythematosus. *Arthritis Rheum* 26:574.

———. 1984. Neurofibromatosis heterogeneity. *J Am Acad Dermatol* 10:518–9.

———. 1992. *Neurofibromatosis: Phenotype, Natural History, and Pathogenesis.* 2nd ed. Baltimore: The Johns Hopkins University Press.

———. 1993. Genotype, malleotype, phenotype, and randomness: lessons from neurofibromatosis-I (NF-I). *Am J Hum Genet* 53:301–4.

Riccardi VM and Eichner JE. 1986. *Neurofibromatosis: Phenotype, Natural History, and Pathogenesis.* Baltimore: The Johns Hopkins University Press.

Riccardi VM and Elder DW. 1986. Multiple cytogenetic aberrations in neurofibrosarcomas complicating neurofibromatosis. *Cancer Genet Cytogenet* 23:199–209.

Riccardi VM and Wald JS. 1987. Discounting an adverse maternal effect on severity of neurofibromatosis. *Pediatrics* 79:386–93.

Riccardi VM, Kleiner B, and Lubs ML. 1979. Neurofibromatosis: variable expression is not instrinsic to the mutant gene. *Birth Defects* 15(5b):283–9.

Ritchie RJ, Mattei MG, and Lalande M. 1998. A large polymorphic repeat in the pericentromeric region of human chromosome 15q contains three partial gene duplications. *Hum Mol Genet* 7:1253–60.

Riva P, Castorina P, Manoukian S, Dalprà L, Doneda L, Marini G, den Dunnen J, and Larizza L. 1996. Characterization of a cytogenetic 17q11.2 deletion in an NF1 patient with a contiguous gene syndrome. *Hum Genet* 98:646–50.

Roth RR, Martines R, and James WD. 1987. Segmental neurofibromatosis. *Arch Dermatol* 123:917–20.

Rubenstein AE, Bader JL, Aron AA, and Wallace S. 1983. Familial transmission of segmental neurofibromatosis. *Neurology* 33(Suppl 2):76.

Rubenstein AE, Halperin JC, Mindel J, Wallace S, and Aron A. 1990. Lisch nodules in neurofibromatosis-1 are not dependent on sympathetic innervation. *Am J Hum Genet* 47:A76.

Samuelsson B and Axelsson R. 1981. Neurofibromatosis: a clinical and genetic study of 96 cases in Gothenburg, Sweden. *Acta Derm Venereol Suppl (Stockh)* 95:67–71.

Samuelsson B and Samuelsson S. 1989. Neurofibromatosis in Gothenburg, Sweden. I. Background, study design and epidemiology. *Neurofibromatosis* 2:6–22.

Saul RA and Stevenson RG. 1984. Segmental neurofibromatosis: a distinct type of neurofibromatosis? *Proc Greenwood Genet Ctr* 3:3–6.

———. 1986. Are Bannayan syndrome and Ruvalcaba-Myhre-Smith syndrome discrete entities? *Proc Greenwood Genet Ctr* 5:3–7.

Sawada S, Florell S, Purandare SM, Ota M, Stephens K, and Viskochil D. 1996. Identification of *NF1* mutations in both alleles of a dermal neurofibroma. *Nat Genet* 14:110–2.

Seizinger BR, Rouleau GA, Ozelius LJ, Lane AH, Faryniarz AG, Chao MV, Huson S, et al. 1987. Genetic linkage of von Recklinghausen neurofibromatosis to the nerve growth factor receptor gene. *Cell* 49:589–94.

Sergeyev AS. 1975. On the mutation rate of neurofibromatosis. *Hum Genet* 28:129–38.

Sharland M, Burch M, McKenna WM, and Paton MA. 1992a. A clinical study of Noonan syndrome. *Arch Dis Child* 67:178–83.

Sharland M, Taylor R, Patton MA, and Jeffery S. 1992b. Absence of linkage of Noonan syndrome to the neurofibromatosis type 1 locus. *J Med Genet* 29:188–90.

Shearer P, Parham D, Kovnar E, Kun L, Rao B, Lobe T, and Pratt C. 1994. Neurofibromatosis type I and malignancy: review of 32 pediatric cases treated at a single institution. *Med Pediatr Oncol* 22:78–83.

Shekitka KM and Sobin LH. 1994. Ganglioneuromas of the gastrointestinal tract: relation to von Recklinghausen disease and other multiple tumor syndromes. *Am J Surg Pathol* 18:250–7.

Sinha RP, Ducker TB, and Balentine JD. 1973. Neurofibromatosis (von Recklinghausen's disease) and juxtamedullary spinal lipoma. *Surg Neurol* 1:281–3.

Skuse GR and Cappione AJ. 1997. RNA processing and clinical variability in neurofibromatosis type I (NF1). *Hum Molec Genet* 6:1707–12.

Sørensen SA, Mulvihill JJ, and Nielsen A. 1986a. On the natural history of von Recklinghausen neurofibromatosis. *Ann NY Acad Sci* 486:30–7.

———. 1986b. Long-term follow-up of von Recklinghausen neurofibromatosis: survival and malignant neoplasms. *N Engl J Med* 314:1010–5.

Stern HJ, Saal HM, Lee JS, Fain PR, Goldgar DE, Rosenbaum KN, and Barker DF. 1992. Clinical variability of type 1 neurofibromatosis: Is there a neurofibromatosis-Noonan syndrome? *J Med Genet* 29:184–7.

Tassabehji M, Strachan T, Sharland M, Colley A, Donnai D, Harris R, and Thakker N. 1993. Tandem duplication within a neurofibromatosis type I (NFI) gene exon in a family with features of Watson syndrome and Noonan syndrome. *Am J Hum Genet* 53:90–5.

Taylor RG, Rab GT, Liberman JS, and Setoguchi Y. 1984. Neurofibromatosis and Ehlers-Danlos syndrome in a young amputee. *Arch Phys Med Rehabil* 65:645–6.

Tonsgard JH, Kwak SM, Short MP, and Dachman AH. 1998. CT imaging in adults with neurofibromatosis-1: frequent asymptomatic plexiform lesions. *Neurology* 50: 1755–60.

Tonsgard JH, Yelavarthi KK, Cushner S, Short MP, and Lindgren V. 1997. Do NF1 gene deletions result in a characteristic phenotype? *Am J Med Genet* 73:80–6.

Tung T-C, Chen Y-R, Chen K-T, Chen C-T, and Bendor-Samuel R. 1997. Massive intratumor hemorrhage in facial plexiform neurofibroma. *Head Neck* 19:158–62.

Turkington RW and Grode HE. 1964. Ehlers-Danlos syndrome and multiple neurofibromatosis. *Ann Intern Med* 61:1142–3.

Upadhyaya M, Ruggieri M, Maynard J, Osborn M, Hartog C, Mudd S, Penttinen M, Cordeiro I, Ponder M, Ponder BAJ, Krawczak M, and Cooper DN. 1998. Gross deletions of the neurofibromatosis type 1 (*NF1*) gene are predominantly of maternal origin and commonly associated with a learning disability, dysmorphic features and developmental delay. *Hum Genet* 102:591–7.

Upadhyaya M, Shen M, Cherryson A, Farnham J, Maynard J, Huson SM, and Harper PS. 1992. Analysis of mutations at the neurofibromatosis (NF1) locus. *Hum Mol Genet* 1:735–40.

Valero MC, Pascual-Castroviejo I, Velasco E, Moreno F, Hernádez-Chico C. 1997. Identification of de novo deletions at the NF1 gene: no preferential paternal origin and phenotypic analysis of patients. *Hum Genet* 99:720–6.

van Asperen CJ, Overweg-Plandsoen WCG, Cnossen MH, van Tijn DA, and Hennekam RCM. 1998. Familial neurofibromatosis type 1 associated with an overgrowth syndrome resembling Weaver syndrome. *J Med Genet* 35:323–7.

Verhest A, Heimann R, Verschraegen J, Vamos E, and Hecht F. 1988. Hereditary intestinal neurofibromatosis. II. Translocation between chromosomes 12 and 14. *Neurofibromatosis* 1:33–6.

Viskochil D and Carey JC. 1994. Alternate and related forms of the neurofibromatoses. In: Huson SM, Hughes RAC, eds. *The Neurofibromatoses: A Pathogenic and Clinical Overview.* London: Chapman & Hall, pp. 445–74.

Viskochil D, Cawthon R, O'Connell P, Xu G, Stevens J, Culver M, Carey J, and White R. 1991. The gene encoding the oligodendrocyte-myelin glycoprotein is embedded within the neurofibromatosis type 1 gene. *Mol Cell Biol* 11:906–12.

Vivot N, Kizlansky V, Lynch P, Barragan ME, Greiner H, and Frola P. 1986. [Recklinghausen's disease with liposarcoma]. *Rev Argent Dermatol* 67:266–75.

Watson GH. 1967. Pulmonary stenosis, café-au-lait spots, and dull intelligence. *Arch Dis Childh* 42:303–7.

Waxman BP, Buzzard AJ, Cox J, and Stephens MJ. 1986. Gastric and intestinal bleeding in multiple neurofibromatosis with cardiomyopathy. *Aust NZ J Surg* 56:171–3.

Weleber RG and Zonana J. 1983. Iris hamartomas (Lisch nodules) in a case of segmental neurofibromatosis. *Am J Ophtahlmol* 96:740–3.

Westerhof W, Delleman JW, Wolters E, and Dijkstra P. 1984. Neurofibromatosis and hypertelorism. *Arch Dermatol* 120:1579–81.

Wheeler MH, Curley IR, and Williams ED. 1986. The association of neurofibromatosis, pheochromocytoma, and somatostatin-rich duodenal carcinoid tumor. *Surgery* 100: 1163–9.

Whitehouse D. 1966. Diagnostic value of the café-au-lait spot in children. *Arch Dis Child* 41:316–9.

Wolpert L, Beddington R, Brockes J, Jessell T, Lawrence P, and Meyerowitz E. 1998. *Principles of Development.* London: Current Biology.

Wong V C-N. 1994. Clinical manifestations of neurofibromatosis-1 in Chinese children. *Pediatr Neurol* 11:301–7.

Woodruff JM, Marshall ML, Godwin TA, Funkhouser JW, Thompson NJ, and Erlandson RA. 1983. Plexiform (multinodular) schwannoma: a tumor simulating the plexiform neurofibroma. *Am J Surg Pathol* 7:691–7.

Wu B-L, Austin MA, Schneider GH, Boles RG, and Korf BR. 1995. Deletion of the entire *NF1* gene detected by FISH: four deletion patients associated with severe manifestations. *Am J Med Genet* 59:528–35.

Wu B-L, Boles RG, Yaari H, Weremowicz S, Schneider GH, and Korf BR. 1997a. Somatic mosaicism for deletion of the entire *NF1* gene identified by FISH. *Hum Genet* 99:209–13.

Wu B-L, Schneider GH, Korf BR. 1997b. Deletion of the entire *NF1* gene causing distinct manifestations in a family. *Am J Med Genet* 69:98–101.

Xu W, Mulligan LM, Pander MA, Liu L, Smith BA, Mathew CG, and Ponder BA. 1992. Loss of NF1 alleles in phaeochromocytomas from patients with type I neurofibromatosis. *Genes Chromosomes Cancer* 4:337–342.

Zehavi C, Romano A, and Goodman RM. 1986. Iris (Lisch) nodules in neurofibromatosis. *Clin Genet* 29:51–5.

Zlotogora J. 1993. Mutations in von Recklinghausen neurofibromatosis: an hypothesis. *Am J Med Genet* 46:182–4.

Zöller M, Rembeck B, Åkesson HO, and Angervall L. 1995. Life expectancy, mortality and prognostic factors in neurofibromatosis type 1: a twelve-year follow-up of an epidemiological study in Göteborg, Sweden. *Acta Derm Venerol (Stockh)* 75:136–40.

Zöller M, Rembeck B, and Bäckman L. 1997a. Neuropsychological deficits in adults with neurofibromatosis type 1. *Acta Neurol Scand* 95:225–32.

Zöller M, Rembeck B, Odén A, Samuelsson M, and Agervall L. 1997b. Malignant and benign tumors in patients with neurofibromatosis type 1 in a defined Swedish population. *Cancer* 79:2125–31.

Zvulunov A, Barak Y, and Metzker A. 1995. Juvenile xanthogranuloma, neurofibromatosis, and juvenile chronic myelogenous leukemia: world statistical analysis. *Arch Derm* 131:904–8.

Zvulunov A, Weitz R, and Metzker A. 1998. Neurofibromatosis type 1 in childhood: evaluation of clinical and epidemiological features as predictive factors for severity. *Clin Pediatr* 37:295–300.

3

Evaluation and Management

J. M. Friedman, M.D., Ph.D.

EVALUATION AND DIAGNOSTIC STRATEGIES

NIH DIAGNOSTIC CRITERIA

Neurofibromatosis type 1 (NF1) was well described as a clinical entity in 1882 (von Recklinghausen 1882), but generally accepted diagnostic criteria were not established until a U.S. National Institutes of Health Consensus Development Conference did so in 1987 (Table 3-1). Although the *NF1* gene was subsequently identified and sequenced (Cawthon et al. 1990; Viskochil et al. 1990; Wallace et al. 1990), NF1 remains a clinical diagnosis based on the NIH criteria. These criteria were reevaluated in 1997 by a group of physicians with extensive experience in the diagnosis and management of NF1. This group recommended continued use without modification of the NIH diagnostic criteria for NF1 (Gutmann et al. 1997).

Despite their widespread use, no formal studies of the specificity or sensitivity of the NIH diagnostic criteria have been reported. Such studies will be very difficult until a reliable method for detecting all pathogenic *NF1* mutations is available to provide an independent "gold standard." Nevertheless, clinical experience indicates that the NIH diagnostic criteria are both highly specific and highly sensitive in adults with NF1 (Gutmann et al. 1997). The NIH diagnostic criteria are also very specific in children, but many children who later are shown unequivocally to have NF1 do not meet the NIH diagnostic criteria in the first years of life (Fois et al. 1993; Goldberg et al. 1996; Huson et al. 1989b; Obringer et al. 1989; Riccardi 1981). Figure 3-1 shows that two or more of the clinical features listed as NIH diagnostic criteria are apparent in about 90% of children with NF1 by 6 years of age but that the diagnosis cannot be made with certainty in many younger children with a negative family history.

The appearance of most signs of NF1 is age-dependent (Friedman and Birch 1997; Huson 1994; Huson et al. 1989b; Korf 1992; Niimura 1990; Obringer et al. 1989; Wolkenstein et al. 1996). Cardinal features of NF1, such as Lisch nodules and cutaneous and subcutaneous neurofibromas, are uncommon in young children and do not reach maximum frequencies until adulthood (Figs. 3-2 and

Table 3-1. NIH diagnostic criteria for NF1

NF1 is present in a patient who has two or more of the following signs:
Six or more café-au-lait macules > 5 mm in greatest diameter in prepubertal individuals or
  > 15 mm in greatest diameter after puberty.
Two or more neurofibromas of any type or one or more plexiform neurofibromas.
Freckling in the axilla or inguinal region (Crowe sign).
A tumor of the optic pathway.
Two or more Lisch nodules (iris hamartomas).
A distinctive osseous lesion, such as sphenoid wing dysplasia or thinning of the cortex of
  the long bones (with or without pseudarthrosis).
A first-degree relative (parent, sib, or offspring) with NF1 by the above criteria.

Source: National Institutes of Health Consensus Development Conference 1988; Gutmann et al. 1997.

3-3). The frequencies of many of other signs increase rapidly during childhood, so that the reliability of the NIH diagnostic criteria improves every year as a child grows older. For example, the prevalence of intertriginous freckling among 912 NF1 probands from the NNFF International Database is 26.7% in children less than 1 year old but increases to more than 80% by age 4 (Fig. 3-4). Optic glioma also reaches its maximum frequency by about age 4 but is much less common than intertriginous freckling (Niimura 1990; Huson 1994; Listernick et al. 1994, 1995, 1997) (see Fig. 3-2C).

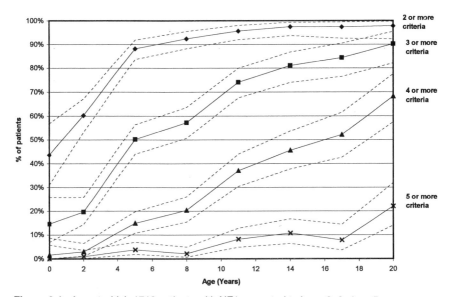

Figure 3-1. Age at which 1713 patients with NF1 are noted to have 2, 3, 4, or 5 or more NIH diagnostic criteria. The error bars indicate 95% confidence intervals. Only physical features were considered in this analysis; a positive family history was not. *Source:* Data from the National Neurofibromatosis Foundation International Database. This analysis was performed by Kimberly DeBella, and is used with her permission.

A) Cutaneous Neurofibromas

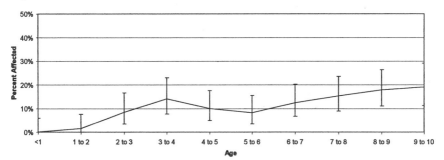

B) Subcutaneous Neurofibromas

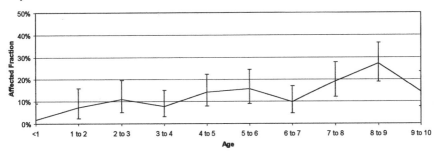

C) Symptomatic Optic Glioma

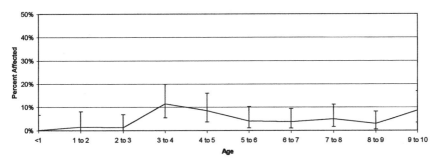

Figure 3-2. Prevalence by age of (A) two or more cutaneous neurofibromas, (B) two or more subcutaneous neurofibromas, or (C) symptomatic optic glioma among NF1 probands. Information was available on 866, 904, and 900 probands, respectively. The error bars indicate 95% confidence intervals. *Source:* Data from the National Neurofibromatosis Foundation International Database. This analysis was performed by Kimberly DeBella, and is used with her permission.

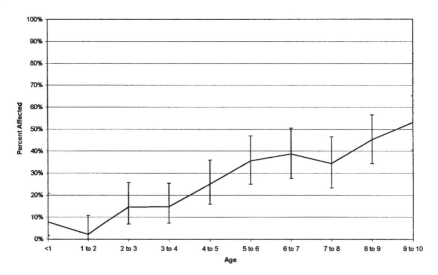

Figure 3-3. Prevalence by age of Lisch nodules among 674 probands with NF1 who had ophthalmologic examinations. The error bars indicate 95% confidence intervals.
Source: Data from the National Neurofibromatosis Foundation International Database. This analysis was performed by Kimberly DeBella, and is used with her permission.

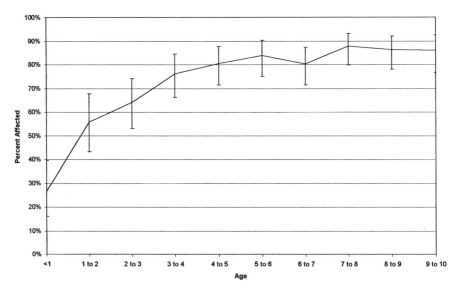

Figure 3-4. Prevalence by age of intertriginous freckling among 912 probands with NF1. The error bars indicate 95% confidence intervals. *Source:* Data from the National Neurofibromatosis Foundation International Database. This analysis was performed by Kimberly DeBella, and is used with permission.

Children who have inherited NF1 from an affected parent can usually be diagnosed within the first year of life because the diagnosis requires just one clinical sign in addition to the positive family history. That clinical sign is usually multiple café-au-lait spots, a feature that is seen in most patients with NF1 at or shortly after birth (Fig. 3-5) (Fois et al. 1993; Huson 1994; Huson et al. 1989b; Obringer et al. 1989; Riccardi 1981; Wolkenstein et al. 1996). Less frequently, the first feature noted is a plexiform neurofibroma or anterior tibial bowing, which may also present early in life (Fig. 3-6). Plexiform neurofibromas and anterior tibial bowing are particularly useful in diagnosing NF1 in young patients because such features are rarely seen in children who do not have NF1.

Other clinical or radiologic features have been suggested as additional criteria to improve diagnostic sensitivity for NF1 in young children. For example, some authors consider the focal areas of signal hyperintensity ("unidentified bright objects," or UBOs) seen on T_2-weighted MRI brain scans to be useful diagnostically (Balestri et al. 1993; Curless et al. 1998; DiMario et al. 1993; Duffner et al. 1989; Goldstein et al. 1989; Van Es et al. 1996). Expert consensus does not support this position, however, because specificity of MRI hyperintensities for NF1 has not been established (Gutmann et al. 1997). Macrocephaly and short stature are frequently seen among patients with NF1 (Goldberg et al. 1996; Hughes 1994; Huson 1994; North 1993; Riccardi 1981), but neither sign has sufficient specificity to be useful as a diagnostic criterion (Gutmann et al. 1997). Dysplastic scoliosis is a much less frequent but much more distinctive finding (Holt 1978; Fairbank 1994; Gabriel 1996), but it is not considered sufficient by itself for diagnosis of NF1 (Gutmann et al. 1997).

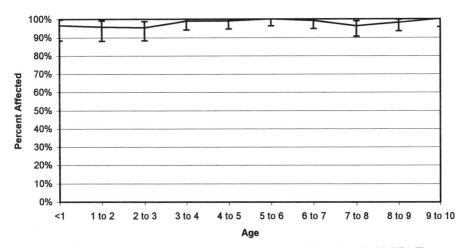

Figure 3-5. Prevalence by age of café-au-lait spots among 907 probands with NF1. The error bars indicate 95% confidence intervals. *Source:* Data from the National Neurofibromatosis Foundation International Database. This analysis was performed by Kimberly De-Bella, and is used with her permission.

A) Plexiform neurofibromas

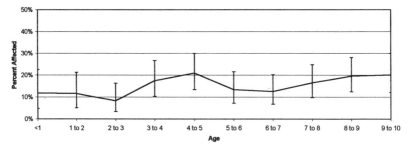

B) Anterior Tibial Bowing

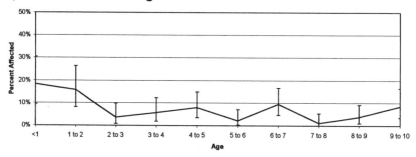

Figure 3-6. Prevalence by age of (A) plexiform neurofibromas or (B) anterior tibial bowing among 908 probands with NF1. The error bars indicate 95% confidence intervals.
Source: Data from the National Neurofibromatosis Foundation International Database. This analysis was performed by Kimberly DeBella, and is used with her permission.

INITIAL DIAGNOSTIC ASSESSMENT FOR NF1

An approach to the evaluation of a patient in whom a diagnosis of NF1 is being considered or confirmed is described below and summarized in Table 3-2. This approach is designed to establish or rule out NF1 using the NIH diagnostic criteria and to identify serious manifestations and complications of the disease if present. A more extensive diagnostic protocol recommended in previous editions of this book (Riccardi 1992; Riccardi and Eichner 1986) is valuable for clinical research studies but is not necessary for routine clinical care of patients with NF1.

History

The medical history of a patient in whom a diagnosis of NF1 is being considered should provide a general assessment of health, focusing on symptoms known to be associated with NF1. The time of appearance and subsequent behavior of any pigmented skin lesions and dermal tumors are important. A history of learning problems, abnormalities of vision, seizures, headaches, scoliosis, other skeletal anomalies, or hypertension should also be elicited. Obtaining records of prior medical evaluations is often useful. Pathology reports on tumors that have been

Table 3-2. Initial diagnostic assessment for NF1

Medical history focusing on symptoms of NF1
  Pigmented skin lesions
  Dermal tumors
  Learning disabilities
  Visual abnormalities
  Seizures
  Headaches
  Scoliosis
  Other skeletal abnormalities
  Hypertension
  Review of previous medical reports
Physical examination
  Measurement of height, weight, and head circumference
  Measurement of blood pressure
  Thorough examination of skin (with a Wood light, if necessary) for café-au-lait spots, in-
    tertriginous freckling, and dermal tumors
  Inspection of long bones for hypertrophy or bowing, especially anterolateral bowing of the
    tibia
  Examination of the back for scoliosis
  Age-appropriate neurologic examination, with emphasis on assessment of eyes for prop-
    tosis or strabismus and of limbs for weakness or decreased deep tendon reflexes
Ophthalmologic examination
  Complete examination for signs of optic glioma
  Slit-lamp examination for Lisch nodules
Evaluation of family members
  Family history for signs and symptoms of NF1
  Full assessment of any relative reported or suspected to have NF1
  Full assessment of both parents and all children of an affected individual
Laboratory and imaging studies
  Only to identify specific complications suspected because of the medical history, physical
    examination, or ophthalmologic examination

removed and reports of previous ophthalmologic examinations, skeletal radiographs, and cranial imaging studies are often especially valuable.

Physical Examination

Examination of the patient in whom NF1 is suspected should include measurement of the height, weight, and head circumference, with comparison to age- and gender-appropriate standards. The blood pressure should be checked with a cuff of the proper size for the patient. Careful skin examination of the fully disrobed patient is especially important. Examination with a Wood light in a darkened room is useful in identifying café-au-lait spots, freckling, and other pigmentary alterations, especially when the lesions and unaffected skin are similar in color. Wood lamp examination should be performed on any patient in whom café-au-lait spots and freckling characteristic of NF1 are not unequivocally present on routine examination. The examiner should pay special attention to freckling in the axillae, groin, neck, and area under pendulous breasts because sparse lesions are easily overlooked. The skin should also be thoroughly examined for cutaneous, subcutaneous, and plexiform tumors, which may vary considerably in number, size, and location. Discrete dermal neurofibromas are typically soft to rubbery in consistency and may be underneath the skin, sessile, or pedunculated. The overlying skin may appear normal, reddened, bluish, or hyperpigmented. Viewing the skin surface tangentially, in addition to looking at it directly, is often useful in recognizing diffuse involvement with innumerable tiny tumors. These may produce a pebbly appearance over the abdomen or on the surface of a limb. The examiner should also look specifically for nipple neurofibromas, which are very common in women with NF1. The characteristics of all tumors should be noted, and those that appear to be neurofibromas should be differentiated from any others identified. The patient and family should be asked to point out any tumors that the examiner may have missed.

In addition, the examiner should look for more serious manifestations and complications of NF1. It is especially important in young children to identify signs of osseous dysplasia that may lead to pathologic fracture and pseudarthrosis. Involvement of the tibia, the most frequently affected long bone, presents as anterolateral bowing of the leg. When severe, this lesion is obvious on inspection, but identification of milder manifestations requires careful comparison of the legs for asymmetry or subtle protrusion of one shin when viewed from the side. Asymmetry of part or all of a limb may also occur when a plexiform neurofibroma occurs in the area. In some cases, the asymmetry is apparent even though there is no other sign of the tumor on the surface. Scoliosis in patients with NF1 may be diagnosed in late childhood or early adolescence but is usually seen earlier when there is vertebral dysplasia. Asymmetry of the upper face is sometimes seen in association with sphenoid wing dysplasia. A careful neurologic examination, conducted in a manner appropriate for the patient's age, is also important. Proptosis, strabismus, and other abnormalities of visual function may be signs of optic glioma in a child with NF1. Limb weakness or areflexia may indicate involvement of a spinal nerve root by neurofibromas.

Ophthalmologic Examination
A thorough ophthalmologic examination, including a slit-lamp examination, is necessary for any patient in whom NF1 is suspected. Lisch nodules, one of the most frequently observed diagnostic features (Huson et al. 1987; Lubs et al. 1991; Ragge et al. 1993), can usually be identified unequivocally on slit-lamp examination. Lisch nodules can be seen to be elevated above the surface of the iris on slit-lamp examination, but they may be confused on routine ophthalmoscopic examination with flat iris freckles, which have no diagnostic significance. In addition, the ophthalmologist should look for lid neurofibromas, choroidal hamartomas, abnormalities of pupillary function, deficits of extraocular muscle function, decreased color vision, visual-field disturbances, glaucoma, optic atrophy, and papilledema (Huson et al. 1987; Kuenzle et al. 1994; Listernick et al. 1994, 1995, 1997; Lund and Skovby 1991; Massry et al. 1997; Purvin and Dunn

1994). Intracranial imaging studies should be performed if any sign of optic tract glioma or brain tumor is found.

Evaluation of Family Members

The initial evaluation of a patient in whom NF1 is suspected should include a careful family history for signs and symptoms of NF1. A medical pedigree should be constructed that shows the proband and all of his or her first- and second-degree relatives. If any relative is reported or suspected to have NF1, the pedigree should be extended as necessary to incorporate more distant relatives. More extensive pedigrees are not necessary in apparently sporadic cases because the penetrance of NF1 is complete or very nearly so (see Chapter 4).

If the information obtained from the family history suggests that one or more relatives of the proband may also have NF1, the diagnosis must be confirmed. A positive family history cannot be used to establish the diagnosis of NF1 in an individual unless at least one first-degree relative is known to meet the NIH diagnostic criteria. The best way to confirm the diagnosis in other relatives is to evaluate them thoroughly, as described above. If this has already been done, it is necessary only to obtain a copy of the medical record describing the assessment. If the diagnosis of NF1 has not been fully established in a relative who is unavailable for complete evaluation, obtaining other medical records (e.g., pathology reports of dermal tumor biopsies or autopsy reports) may be helpful. Both parents of a child with suspected or established NF1 should routinely be evaluated by history, physical examination, and ophthalmologic examination. Establishing the diagnosis in a parent is important for genetic counseling and may allow a firm diagnosis to be made in a young child who has just one other cardinal feature of NF1. Similarly, full assessment for NF1 is indicated in all children of an affected parent.

MOLECULAR GENETIC TESTING

Routine molecular genetic testing of patients in whom NF1 is suspected is not currently recommended for several reasons (Gutmann et al. 1997). A definitive diagnosis can be made on the basis of clinical and ophthalmologic examinations in most patients, especially in those who are over 6 years of age (Huson 1994; Korf 1992; Obringer et al. 1989; see Fig. 3-1). The wide range of NF1 mutations that occur and the large size of the gene have made mutation analysis very difficult (Gutmann et al. 1997; Huson and Upadhyaya 1994; Shen et al. 1996). The protein truncation test identifies more than half of such mutations (Heim et al. 1994, 1995), but the sensitivity and specificity of this test have not been established (Gutmann et al. 1997). False positive and false negative test results can have very serious adverse repercussions in a disease like NF1, and routine use of a genetic test is inappropriate until its validity and precision have been clearly established. At present, molecular genetic testing of patients with NF1 is indicated only as part of a research protocol, to permit prenatal diagnosis in the fetus of an affected parent, or for identification of suspected deletions of the entire *NF1* gene, which have been associated with an unusually severe phenotype

(Kayes et al. 1992, 1994; Leppig et al. 1996, 1997; Riva et al. 1996; Tonsgard et al. 1997; Upadhyaya et al. 1998; Valero et al. 1997; Wu et al. 1995, 1997b).

OTHER STUDIES

Additional laboratory and radiologic tests should be performed to identify specific complications that are suspected on the basis of the medical history, physical examination, or ophthalmologic examination. No radiographic or laboratory study is routinely recommended unless it is clinically indicated because none has been shown to be useful (Cnossen et al. 1998; Gutmann et al. 1997; Huson and Upadhyaya 1994; Wolkenstein et al. 1996).

There has been considerable controversy over the value of routine cranial MRI studies in patients with NF1 (Balestri et al. 1993; Bognanno et al. 1988; Carey 1992; Cnossen et al. 1998; Curless et al. 1998; DiMario and Ramsby 1998; Ferner et al. 1993; Huson and Upadhyaya 1994; Listernick et al. 1989, 1994; North et al. 1994; O'Connor 1997; Pollack et al. 1996; Rossi et al. 1994; Truhan and Filipek 1993; Wolkenstein et al. 1996). The current expert consensus is that routine cranial MRI does not improve the management of children with NF1 who have undergone complete neurologic and ophthalmologic examinations (Gutmann et al. 1997; Listernick et al. 1997; Seashore et al. 1995). Patients with neurologic abnormalities, including children whose head growth is crossing centiles, should be referred immediately to a specialist for appropriate imaging studies (Bilaniuk et al. 1997; Broniscer et al. 1997; Gower et al. 1990; Kuenzle et al. 1994; Pollack et al. 1996; Van Es et al. 1996). Neurologic consultation is also indicated for any child found on incidental cranial imaging studies to have an enhancing lesion or a major structural anomaly of the brain.

Radiographic studies are necessary for all children with NF1 in whom osseous dysplasia or scoliosis is suspected. There is no evidence that routine imaging of the chest, skeleton, or abdomen improves the management of asymptomatic patients with NF1, but MRI imaging can be very useful in determining the anatomic involvement and extent of plexiform neurofibromas (Biondetti et al. 1983; Daneman et al. 1983; Glasier et al. 1989; Inoue et al. 1997; Matsuki et al. 1997; Nguyen 1997; Pivnick et al. 1997; Seppala et al. 1997; Shu et al. 1993). Such studies are particularly important if surgical treatment is being considered. Ultrasonography has also been used to visualize neurofibromas within soft tissues (Bauer et al. 1992), but studies comparing the utility of ultrasound imaging and MRI scanning have not been reported.

A number of other studies may be valuable for further assessment of particular problems and complications found on routine evaluation of patients with NF1. Pathologic examination is necessary to characterize tumors that are removed from a patient with NF1, especially if malignancy is suspected. Identification of hypertension in a patient with NF1 requires evaluation for vascular dysplasia such as renal artery stenosis or coarctation of the aorta (see Chapter 12). In adult patients, pheochromocytoma also needs to be considered (see Chapter 12). Learning disabilities are very frequent in children with NF1 but may be subtle and present in a variety of ways. Complete developmental assessment should be performed on any child with NF1 in whom learning problems are suspected (North et al. 1997; see Chapter 7).

DIFFERENTIAL DIAGNOSIS

Use of the NIH diagnostic criteria usually permits unequivocal diagnosis of patients who have NF1 and exclusion of the diagnosis in those who do not have the disease. For example, otherwise normal adults who have a single cardinal feature—pseudarthrosis or one plexiform neurofibroma or a large café-au-lait spot—clearly can be said not to have NF1. Differential diagnosis is usually not difficult, either.

The most frequent alternative diagnosis considered in the young child is multiple café-au-lait spots, which can be transmitted as an autosomal dominant trait without other characteristic features of NF1 (Arnsmeier et al. 1994; Charrow et al. 1993; Riccardi 1980, 1982; Whitehouse 1966). In most families that have been studied, this trait is not linked to the *NF1* locus (Brunner et al. 1993; Charrow et al. 1993), although linkage to *NF1* appears likely in one large kindred (Abeliovich et al. 1995). Isolated multiple café-au-lait spots are rare and almost always familial. Examination of the parents is, therefore, critical to establishing a diagnosis of dominantly inherited multiple café-au-lait spots. Adults who are affected with this condition have many café-au-lait spots but no other features of NF1. If a young child has six or more café-au-lait spots greater than 5 mm in diameter and neither of the biologic parents has such spots, sporadic NF1 is a much more likely diagnosis than familial multiple café-au-lait spots (Fois et al. 1993; Huson et al. 1989b; Korf 1992; Riccardi 1982, 1991). It is important to conduct a complete ophthalmologic examination of young children with multiple café-au-lait spots and to follow these children as if they have NF1 until the diagnosis is either established or ruled out. Usually, the uncertainty remains only for a few years (Korf 1992; Huson 1994; Obringer et al. 1989).

Several other entities that have some similarities to NF1 can cause confusion in an occasional patient. These include NF2, McCune–Albright syndrome, LEOPARD syndrome, Bannayan–Riley–Ruvalcaba syndrome, multiple endocrine neoplasia syndrome type 2B, Klippel–Trenaunay–Weber syndrome, multiple lipomatosis, congenital generalized fibromatosis, juvenile hyaline fibromatosis, multiple intradermal nevi, and Proteus syndrome.

Development of the NIH diagnostic criteria for NF1 and NF2 (National Institutes of Health 1988; Gutmann et al. 1997) has done a great deal to resolve the confusion that previously existed between these two different diseases. NF2 is described in detail in Chapter 13. Patients with NF1 rarely have vestibular schwannomas, the most consistent and characteristic feature of NF2 (Martuza and Ojemann 1992; Michels et al. 1989). Diagnostic confusion is most likely in patients with NF2 who have multiple dermal tumors (Reith and Goldblum 1996) or multiple spinal cord tumors. Although cutaneous tumors in patients with NF1 and NF2 usually differ clinically (see Chapter 13), the subcutaneous and spinal cord tumors may be impossible to distinguish on clinical or radiologic grounds alone. Biopsy may be helpful in these cases because the pathology of both dermal and spinal cord tumors in patients with NF1 is schwannoma, not neurofibroma. Patients with NF2 may have more café-au-lait spots than most people in the general population, but patients with NF2 rarely meet the NIH criterion for café-au-lait spots in NF1 (Parry et al. 1994). Lisch nodules and intertriginous freckling are not features of NF2. Finding more typical features of NF2 (and not NF1) in other family members is often a useful way of confirming the diagnosis of NF2 when diagnostic uncertainty exists.

Multiple café-au-lait spots occur in patients with McCune–Albright syndrome, but the macules tend to be fewer in number and to have more irregular margins than in patients with NF1 (Mauras and Blizzard 1986). Bony abnormalities are typically much more extensive in McCune–Albright syndrome than in NF1; the characteristic abnormality is polyostotic fibrous dysplasia. Most patients with McCune–Albright syndrome lack cutaneous tumors, intertriginous freckling, or Lisch nodules. McCune–Albright syndrome is usually sporadic, resulting from somatic mosaicism for activating mutations of the adenyl cyclase stimulatory G protein gene (Schwindinger et al. 1992; Weinstein et al. 1991).

Patients with LEOPARD syndrome have diffuse, darkly pigmented lentigines rather than typical café-au-lait spots and generally do not have cutaneous tumors or Lisch nodules (Coppin and Temple 1997). The lentigines in LEOPARD syndrome may occur anywhere on the body, but are especially frequent on the neck and trunk. Other characteristic features include mild to moderate deafness, pulmonic stenosis, and hypertrophic cardiomyopathy, all of which are infrequent among patients with NF1. LEOPARD syndrome is transmitted as an autosomal dominant trait. It was not linked to the *NF1* locus in one family that has been studied (Edman Ahlbom et al. 1995).

Multiple subcutaneous tumors, macrocephaly, and skin pigmentation are all features of both Bannayan–Riley–Ruvalcaba syndrome and NF1, but the conditions are nevertheless quite distinct (Gorlin et al. 1992). The presenting feature in children with Bannayan–Riley–Ruvalcaba syndrome is usually mental retardation, an infrequent manifestation of NF1. The subcutaneous tumors are usually lipomas or hemangiomas, not the neurofibromas characteristic of NF1. Boys with Bannayan–Riley–Ruvalcaba syndrome typically have pigmentation of the glans and shaft of the penis; café-au-lait spots occur but are not numerous or widely distributed, as in NF1. Patients with Bannayan–Riley–Ruvalcaba syndrome do not usually have intertriginous freckling, Lisch nodules, or other features typical of NF1. Bannayan–Riley–Ruvalcaba syndrome results from dominantly transmitted mutations of the *PTEN* gene (Marsh et al. 1997).

Although patients with multiple endocrine neoplasia syndrome type 2B (MEN2B) occasionally have café-au-lait spots or neurofibromas, the predominant clinical features are multiple mucosal neuromas and endocrine tumors, especially medullary thyroid carcinoma or pheochromocytoma (Morrison and Nevin 1996; Raue et al. 1994). Other features characteristic of NF1 are lacking, and most patients with MEN2B have a marfanoid body habitus. MEN2B results from a constitutional mutation of the *RET* proto-oncogene that is transmitted as an autosomal dominant trait (Carlson et al. 1994; Hofstra et al. 1994).

Patients with Klippel–Trenaunay–Weber syndrome often have overgrowth of affected body parts (Samuel and Spitz 1995; Viljoen 1988). The hemangiomas that characterize Klippel–Trenaunay–Weber syndrome are not usually a prominent component of NF1, and other features of the two conditions differ.

NF1 is sometimes a diagnostic consideration in patients who have large numbers of dermal tumors of other kinds. These conditions include multiple lipomatosis (Rabbiosi et al. 1977), juvenile hyaline fibromatosis (Aldred and Crawford 1987; Fayad et al. 1987), congenital generalized fibromatosis (Bracko et al. 1992; Chung and Enzinger 1981), and multiple intradermal nevi (Lycka et al. 1991). The histopathology of the tumors in each of these disorders is clearly different from that in NF1, and affected patients do not have other features of NF1. The family described by Gorlin and Koutlas (1998) appears to represent a previously undescribed entity in which multiple nevi, multiple deep schwannomas, and multiple vaginal leiomyomas are inherited as a dominant trait.

The most notorious misdiagnosis of NF1 occurred in Joseph Merrick, the "elephant man," who actually had Proteus syndrome (Clark 1994; Cohen 1988, 1993; Seward 1994). Multiple cutaneous tumors and hyperpigmented skin lesions are typical features of Proteus syndrome, but the tumors are usually lipomas, lymphangiomas, or hemangiomas, not neurofibromas, and the hyperpigmented lesions are epidermal nevi, not café-au-lait spots. Bizarre areas of thickened skin over the soles and hypertrophy of various body parts are characteristic of Proteus syndrome but uncommon in NF1. Because almost all cases of Proteus syndrome are sporadic, and because patients are often severely but asymmetrically affected, mosaicism for a mutation that would be lethal if present in all cells has been postulated (Biesecker et al. 1998). Further work is needed to elucidate the molecular pathogenesis of this disorder.

A few patients who have mutations of the *NF1* locus do not meet the NIH diagnostic criteria for NF1. Examples include some patients with segmental NF1, Watson syndrome, or familial café-au-lait spots. These and other uncommon clinical variants are described in Chapter 2.

GENERAL PRINCIPLES OF FOLLOW-UP AND MANAGEMENT

Current recommendations for routine management of patients with NF1 are based on clinical experience and expert consensus (Carey 1992; Huson and Upadhyaya 1994; Seashore et al. 1995; Gutmann et al. 1997). The validity of these recommendations has not been rigorously assessed. A multidisciplinary neurofibromatosis clinic can often provide expert consultation for patients with NF1. Referral should be considered for all patients newly diagnosed with NF1 when such a clinic is available locally. All patients with NF1 should be seen at least annually by a physician who is familiar with them and with the disease. The annual assessment should include an interval history and physical examination, with particular attention paid to any signs or symptoms of problems associated with NF1. The blood pressure should be checked in a patient with NF1 whenever he or she is seen by a physician because of the frequency and sometimes intermittent nature of hypertension in this disease (see Chapter 12).

An important component of the annual visit is providing anticipatory guidance regarding features of NF1 that are developing or are likely to develop at the patient's current age (Riccardi 1981; Huson and Upadhyaya 1994; Goldberg et al. 1996). In infants and young children, plexiform neurofibromas, congenital glaucoma, and osseous dysplasia are of particular concern. Recognition of anterolateral tibial bowing early may prevent fractures and subsequent pseudarthrosis (see Chapter 11) (Goldberg et al. 1996). Learning disability is the most frequent problem is school-age children, and the annual assessment of every school-age child with NF1 should include a review of academic performance and a discussion of the possibility of learning disabilities. Any child with NF1 in whom learning disabilities are suspected should be thoroughly assessed (North et al. 1997; see Chapter 7), and appropriate educational interventions should be instituted, if necessary. Scoliosis in patients with NF1 is most often diagnosed in late childhood or adolescence, but dysplastic scoliosis typically presents between 6 and 10 years of age (see Chapter 11). Early referral to an orthopedic specialist and appropriate treatment is important for patients with NF1 who have scoliosis, especially those with the dysplastic form.

Dermal tumors at any time in the life may develop in patients with NF1, but such tumors most often begin to appear in late childhood or adolescence (see Fig. 3-2). Additional tumors may occur throughout life. They may become much more numerous in some parts of the body than in others. The rate of tumor development may vary from year to year, and patients who are experiencing a period of rapid tumor development can often be reassured that this will not continue throughout their life. Women with NF1 may experience a rapid increase in the number and size of their dermal neurofibromas during pregnancy (see Chapter 12). It is impossible to predict how many dermal neurofibromas will develop in a particular patient with NF1 before the tumors appear. Patients who have deletions of the entire *NF1* locus (see Chapter 2) may be an exception to this rule. Such patients often have an unusually large number of dermal tumors early in life (Kayes et al. 1992, 1994; Leppig et al. 1996, 1997; Riva et al. 1996; Tonsgard et al. 1997; Valero et al. 1997; Wu et al. 1995, 1997b). Dermal neurofibromas can be removed surgically by conventional excision, with a laser, or by other means (Goldberg et al. 1996; Spira and Riccardi 1987). No particular method has been shown to be substantially better than any other. Many patients choose to have skin tumors removed if they are unsightly or in an inconvenient location (e.g., where clothes rub or where the lesions are frequently bumped). Pedunculated tumors are subject to being ripped off inadvertently, and some patients prefer to have larger ones removed to prevent this from happening. Discrete dermal neurofibromas rarely, if ever, undergo malignant degeneration in patients with NF1, but malignant peripheral nerve sheath tumors may arise in deep nodular or plexiform neurofibromas (McCarron and Goldblum, 1998; see Chapter 6). Patients with deep nodular or plexiform neurofibromas should be instructed to consult their physician immediately if these lesions become painful, grow rapidly, bleed, or become infected.

Annual ophthalmologic evaluation is recommended for all children with NF1 for the first 6 years of life, with less frequent eye exams thereafter (Listernick et al. 1997). Optic pathway gliomas usually present between 4 and 6 years of age (Listernick et al. 1989, 1994, 1995, 1997). Cranial MRI is indicated in any child with NF1 who has signs or symptoms of optic pathway glioma. Many of these tumors are asymptomatic, but even if symptoms occur, optic gliomas are infrequently progressive in patients with NF1 (Listernick et al. 1989, 1994, 1995, 1997). The natural history, diagnosis, and management of optic pathway gliomas and other, less common, central nervous system tumors in patients with NF1 are discussed in Chapters 9 and 10.

Many other clinical problems may occur in patients with NF1. Some of these problems, such as pheochromocytoma (see Chapter 10) and vasculopathy (see Chapter 12), may be very serious but are uncommon among patients with NF1. Other problems, such as spinal nerve tumors, are much more common but are infrequently symptomatic (Tonsgard et al. 1998). Patients who are found to have such problems should be referred promptly to appropriate specialists for evaluation and possible treatment. Consultation with a multidisciplinary neurofibromatosis clinic may help to ensure optimal management. All these conditions are discussed in other chapters of this book.

GENETIC COUNSELING

Genetic counseling should be offered to every family in which one or more members have been diagnosed with NF1. The genetic issues faced by members of an affected family differ at various times of life, and it is useful to readdress these concerns briefly during regular follow-up visits and to refer the family for further genetic counseling if needed. Many families with NF1 benefit from referral to a support group or from reading patient education materials on the disease. The Appendix provides information on these resources.

Once a diagnosis of NF1 has been established in a family, adults and most children who are affected can be distinguished from those who are not by clinical and ophthalmologic evaluation using the NIH diagnostic criteria (see Table 3-1). Because the penetrance of NF1 is complete in adults (see Chapter 4), unaffected adult relatives such as the aunts or uncles of a sporadic proband with NF1 are at no greater risk to have children with NF1 themselves than members of the general population. The risk of NF1 in each child of a person with NF1 is 50%. The risk to the child of an affected man is the same as the risk to the child of an affected woman, and the risk is the same for boys and girls. The suggestion that NF1 is more severe when inherited from the mother than when inherited from the father (Hall 1981; Miller and Hall 1978) appears to be incorrect (Huson et al. 1989a; Riccardi and Wald 1987; Rodenhiser et al. 1991).

Our inability to predict the severity of NF1 in an affected child is one of the most difficult aspects of genetic counseling for both families and counsellors (Huson et al. 1989b). The extreme variability that can occur in the NF1 phenotype even within a family is discussed in Chapter 2. One circumstance in which the disease can be expected to be more severe in an affected child than in his or her parent is when the parent has somatic mosaicism for an *NF1* mutation (Ainsworth et al. 1997; Colman et al. 1996; Tonsgard et al. 1997; Wu et al. 1997a). A patient who has somatic mosaicism would be expected, on average, to have less severe NF1 than an individual who has the same mutation in all of his or her cells. Germline mosaicism may occur in patients who have somatic mosaicism (Edwards 1989). A child who inherits an *NF1* mutation from a mosaic parent would have that mutation in all cells and would, therefore, usually be more severely affected than his or her mosaic parent. Segmental NF1 is presumed (but has not yet been proven) to represent somatic mosaicism for a pathogenic *NF1* mutation (Crowe et al. 1956; Hager et al. 1997; Miller and Sparkes 1977; Nicholls 1969; Riccardi 1981, 1982). Several families have been reported in which a parent with segmental NF1 has had a child with typical NF1 (Rubenstein et al. 1983; Boltshauser et al. 1989; Huson 1994; Moss and Green 1994).

PRENATAL AND PRESYMPTOMATIC DIAGNOSIS

Presymptomatic diagnosis by molecular testing, although sometimes possible, is rarely indicated in NF1. Adults can be diagnosed clinically, and it is difficult to envision a circumstance that would justify presymptomatic testing for NF1 in a child. Neither population screening nor newborn screening is available for NF1, but neither seems likely to be worthwhile even if a practical test were available (Shen et al. 1996). NF1 can usually be diagnosed clinically during childhood, and no method is known to prevent serious complications before they become apparent clinically.

Prenatal diagnosis is usually available for pregnancies in which one of the parents has NF1. Prenatal diagnosis can be done by direct analysis if a specific mutation has been identified in the family (Shen et al. 1996). Alternatively, prenatal diagnosis can be provided by linkage if enough family members are available for testing (Elyakim et al. 1994; Hofman and Boehm 1992; Huson and Upadhyaya 1994; Lazaro et al. 1992, 1995; Rodenhiser et al. 1993; Spiegel et al. 1991; Upadhyaya et al. 1992; Vivarelli et al. 1991, 1993; Ward et al. 1990). The fetal DNA specimen may be obtained by amniocentesis or chorionic villus sampling. Some manifestations of NF1 have been identified prenatally by detailed ultrasound examination in an exceptionally severe case (Drouin et al. 1997), but prenatal ultrasound examination is not a reliable means of diagnosing most instances of fetal NF1.

Despite the availability of prenatal molecular diagnosis for NF1, few families request it (Huson and Upadhyaya 1994; Shen et al. 1996). There are several reasons for the lack of popularity of prenatal testing. Some families oppose prenatal diagnosis in general and would not consider having it under any circumstances. Other families do not consider NF1 to be sufficiently severe to justify the risk of the procedure. Perhaps the most important limitation of prenatal testing is our current inability to predict the severity of NF1 in an affected fetus. This limitation leads many families to believe that prenatal diagnosis is simply not informative enough to meet their needs.

REFERENCES

Abeliovich D, Gelman-Kohan Z, Silverstein S, Lerer I, Chemke J, Merlin S, and Zlotogora J. 1995. Familial café au lait spots: a variant of neurofibromatosis type 1. *J Med Genet* 32:985–6.

Ainsworth PJ, Charkraborty PK, and Weksberg R. 1997. Example of somatic mosaicism in a series of de novo neurofibromatosis type 1 cases due to a maternally derived deletion. *Hum Mutat* 9:452–7.

Aldred MJ and Crawford PJM. 1987. Juvenile hyaline fibromatosis. *Oral Surg Oral Med Oral Pathol* 63:71–7.

Arnsmeier SL, Riccardi VM, and Paller AS. 1994. Familial multiple café au lait spots. *Arch Dermatol* 130:1425–6.

Balestri P, Calistri L, Vivarelli R, Bartalini G, Mancini L, Berardi A, and Fois A. 1993. Central nervous system imaging in reevaluation of patients with neurofibromatosis type 1. *Child Nerv Syst* 9:448–51.

Bauer F-P, Kehrl W, and Leuwer R. 1992. Ultraschalldiagnostik eines isolierten Vagusneurofibroms bei Morbus Recklinghausen. *Bilkgebung* 59:40–2.

Biesecker LG, Peters KF, Darling TN, Choyke P, Hill S, Schimke N, Cunningham M, Meltzer P, and Cohen MM Jr. 1998. Clinical differentiation between Proteus syndrome and hemihyperplasia: description of a distinct form of hemihyperplasia. *Am J Med Genet* 79:311–8.

Bilaniuk LT, Molloy PT, Zimmerman RA, Phillips PC, Vaughan SN, Liu GT, Sutton LN, and Needle M. 1997. Neurofibromatosis type 1: brain stem tumours. *Neuroradiology* 39:642–53.

Biondetti PR, Vigo M, Fiore D, De Faveri D, Ravasini R, and Benedetti L. 1983. CT appearance of generalized von Recklinghausen neurofibromatosis. *J Comput Assist Tomogr* 7:866–9.

Bognanno JR, Edwards MK, Lee TA, Dunn DW, Roos KL, and Klatte EC. 1988. Cranial MR imaging in neurofibromatosis. *AJR Am J Roentgenol* 151:381–8.

Boltshauser E, Stocker H, and Machler M. 1989. Neurofibromatosis type 1 in a child of a parent with segmental neurofibromatosis (NF-5). *Neurofibromatosis* 2:244–5.

Bracko M, Cindro L, and Golouh R. 1992. Familial occurrence of infantile myofibromatosis. *Cancer* 69:1294–9.

Broniscer A, Gajjar A, Bhargava R, Langston JW, Heideman R, Jones D, Kun LE, and Taylor J. 1997. Brain stem involvement in children with neurofibromatosis type 1: role of magnetic resonance imaging and spectroscopy in the distinction from diffuse pontine glioma. *Neurosurgery* 40:331–8.

Brunner HG, Hulsebos T, Steijlen PM, der Kinderen DJ, van den Steen A, and Hamel BCJ. 1993. Exclusion of the neurofibromatosis 1 locus in a family with inherited café-au-lait spots. *Am J Med Genet* 46:472–4.

Carey JC. 1992. Health supervision and anticipatory guidance for children with genetic disorders (including specific recommendations for trisomy 21, trisomy 18, and neurofibromatosis I). *Pediat Clin N Am* 39:25–53.

Carlson KM, Dou S, Chi D, Scavarda N, Toshima K, Jackson CE, Wells SA, Goodfellow PJ, and Donis-Keller H. 1994. Single missense mutation in the tyrosine kinase catalytic domain of the *RET* protooncogene is associated with multiple endocrine neoplasia type 2B. *Proc Nat Acad Sci* 91:1579–83.

Cawthon RM, Weiss R, Xu G, Viskochil D, Culver M, Stevens J, Robertson M, Dunn D, Gesteland R, O'Connell P, and White R. 1990. A major segment of the neurofibromatosis type 1 gene: cDNA sequence, genomic structure, and point mutations. *Cell* 62:193–201.

Charrow J, Listernick R, and Ward K. 1993. Autosomal dominant multiple café-au-lait spots and neurofibromatosis-1: evidence of non-linkage. *Am J Med Genet* 45:606–8.

Chung EB and Enzinger FM. 1981. Infantile myofibromatosis. *Cancer* 48:1807–18.

Clark RD. 1994. Proteus syndrome. In: Huson SM, and Hughes RAC, eds. *The Neurofibromatoses: A Pathogenic and Clinical Overview.* London: Chapman & Hall, pp. 402–13.

Cnossen MH, de Goede-Bolder A, van den Broek KM, Waasdorp CME, Oranje AP, Stroink H, Simonsz HJ, van den Ouweland AMW, Halley DJJ, and Niermeijer MF. 1998. A prospective 10 year follow up study of patients with neurofibromatosis type 1. *Arch Dis Child* 78:408–12.

Cohen MM Jr. 1988. Understanding Proteus syndrome, unmasking the elephant man, and stemming elephant fever. *Neurofibromatosis* 1:260–80.

———. 1993. Proteus syndrome: clinical evidence for somatic mosaicism and selective review. *Am J Med Genet* 47:645–52.

Colman SD, Rasmussen SA, Ho VT, Abernathy CR, and Wallace MR. 1996. Somatic mosaicism in a patient with neurofibromatosis type 1. *Am J Hum Genet* 58:484–90.

Coppin BD and Temple IK. 1997. Multiple lentigines syndrome (LEOPARD syndrome or progressive cardiomyopathic lentiginosis). *J Med Genet* 34:582–6.

Crowe FW, Schull WJ, and Neel JV. 1956. *A Clinical, Pathological, and Genetic Study of Multiple Neurofibromatosis.* Springfield, Ill.: Charles C Thomas.

Curless RG, Siatkowski M, Glaser JS, and Shatz NJ. 1998. MRI diagnosis of NF-1 in children without café-au-lait skin lesions. *Pediatr Neurol* 18:269–71.

Daneman A, Mancer K, and Sonley M. 1983. CT appearance of thickened nerves in neurofibromatosis. *AJR Am J Roentgenol* 141:899–900.

DiMario FJ and Ramsby G. 1998. Magnetic resonance imaging lesion analysis in neurofibromatosis type 1. *Arch Neurol* 55:500–5.

DiMario FJ, Ramsby G, Greenstein R, Langshur S, and Dunham B. 1993. Neurofibromatosis type 1: magnetic resonance imaging findings. *J Child Neurol* 8:32–9.

Drouin V, Marret S, Petitcolas J, Eurin D, Vannier JP, Fessard C, and Tron P. 1997. Prenatal ultrasound abnormalities in a patient with generalized neurofibromatosis type 1. *Neuropediatrics* 28:120–1.

Duffner PK, Cohen ME, Seidel FG, and Shucard DW. 1989. The significance of MRI abnormalities in children with neurofibromatosis. *Neurology* 39:373–8.

Edman Ahlbom B, Dahl N, Zetterqvist P, and Annerén G. 1995. Noonan syndrome with café-au-lait spots and multiple lentigines syndrome are not linked to the neurofibromatosis type 1 locus. *Clin Genet* 48:85–9.

Edwards JH. 1989. Familiarity, recessivity and germline mosaicism. *Ann Hum Genet* 53:33–47.

Elyakim S, Lerer I, Zlotogora J, Sagi M, Gelman-Kohan Z, Merin S, and Abeliovich D. 1994. Neurofibromatosis type I (NFI) in Israeli families: linkage analysis as a diagnostic tool. *Am J Med Genet* 53:325–34.

Fairbank J. 1994. Orthopedic manifestations of neurofibromatosis. In: Huson SM and Hughes RAC, eds. *The Neurofibromatoses: A Pathogenic and Clinical Overview.* London: Chapman & Hall, pp. 275–304.

Fayad MN, Yacoub A, Salman S, Khudr A, and Der Kaloustian VM. 1987. Juvenile hyaline fibromatosis: two new patients and review of the literature. *Am J Med Genet* 26:123–31.

Ferner RE, Chaudhuri R, Bingham J, Cox T, and Hughes RAC. 1993. MRI in neurofibromatosis 1: the nature and evolution of increased intensity T2 weighted lesions and their relationship to intellectual impairment. *J Neurol Neurosurg Psychiatry* 56:492–5.

Fois A, Calistri L, Balestri P, Vivarelli R, Bartalini G, Mancini L, Berardi A, and Vanni M. 1993. Relationship between café-au-lait spots as the only symptom and peripheral neurofibromatosis (NF1): a followup study. *Eur J Pediatr* 152:500–4.

Friedman JM and Birch PH. 1997. Type 1 neurofibromatosis: a descriptive analysis of the disorder in 1,728 patients. *Am J Med Genet* 70:138–43.

Gabriel KR. 1996. Neurofibromatosis. *Curr Opin Pediatr* 9:89–93.

Glasier CM, Williamson MR, and Lange TA. 1989. MRI of peripheral neurofibromas in children. *Orthopedics* 12:269–72.

Goldberg Y, Dibbern K, Klein J, Riccardi VM, and Graham JM. 1996. Neurofibromatosis type 1: an update and review for the primary pediatrician. *Clin Pediatr (Phila)* 35:545–61.

Goldstein SM, Curless RG, Donovan Post MJ, and Quencer RM. 1989. A new sign of neurofibromatosis on magnetic resonance imaging of children. *Arch Neurol* 46:1222–4.

Gorlin RJ, Cohen MM Jr, Condon LM, and Burke BA. 1992. Bannayan-Riley-Ruvalcaba syndrome. *Am J Med Genet* 44:307–14.

Gorlin RJ and Koutlas IG. 1998. Multiple schwannomas, multiple nevi, and multiple vaginal leiomyomas: a new dominant syndrome. *Am J Med Genet* 78:76–81.

Gower DJ, Pollay M, Shuman RM, and Brumback RA. 1990. Cystic optic glioma. *Neurosurgery* 26:133–7.

Gutmann DH, Aylsworth A, Carey JC, Korf B, Marks J, Pyeritz RE, Rubenstein A, and Viskochil D. 1997. The diagnostic evaluation and multidisciplinary management of neurofibromatosis 1 and neurofibromatosis 2. *JAMA* 278:51–7.

Hager CM, Cohen PR, and Tschen JA. 1997. Segmental neurofibromatosis: case reports and review. *J Am Acad Dermatol* 37:864–9.

Hall JG. 1981. Possible maternal and hormonal factors in neurofibromatosis. *Adv Neurol* 29:125–31.

Heim RA, Kam-Morgan LNW, Binnie CG, Corns DD, Cayouette MC, Farber RA, Aylsworth AS, Silverman LM, and Luce MC. 1995. Distribution of 13 truncating mutations in the neurofibromatosis 1 gene. *Hum Mol Genet* 4:975–81.

Heim RA, Silverman LM, Farber RA, Kam-Morgan LNW, and Luce MC. 1994. Screening for truncated NF1 proteins. *Nat Genet* 8:218–9.

Hofman KJ and Boehm CD. 1992. Familial neurofibromatosis type 1: clinical experience with DNA testing. *J Pediatr* 120:394–8.

Hofstra RMW, Landsvater RM, Ceccherini I, Stulp RP, Stelwagen T, Luo Y, Pasini B, Höppener JWM, Ploos van Amstel HK, Romeo G, Lips CJM, and Buys CHCM. 1994. A mutation in the *RET* protoconcogene associated with multiple endocrine neoplasia type 2B and sporadic medullary thyroid carcinoma. *Nature* 367:375–6.

Holt JF. 1978. Neurofibromatosis in children. *AJR Am J Roentgenol* 130:615–39.

Hughes RAC. 1994. Neurological complications of neurofibromatosis 1. In: Huson SM and Hughes RAC, eds. *The Neurofibromatoses: A Pathogenic and Clinical Overview.* London: Chapman & Hall, pp. 204–32.

Huson SM. 1994. Neurofibromatosis 1: a clinical and genetic overview. In: Huson SM and Hughes RAC, eds. *The Neurofibromatoses: A Pathogenic and Clinical Overview.* London: Chapman & Hall, pp. 160–203.

Huson SM, Compston DAS, Clark P, and Harper PS. 1989a. A genetic study of von Recklinghausen neurofibromatosis in south east Wales. I. Prevalence, fitness, mutation rate, and effect of parental transmission on severity. *J Med Genet* 26:704–11.

Huson SM, Compston DAS, and Harper PS. 1989b. A genetic study of von Recklinghausen neurofibromatosis in south east Wales. II. Guidelines for genetic counselling. *J Med Genet* 26:712–21.

Huson S, Jones D, and Beck L. 1987. Ophthalmologic manifestations of neurofibromatosis. *Br J Ophthalmol* 71:235–8.

Huson SM and Upadhyaya M. 1994. Neurofibromatosis 1: clinical management and genetic counselling. In: Huson SM and Hughes RAC, eds. *The Neurofibromatoses: A Pathogenic and Clinical Overview.* London: Chapman & Hall, pp. 355–81.

Inoue Y, Nemoto Y, Tashiro T, Nakayama K, Nakayama T, and Daikokuya H. 1997. Neurofibromatosis type 1 and type 2: review of the central nervous system and related structures. *Brain Dev* 19:1–12.

Kayes LM, Burke W, Riccardi VM, Bennett R, Ehrlich P, Rubenstein A, and Stephens K. 1994. Deletions spanning the neurofibromatosis I gene: Identification and phenotype of five patients. *Am J Hum Genet* 54:424–36.

Kayes LM, Riccardi VM, Burke W, Bennett RL, and Stephens K. 1992. Large de novo DNA deletion in a patient with sporadic neurofibromatosis 1, mental retardation, and dysmorphism. *J Med Genet* 29:686–90.

Korf BF. 1992. Diagnostic outcome in children with multiple café-au-lait spots. *Pediatrics* 90:924–7.

Kuenzle C, Weissert M, Roulet E, Bode H, Schefer S, Huisman T, Landau K, and Boltshauser E. 1994. Follow-up of optic pathway gliomas in children with neurofibromatosis type 1. *Neuropediatrics* 25:295–300.

Lazaro C, Gaona A, Ravella A, Volpini V, and Estivill X. 1995. Prenatal diagnosis of neurofibromatosis type 1: from flanking RFLPs to intragenic microsatellite markers. *Prenat Diagn* 15:129–34.

Lazaro C, Ravella A, Casals C, Volpini V, and Estivill X. 1992. Prenatal diagnosis of sporadic neruofibromatosis 1. *Lancet* 339:119–20.

Leppig KA, Kaplan P, Viskochil D, Weaver M, Ortenberg J, and Stephens K. 1997. Familial neurofibromatosis 1 microdeletions: cosegregation with distinct facial phenotype and early onset of cutaneous neurofibromata. *Am J Med Genet* 73:197–204.

Leppig KA, Viskochil D, Neil S, Rubenstein A, Johnson VP, Zhu XL, Brothman AR, and Stephens K. 1996. The detection of contiguous gene deletions at the neurofibromatosis 1 locus with fluorescence in situ hybridization. *Cytogenet Cell Genet* 72:95–8.

Listernick R, Charrow J, Greenwald MJ, and Esterly NB. 1989. Optic gliomas in children with neurofibromatosis type 1. *J Pediatr* 114:788–92.

Listernick R, Charrow J, Greenwald M, and Mets M. 1994. Natural history of optic pathway tumors in children with neurofibromatosis type 1: a longitudinal study. J Pediatr 125:63–6.

Listernick R, Darling C, Greenwald M, Strauss L, and Charrow J. 1995. Optic pathway tumors in children: the effect of neurofibromatosis type 1 on clinical manifestations and natural history. *J Pediatr* 127:718–22.

Listernick R, Louis DN, Packer RJ, and Gutmann DH. 1997. Optic pathway gliomas in children with neurofibromatosis 1: consensus statement from the NF1 Optic Pathway Glioma Task Force. *Ann Neurol* 41:143–9.

Lubs M-LE, Bauer MS, Formas ME, and Djokic B. 1991. Lisch nodules in neurofibromatosis type 1. *N Engl J Med* 324:1264–6.

Lund AM and Skovby F. 1991. Optic gliomas in children with neurofibromatosis type 1. *Eur J Pediatr* 150:835–8.

Lycka B, Krywonis N, and Hordinsky M. 1991. Abnormal nevoblast migration mimicking neurofibromatosis. *Arch Dermatol* 127:1702–4.

Marsh DJ, Dahia PLM, Zheng Z, Liaw D, Parsons R, Gorlin RJ, and Eng C. 1997. Germline mutations of *PTEN* are present in Bannayan-Zonana syndrome. *Nat Genet* 16:333–4.

Martuza RL and Ojemann RG. 1982. Bilateral acoustic neuromas: clinical aspects, pathogenesis, and treatment. *Neurosurgery* 10:1–12.

Massry GG, Morgan CF, and Chung SM. 1997. Evidence of optic pathway gliomas after previously negative neuroimaging. *Ophthalmology* 104:930–5.

Matsuki K, Kakitsubata Y, Watanabe K, Tsukino H, and Nakajima K. 1997. Mesenteric plexiform neurofibroma associated with Recklinghausen's disease. *Pediatr Radiol* 27:255–6.

Mauras N and Blizzard RM. 1986. The McCune-Albright syndrome. *Acta Endocrinol Suppl* 279:207–17.

McCarron KF and Goldblum JR. 1998. Plexiform neurofibroma with and without associated malignant peripheral nerve sheath tumor: a clinicopathologic and immunohistochemical analysis of 54 cases. *Mod Pathol* 11:612–7.

Michels VV, Whisant JP, Garrity JA, and Miller GM. 1989. Neurofibromatosis type 1 with bilateral acoustic neuromas. *Neurofibromatosis* 2:213–7.

Miller M and Hall JG. 1978. Possible maternal effect on severity of neurofibromatosis. *Lancet* 2:1071–3.

Miller RM and Sparkes RS. 1977. Segmental neurofibromatosis. *Arch Dermatol* 113:837–8.

Morrison PJ and Nevin NC. 1996. Multiple endocrine neoplasia type 2B (mucosal neuroma syndrome, Wagenmann-Froboese syndrome). *J Med Genet* 33:779–82.

Moss C and Green SH. 1994. What is segmental neurofibromatosis? *Br J Dermatol* 130:106–10.

National Institutes of Health Consensus Development Conference. 1988. Neurofibromatosis: conference statement. *Arch Neurol* 45:575–8.

Nguyen BD. 1997. Tc-99m DTPA delayed SPECT imaging of neurofibromatosis. *Clin Nucl Med* 22:132.

Nicholls EM. 1969. Somatic variation and multiple neurofibromatosis. *Hum Hered* 19:473–9.

Niimura M. 1990. Neurofibromatosis in Japan. In: Ishibashi Y, and Hori Y, eds. *Tuberous Sclerosis and Neurofibromatosis: Epidemiology, Pathophysiology, Biology, and Management.* Amsterdam: Elsevier, pp. 23–31.

North K. 1993. Neurofibromatosis type 1: review of the first 200 patients in an Australian clinic. *J Child Neurol* 8:395–402.

North K, Cochineas C, Tang E, and Fagan E. 1994. Optic gliomas in neurofibromatosis type 1: role of visual evoked potentials. *Pediatr Neurol* 10:117–23.

North KN, Riccardi V, Samango-Sprouse C, Ferner R, Moore B, Legius E, Ratner N, and Denckla MB. 1997. Cognitive function and academic performance in neurofibromatosis 1: consensus statement from the NF1 Cognitive Disorders Task Force. *Neurology* 48:1121–7.

Obringer AC, Meadows AT, and Zackai EH. 1989. The diagnosis of neurofibromatosis-1 in the child under the age of 6 years. *Am J Dis Child* 143:717–9.

O'Connor WJ. 1997. Screening in neurofibromatosis type 1. *Arch Dermatol* 133:655–6.

Parry DM, Eldridge R, Kaiser-Kupfer MI, Bouzas EA, Pikus A, and Patronas N. 1994. Neurofibromatosis 2 (NF2): clinical characteristics of 63 affected individuals and clinical evidence for heterogeneity. *Am J Med Genet* 52:450–61.

Pivnick EK, Lobe TE, Fitch SJ, and Riccardi VM. 1997. Hair whorl as an indicator of a mediastinal plexiform neurofibroma. *Pediatr Dermatol* 14:196–8.

Pollack IF, Shultz B, and Mulvihill JJ. 1996. The management of brainstem gliomas in patients with neurofibromatosis 1. *Neurology* 46:1652–60.

Purvin VA and Dunn DW. 1994. Ophthalmological manifestations of neurofibromatosis 1 and 2. In: Huson SM and Hughes RAC, eds. *The Neurofibromatoses: A Pathogenic and Clinical Overview.* London: Chapman & Hall, pp. 253–74.

Rabbiosi G, Borroni G, and Scuderi N. 1977. Familial multiple lipomatosis. *Acta Derm Venerol* 57:265–7.

Ragge NK, Falk RE, Cohen WE, and Murphree AL. 1993. Images of Lisch nodules across the spectrum. *Eye* 7:95–101.

Raue F, Frank-Raue K, and Grauer A. 1994. Multiple endocrine neoplasia type 2: clinical features and screening. *Endocrinol Metabol Clin North Am* 23:137–56.

Reith JD and Goldblum JR. 1996. Multiple cutaneous plexiform schwannomas: report of a case and review of the literature with particular reference to the association with types 1 and 2 neurofibromatosis and schwannomatosis. *Arch Pathol Lab Med* 120:399–401.

Riccardi VM. 1980. Pathophysiology of neurofibromatosis. IV. Dermatologic insights into heterogeneity and pathogenesis. *J Am Acad Dermatol* 3:157–66.

———. 1981. Von Recklinghausen neurofibromatosis. *N Engl J Med* 305:1617–27.

————. 1982. Neurofibromatosis: Clinical heterogeneity. *Curr Probl Cancer* 7(2):1–34.

————. 1991. Neurofibromatosis mimicry. *Arch Dermatol* 127:1714–5.

————. 1992. *Neurofibromatosis: Phenotype, Natural History, and Pathogenesis,* 2nd ed. Baltimore: Johns Hopkins University Press.

Riccardi VM and Eichner JE. 1986. *Neurofibromatosis: Phenotype, Natural History, and Pathogenesis.* Baltimore: Johns Hopkins University Press.

Riccardi VM and Wald JS. 1987. Discounting an adverse maternal effect on severity of neurofibromatosis. *Pediatrics* 79:386–93.

Riva P, Castorina P, Manoukian S, Dalprà L, Doneda L, Marini G, den Dunnen J, and Larizza L. 1996. Characterization of a cytogenetic 17q11.2 deletion in an NF1 patient with a contiguous gene syndrome. *Hum Genet* 98:646–50.

Rodenhiser DI, Ainsworth PJ, Coulter-Mackie MB, Singh SM, and Jung JH. 1993. A genetic study of neurofibromatosis type 1 (NF1) in south-western Ontario. II. A PCR based approach to molecular and prenatal diagnosis using linkage. *J Med Genet* 30:363–8.

Rodenhiser DI, Coulter-Mackie MB, Jung JH, and Singh SM. 1991. A genetic study of neurofibromatosis 1 in south-western Ontario. I. Population, familial segregation of phenotype, and molecular linkage. *J Med Genet* 28:746–51.

Rossi LN, Pastorino G, Scotti G, Gazocchi M, Maninetti MM, Zanolini C, and Chiodi A. 1994. Early diagnosis of optic glioma in children with neurofibromatosis type 1. *Child Nerv Syst* 10:426–9.

Rubenstein AE, Bader JL, Aron AA, and Wallace S. 1983. Familial transmission of segmental neurofibromatosis. *Neurology* 33 (Suppl 2):76.

Samuel M and Spitz L. 1995. Klippel-Trenaunay syndrome: clinical features, complications, and management in children. *Br J Surg* 82:757–61.

Schwindinger WF, Francomano CA, and Levine MA. 1992. Identification of a mutation in the gene encoding the subunit of the stimulatory G protein of adenyl cyclase in McCune-Albright syndrome. *Proc Natl Acad Sci USA* 89:5152–6.

Seashore MR, Cho S, Deposito F, Sherman J, Wappner RS, and Wilson MG. 1995. Health supervision for children with neurofibromatosis. *Pediatrics* 96:368–72.

Seppala R, Préfontaine M, and Mikhael NZ. 1997. Mesenteric small-bowel polyposis: a diagnostic radiographic sign of neurofibromatosis. *AJR Am J Roentgenol* 168:434–6.

Seward GR. 1994. Did the Elephant Man have neurofibromatosis 1? In: Huson SM and Hughes RAC, eds. *The Neurofibromatoses: A Pathogenic and Clinical Overview.* London: Chapman & Hall, pp. 382–401.

Shen MH, Harper PS, and Upadhyaya M. 1996. Molecular genetics of neurofibromatosis type 1 (NF1). *J Med Genet* 33:2–17.

Shu HH, Mirowitz SA, and Wippold FJ. 1993. Neurofibromatosis: MR imaging findings involving the head and spine. *AJR Am J Roentgenol* 160:159–64.

Spiegel R, Mächler M, Stocker HP, Boltshauser E, and Schmid W. 1991. Neurofibromatose Typ 1: Genetische Untersuchungen mit DNA-Markern bei 38 Familien. *Schweiz Med Wochenschr* 121:1445–52.

Spira M and Riccardi V. 1987. Neurofibromatosis. *Clin Plastic Surg* 14:315–25.

Tonsgard JH, Kwak SM, Short MP, and Dachman AH. 1998. CT imaging in adults with neurofibromatosis-1: frequent asymptomatic plexiform lesions. *Neurology* 50:1755–60.

Tonsgard JH, Yalavarthi KK, Cushner S, Short MP, and Lindgren V. 1997. Do NF1 gene deletions result in a characteristic phenotype? *Am J Med Genet* 73:80–6.

Truhan AP and Filipek PA. 1993. Magnetic resonance imaging: its role in the neuroradiologic evaluation of neurofibromatosis, tuberous sclerosis, and Sturge-Weber syndrome. *Arch Dermatol* 129:219–26.

Upadhyaya M, Fryer A, MacMillan J, Broadhead W, Huson SM, and Harper PS. 1992. Prenatal diagnosis and presymptomatic detection of neurofibromatosis type 1. *J Med Genet* 29:180–3.

Upadhyaya M, Ruggieri M, Maynard J, Osborn M, Hartog C, Mudd S, Penttinen M, Cordeiro I, Ponder M, Ponder BAJ, Krawczak M, and Cooper DN. 1998. Gross deletions of the neurofibromatosis type 1 (*NF1*) gene are predominantly of maternal origin and commonly associated with a learning disability, dysmorphic features and developmental delay. *Hum Genet* 102:591–7.

Upadhyaya M, Shaw DJ, and Harper PS. 1994. Molecular basis of neurofibromatosis type 1 (NF1): mutation analysis and polymorphisms in the NF1 gene. *Hum Mutat* 4:83–101.

Valero MC, Pascual-Castroviejo I, Velasco E, Moreno F, and Hernádez-Chico C. 1997. Identification of de novo deletions at the NF1 gene: no preferential paternal origin and phenotypic analysis of patients. *Hum Genet* 99:720–6.

Van Es S, North KN, McHugh K, and De Silva M. 1996. MRI findings in children with neurofibromatosis type 1: a prospective study. *Pediatr Radiol* 26:478–87.

Viljoen DL. 1988. Klippel-Trenaunay-Weber syndrome (angio-osteohypertophy syndrome). *J Med Genet* 25:250–2.

Viskochil D, Buchberg AM, Xu G, Cawthon RM, Stevens J, Wolff RK, Culver M, Carey JC, Copeland NG, Jenkins NA, White R, and O'Connell P. 1990. Deletions and a translocation interrupt a cloned gene at the neurofibromatosis type 1 locus. *Cell* 62:187–92.

Vivarelli R, Bartalani G, Berardi A, Calistri L, Balestri P, and Fois A. 1993. Diagnosis of neurofibromatosis type 1 using RFLPs tightly linked to the gene. *Child Nerv Syst* 9:147–9.

Vivarelli R, Bartalini G, Calistri L, Balestri P, Figus A, Pirastu MJ, Cao A, and Fois A. 1991. Molecular study in von Recklinghausen neurofibromatosis (NF1). *Child Nerv Syst* 7:98–9.

von Recklinghausen F. 1882. *Ueber die multiplen Fibrome der Haut und ihre Beziehungen zu den multiplen Neuromen*. Berlin: August Hirschwald.

Wallace MR, Marchuk DA, Andersen LB, Letcher R, Odeh HM, Saulino AM, Fountain JW, Brereton A, Nicholson J, Mitchell AL, Brownstein BH, and Collins FS. 1990. Type 1 neurofibromatosis gene: identification of a large transcript disrupted in three NF1 patients. *Science* 249:181–6.

Ward K, O'Connell PO, Carey JC, Leppert M, Jolley S, Plaetke R, Ogden B, and White R. 1990. Diagnosis of neurofibromatosis I by using tightly-linked flanking DNA markers. *Am J Hum Genet* 46:943–9.

Weinstein LS, Shenker A, Gejman PV, Merino MJ, Friedman E, and Spiegel AM. 1991. Activating mutations of the stimulatory G protein in the McCune-Albright syndrome. *N Engl J Med* 325:1688–95.

Whitehouse D. 1966. Diagnostic value of the café-au-lait spot in children. *Arch Dis Child* 41:316–9.

Wolkenstein P, Frèche B, Zeller J, and Revuz J. 1996. Usefulness of screening investigations in neurofibromatosis type 1: a study of 152 patients. *Arch Dermatol* 132:1333–6.

Wu B-L, Austin MA, Schneider GH, Boles RG, and Korf BR. 1995. Deletion of the entire *NF1* gene detected by FISH: four deletion patients associated with severe manifestations. *Am J Med Genet* 59:528–35.

Wu B-L, Boles RG, Yaari H, Weremowicz S, Schneider GH, and Korf BR. 1997a. Somatic mosaicism for deletion of the entire *NF1* gene identified by FISH. *Hum Genet* 99:209–13.

Wu B-L, Schneider GH, and Korf BR. 1997b. Deletion of the entire *NF1* gene causing distinct manifestations in a family. *Am J Med Genet* 69:98–101.

4

Clinical Genetics

J. M. Friedman, M.D., Ph.D.

The *NF1* gene was identified and sequenced in 1990 (Cawthon et al. 1990; Viskochil et al. 1990; Wallace et al. 1990). There is no evidence of locus heterogeneity; all patients with typical NF1 appear to have mutations at this locus (Collins et al. 1989; Marchuk and Collins 1994; Riccardi 1993; Ward et al. 1990). The structure of the *NF1* locus, the nature of mutations that have been identified, and our knowledge of their functional consequences are discussed in Chapter 5.

NF1 is transmitted as an autosomal dominant disease; affected individuals are heterozygotes for an *NF1* mutation. No convincing example of homozygous NF1 has been reported, despite the relatively high frequency of the disease (Clementi et al. 1990; Huson 1994; Huson et al. 1989; Littler and Morton 1990; Samuelsson and Samuelsson 1989) and known instances of consanguinity in families in which NF1 is segregating (Pericak-Vance et al. 1987; Vance et al. 1989). The fact that homozygosity for mutations of the murine homologue of *NF1* is lethal to embryos (Brannan et al. 1994; Jacks et al. 1994) suggests that at least one functional *NF1* allele is essential for life in humans as well.

PENETRANCE

The penetrance of pathogenic *NF1* mutations is complete or very nearly so. In five clinical studies involving about 200 multigenerational families with NF1, no instance of nonpenetrance was observed among obligate carriers (Crowe et al. 1956; Huson et al. 1989; Riccardi 1992; Riccardi and Lewis 1988; Samuelsson and Åkesson 1989; Sergeyev 1975). A few cases of apparent nonpenetrance of NF1 have been reported (Carey et al. 1979; Spence et al. 1983), but none has been documented with mutation analysis, linkage, or clinical evaluation using the NIH diagnostic criteria. The interpretation of these cases therefore remains uncertain.

In rare instances, germinal mosaicism for an *NF1* mutation may produce nonpenetrance. Germline mosaicism has been demonstrated in an individual who has no clinical features of NF1 but had two affected children (Lázaro et al. 1994, 1995). Germline mosaicism probably accounts for other families in which affected sibs or half-sibs have NF1, but the parents are either unaffected (Berry et al. 1984; Riccardi and Lewis 1988) or have manifestations that are too mild to permit a diagnosis of NF1 (Riccardi and Lewis 1988). Germline mosaicism among individuals who do not exhibit clinical features of NF1 must be rare because the empiric recurrence risk is extremely small in other children of unaffected parents who have had a child with NF1 (Huson 1994; Huson et al. 1989; Riccardi 1981, 1992). One would expect a risk as great as 50% in the children of unaffected parents who have germline mosaicism (Edwards 1989).

Complete or nearly complete penetrance of NF1 implies that if a child with unequivocal NF1 is born to unaffected parents, the child probably represents a new mutation, and the recurrence risk for NF1 in the parents' subsequent children is very small. However, NF1 exhibits considerable clinical variability even within a family (see Chapter 2), and a parent with NF1 may be more mildly affected than his or her child. Both parents must undergo complete clinical and ophthalmologic examination before it can be concluded that they are, in fact, unaffected.

NEW MUTATIONS

A positive family is present in about half of all NF1 cases (Brasfield and Das Gupta 1972; Carey et al. 1979; Clementi et al. 1990; Crowe et al. 1956; Huson et al. 1989; Littler and Morton 1990; North 1993; Poyhonen et al. 1997; Riccardi 1992; Samuelsson and Åkesson 1989; Takano et al. 1992). If one assumes that penetrance is complete, this means that about half of all patients with NF1 represent new mutations. Given the frequency of NF1, this represents one of the highest single-locus mutation rates known in humans. Actual estimates of new mutation rates for the *NF1* locus vary from about 1 in 7800 to 1 in 23,000 gametes (Clementi et al. 1990; Crowe et al. 1956; Huson et al. 1989; Littler and Morton 1990; Samuelsson and Åkesson 1989; Sergeyev 1975; Takano et al. 1992). This range probably reflects differences in diagnosis, ascertainment, and identification of sporadic cases as well as statistical fluctuations and differences in the method used to calculate the mutation rate.

Some new *NF1* mutations have been demonstrated by showing the presence of a pathogenic mutation in an affected child and the absence of this mutation in both unaffected parents (Kayes et al. 1992, 1994; Wallace et al. 1990). As discussed in Chapter 5, a variety of mechanisms cause mutations of the *NF1* locus. Point mutations, large and small deletions, duplications, and gross chromosomal rearrangements, as well as mutations that affect the promoter, enhancers, or splicing have been reported (Shen et al. 1996; Upadhyaya et al. 1994).

The reason for the high mutation rate at the *NF1* locus is not understood. The large size of the *NF1* gene does not appear to be a sufficient explanation (Rodenhiser et al. 1997; Upadhyaya et al. 1994), although this may be one contributing factor. Although most mutations described are unique to a single family, some alterations have been observed repeatedly in unrelated families. The most commonly reported mutation is C5839T, a transition that involves a single CpG site in exon 31 (Shen et al. 1996). Methylated CpG dinucleotides generally show a high mutation rate because of the tendency of 5-methylcytosine to undergo spontaneous deamination to thiamine (Coulondre et al. 1978), but only a small fraction of *NF1* mutations occur at CpG sites (Rodenhiser et al. 1997; Shen et al. 1996). Some deletions and insertions in the *NF1* locus occur within pallindromes, symmetrical elements, or runs of repeated sequences—motifs that have been associated with preferential occurrence of insertions and deletions in other genes (Cooper and Krawczak 1991; Krawczak and Cooper 1991; Rodenhiser et al. 1997). Pathogenic substitutions in the *NF1* gene are often associated with homonucleotide repeats or methylatable CpG dinucleotides (Rodenhiser et al. 1997). Loci with substantial sequence similarity to *NF1* exist on chromosomes 2, 12, 14, 15, 18, 20, 21 and 22 (Gasparini et al. 1993; Legius et al. 1992; Purandare et al. 1995). Gene conversion events may cause some mutations by transfer of a nonfunctional DNA segment from such nonhomologous loci into the *NF1* locus (Purandare et al. 1995; Shen et al. 1996; Upadhyaya et al. 1994). These mechanisms are not mutually exclusive. More than one of them may contribute to the unusually high mutation rate at the *NF1* locus.

It is possible that mutation of the *NF1* locus in a germ-cell precursor provides a proliferative advantage to that cell and its progeny (Rodenhiser et al. 1997). Such an effect would produce germline mosaicism that would increase the likelihood of a given mutation being transmitted to a child. This would increase the apparent (but not the actual) mutation rate for the *NF1* locus. Germline mosaicism has been demonstrated in one individual who has no clinical features of NF1 but who had two affected children (Lázaro et al. 1994, 1995) and is thought to explain several other families in which more than one child with NF1 has been born to unaffected parents (Berry et al. 1984; Riccardi and Lewis 1988).

PARENT OF ORIGIN OF NEW MUTATIONS

More than 80% of new *NF1* mutations are of paternal origin (Elyakim et al. 1994; Jadayel et al. 1990; Lázaro et al. 1996; Spiegel et al. 1991; Stephens et al. 1992; Upadhyaya et al. 1994), but "large" submicroscopic deletions of the *NF1* gene, which account for no more than 5% of all *NF1* mutations, are an exception (Ainsworth et al. 1997; Kayes et al. 1992, 1994; Lázaro et al. 1996; Leppig et al. 1996, 1997; Tonsgard et al. 1997; Upadhyaya et al. 1998; Valero et al. 1997; Wu et al. 1995, 1997). A predominance of paternally derived germline mutations has also been observed for several other genetic diseases that result from diverse mutational mechanisms (Carlson et al. 1994; Dryja et al. 1997; Goldberg et al. 1993; Kato et al. 1994; Kling et al. 1992; Moloney et al. 1996; Palau et al. 1993; Wirth et al. 1997). The predominance of paternal mutations in NF1 is, therefore, unlikely to provide an important clue to the cause of the high mutation rate at the *NF1* locus.

Given the predominance of paternal mutations at the *NF1* locus, one might expect the risk of having a child with sporadic NF1 to increase with paternal age.

Both premeiotic mitosis of spermatogonia and meiosis continue throughout adult life in males, providing a continuing target for mutagens (Crow 1997). However, data regarding a paternal age effect in NF1 are inconsistent (Borberg 1951; Bunin et al. 1997; Clementi et al. 1990; Huson et al. 1989; North 1993; Riccardi et al. 1984; Samuelsson and Åkesson 1989; Sergeyev 1975; Takano et al. 1992). All of the available studies are compromised by at least some of the following problems: uncertainty about the comparability of case and control groups, incomplete ascertainment of NF1 cases, lack of unequivocal demonstration that all cases actually represent new mutations, and small sample size. The largest study of the paternal age effect to date is that of Riccardi et al. (1984), which included 187 patients with NF1 born to apparently unaffected parents. A small but statistically significant increase in the age of the fathers of the cases was observed when compared to the expected paternal age calculated from national averages and weighted by each proband's year of birth. A significant effect was also seen using other methods of analysis that controlled for maternal age. If a paternal age effect does exist for *NF1* mutations, it must be modest.

FITNESS

The fitness of a particular genotype is expressed as a ratio of the reproductive performance of individuals with that genotype to the reproductive performance of the optimal genotype. In NF1, the average number of children produced by affected heterozygotes would be compared to the average number of children produced by people who do not have the disease. When calculated in this manner, fitness can range from 0 to 1. A fitness of 0 means that affected individuals never have children who survive to reproduce; a fitness of 1 means that the reproductive performance of affected individuals is as good as that of unaffected individuals. Crowe et al. (1956) estimated the fitness of patients with NF1 to be 0.53 (i.e., about half of normal). Similar figures (0.47 and 0.54, respectively) were obtained by Huson and associates (1989) and by Takano et al. (1992). Both Crowe et al. and Huson et al. found the fitness to be reduced much more for affected men than for affected women.

Fitness is a function of all factors that affect the ability of a person to have children. Reduced fitness means that people with NF1 have fewer children, on average, than other people. Reduced fitness could occur if individuals who carry a pathogenic *NF1* mutation were more often infertile or subfertile, if NF1 embryos were more often miscarried, if stillbirth were more common in NF1 fetuses, if children with NF1 often died before reaching reproductive maturity, or if adults with NF1 were less likely to have children for medical or social reasons. These possibilities are not mutually exclusive, and several of them may play some role in the reduced fitness of patients with NF1.

Few data are available to assess these various possibilities. Several studies have found that 50% of the children of an affected parent have NF1 (Brasfield and Das Gupta 1972; Clementi et al. 1990; Crow et al. 1956; Huson et al. 1989; Littler and Morton 1990; North 1993; Riccardi 1992; Samuelsson and Åkesson

1989; Sergeyev 1975). If excessive loss of offspring who carry an *NF1* mutation occurred prenatally or in early childhood, fewer children with NF1 than unaffected children would be expected. Riccardi and Eichner (1986) found that the mean number of children of patients with NF1 did not differ significantly from the mean number of children of unaffected sibs, but this analysis was based on a small sample. The average life-span of people with NF1 is reduced by at least 10 to 15 years, but most of the excess mortality occurs after the age at which most people have children (Poyhonen et al. 1997; Samuelsson and Samuelsson 1989; Zöller et al. 1995; see Chapter 2). Crowe et al. (1956) found that about half of the reduced fitness observed among patients with NF1 could be attributed to their lower rates of marriage. This effect was more marked in males than in females.

If the frequency of NF1 remains constant from generation to generation, the loss of mutant *NF1* alleles as a result of reduced fitness must be balanced by the gain of new mutant alleles from some other source. New mutations are the source of these new mutant alleles in a population at genetic equilibrium. This balance between mutation and reduced fitness explains why such a large proportion of NF1 cases result from new mutations.

REFERENCES

Ainsworth PJ, Charkraborty PK, and Weksberg R. 1997. Example of somatic mosaicism in a series of de novo neurofibromatosis type 1 cases due to a maternally derived deletion. *Hum Mutat* 9:452–7.

Berry SA, King RA, Whitley CB, Riccardi VM, and Pierpont MEM. 1984. Familial neurofibromatosis resulting from a probable germinal mutation. *Am J Hum Genet* 36:44s.

Borberg A. 1951. Clinical and genetic investigations into tuberous sclerosis and Recklinghausen's neurofibromatosis: contribution to elucidation of interrelationship and eugenics of the syndromes. *Acta Psychiatr Neurol Scand Suppl* 71:1–239.

Brannan CI, Perkins AS, Vogel KS, Ratner N, Norlund ML, Reid SW, Buchberg AM, Jenkins NA, Parada LF, and Copeland NG. 1994. Targeted disruption of the neurofibromatosis type-1 gene leads to developmental abnormalities in heart and various neural crest-derived tissues. *Genes Dev* 8:1019–29.

Brasfield RD and Das Gupta TK. 1972. von Recklinghausen's disease: a clinicopathological study. *Ann Surg* 175:86–104.

Bunin GR, Needle M, and Riccardi VM. 1997. Paternal age and sporadic neurofibromatosis 1: a case-control study and consideration of methodologic issues. *Genet Epidemiol* 14:507–16.

Carey JC, Laub JM, and Hall BD. 1979. Penetrance and variability in neurofibromatosis: a genetic study of 60 families. *Birth Defects* 15(5B):271–81.

Carlson KM, Bracamontes J, Jackson CE, Clark R, Lacroix A, Wells SA, and Goodfellow PJ. 1994. Parent-of-origin effects in multiple endocrine neoplasia type 2B. *Am J Hum Genet* 55:1076–82.

Cawthon RM, Weiss R, Xu G, Viskochil D, Culver M, Stevens J, Robertson M, Dunn D, Gesteland R, O'Connell P, and White R. 1990. A major segment of the neurofibrmatosis type 1 gene: cDNA sequence, genomic structure, and point mutations. *Cell* 62:193–201.

Clementi M, Barbujani G, Turolla L, and Tenconi R. 1990. Neurofibromatosis-1: a maximum likelihood estimation of mutation rate. *Hum Genet* 84:116–8.

Collins FS, O'Connell P, Ponder BAJ, and Seizinger BR. 1989. Progress towards identifying the neurofibromatosis (NF1) gene. *Trends Genet* 5:217–21.

Cooper DN and Krawczak M. 1991. Mechanisms of insertional mutagenesis in human genes causing genetic disease. *Hum Genet* 87:409–15.

Coulondre C, Miller JH, Farabaugh PJ, and Gilbert W. 1978. Molecular basis of base substitution hotspots in *Escherichia coli*. *Nature* 274:775–80.

Crow JF. 1997. The high spontaneous mutation rate: is it a health risk? *Proc Natl Acad Sci USA* 94:8380–6.

Crowe FW, Schull WJ, and Neel JV. 1956. *A Clinical, Pathological, and Genetic Study of Multiple Neurofibromatosis*. Springfield, Ill.: Charles C Thomas.

Dryja TP, Morrow JF, and Rapaport JM. 1997. Quantification of the paternal allele bias for new germline mutations in the retinoblastoma gene. *Hum Genet* 100:446–9.

Edwards JH. 1989. Familiarity, recessivity and germline mosaicism. *Ann Hum Genet* 53:33–47.

Elyakim S, Lerer I, Zlotogora J, Sagi M, Gelman-Kohan Z, Merin S, and Abeliovich D. 1994. Neurofibromatosis type I (NFI) in Israeli families: linkage analysis as a diagnostic tool. *Am J Med Genet* 53:325–34.

Gasparini P, Grifa A, Origone P, Coviello D, Antonacci R, and Rocchi M. 1993. Detection of a neurofibromatosis type I (NF1) homologous sequence by PCR: implications for the diagnosis and screening of genetic diseases. *Mol Cell Probes* 7:415–8.

Goldberg YP, Kremer B, Andrew SE, Theilmann J, Graham RK, Squitieri F, Telenius H, Adam S, Sajoo A, Starr E, Heiberg A, Wolff G, and Hayden MR. 1993. Molecular analysis of new mutations for Huntington's disease: intermediate alleles and sex of origin effects. *Nat Genet* 5:174–9.

Huson SM. 1994. Neurofibromatosis 1: a clinical and genetic overview. In: Huson SM and Hughes RAC, eds. *The Neurofibromatoses: A Pathogenic and Clinical Overview*. London: Chapman & Hall, pp. 160–203.

Huson SM, Compston DAS, Clark P, and Harper PS. 1989. A genetic study of von Recklinghausen neurofibromatosis in south east Wales. I. Prevalence, fitness, mutation rate, and effect of parental transmission on severity. *J Med Genet* 26:704–11.

Jacks T, Shih TS, Schmitt EM, Bronson RT, Bernards A, and Weinberg RA. 1994. Tumour predisposition in mice heterozygous for targeted mutation of *NF1*. *Nat Genet* 7:353–61.

Jadayel D, Fain P, Upadhyaya M, Ponder MA, Huson SM, Carey J, Fryer A, Mathew CGP, Barker DF, and Ponder BAJ. 1990. Paternal origin of new mutations in von Recklinghausen neurofibromatosis. *Nature* 343:558–9.

Kato MV, Ishizaki K, Shimizu T, Ejima Y, Tanooka H, Takayama J, Kaneko A, Toguchida J, and Sasaki MS. 1994. Parental origin of germ-line and somatic mutations in the retinoblastoma gene. *Hum Genet* 94:31–8.

Kayes LM, Burke W, Riccardi VM, Bennett R, Ehrlich P, Rubenstein A, and Stephens K. 1994. Deletions spanning the neurofibromatosis I gene: Identification and phenotype of five patients. *Am J Hum Genet* 54:424–36.

Kayes LM, Riccardi VM, Burke W, Bennett RL, and Stephens K. 1992. Large de novo DNA deletion in a patient with sporadic neurofibromatosis 1, mental retardation, and dysmorphism. *J Med Genet* 29:686–90.

Kling S, Ljung R, Sjörin E, Montandon J, Green P, Giannelli F, and Nilsson IM. 1992. Origin of mutation in sporadic cases of haemophilia-B. *Eur J Haematol* 48:142–5.

Krawczak M and Cooper DN. 1991. Gene deletions causing human genetic disease: mechanisms of mutagenesis and the role of the local DNA sequence environment. *Hum Genet* 86:425–44.

Lázaro C, Gaona A, Lynch M, Kruyer H, Ravella A, and Estivill X. 1995. Molecular characterization of the breakpoints of a 12-kb deletion in the NF1 gene in a family showing germ-line mosaicism. *Am J Hum Genet* 57:1044–9.

Lázaro C, Gaona A, Ainsworth P, Tenconi R, Vidaud D, Kruyer H, Ars E, Volpini V, and Estivill X. 1996. Sex differences in mutational rate and mutational mechanism in the *NF1* gene in neurofibromatosis type 1 patients. *Hum Genet* 98:696–9.

Lázaro C, Ravella A, Gaona A, Volpini V, and Estivill X. 1994. Neurofibromatosis type 1 due to germ-line mosaicism in a clinically normal father. *N Engl J Med* 331:1403–7.

Legius E, Marchuk DA, Hall BK, Andersen LB, Wallace MR, Collins FS, and Glover TW. 1992. *NF-1* related locus on chromosome 15. *Genomics* 13:1316–8.

Leppig KA, Kaplan P, Viskochil D, Weaver M, Ortenberg J, and Stephens K. 1997. Familial neurofibromatosis 1 microdeletions: cosegregation with distinct facial phenotype and early onset of cutaneous neurofibromata. *Am J Med Genet* 73:197–204.

Leppig KA, Viskochil D, Neil S, Rubenstein A, Johnson VP, Zhu XL, Brothman AR, and Stephens K. 1996. The detection of contiguous gene deletions at the neurofibromatosis 1 locus with fluorescence in situ hybridization. *Cytogenet Cell Genet* 72:95–8.

Littler M and Morton NE. 1990. Segregation analysis of peripheral neurofibromatosis. *J Med Genet* 27:307–10.

Marchuk DA and Collins FS. 1994. Molecular genetics of neurofibromatosis 1. In: Huson SM and Hughes RAC, eds. *The Neurofibromatoses: A Pathogenic and Clinical Overview*. London: Chapman & Hall, pp. 22–49.

Moloney DM, Slaney SF, Oldridge M, Wall SA, Sahlin P, Stenman G, and Wilkie AOM. 1996. Exclusive paternal origin of new mutations in Apert syndrome. *Nat Genet* 13:48–53.

North K. 1993. Neurofibromatosis type 1: review of the first 200 patients in an Australian clinic. *J Child Neurol* 8:395–402.

Palau F, Löfgren A, De Jonghe P, Bort S, Nelis E, Sevilla T, Martin J-J, Vilchez J, Prieto F, and van Broeckhoven C. 1993. Origin of the de novo duplication in Charcot-Marie-Tooth disease type 1A: unequal non-sister chromatid exchange during spermatogenesis. *Hum Mol Genet* 2:2031–5.

Pericak-Vance MA, Yamaoka LH, Vance JM, Small K, Rosenwasser GOD, Gaskell PC, Hung W-Y, Alberts MJ, Haynes CS, Speer MC, Gilbert JR, Herbstreith M, Aylsworth AS, and Roses AD. 1987. Genetic linkage studies on chromosome 17 RFLPs in von Recklinghausen neurofibromatosis (NF-1). *Genomics* 1:349–52.

Poyhonen M, Niemela S, and Herva R. 1997. Risk of malignancy and death in neurofibromatosis. *Arch Pathol Lab Med* 121:139–43.

Purandare SM, Breidenbach HH, Li Y, Zhu XL, Sawada S, Neil SM, Brothman A, White R, Cawthon R, and Viskochil D. 1995. Identification of neurofibromatosis 1 (*NF1*) homologous loci by direct sequencing, fluorescence *in situ* hybridization, and PCR amplification of somatic cell hybrids. *Genomics* 30:476–85.

Riccardi VM. 1981. von Recklinghausen neurofibromatosis. *N Engl J Med* 305:1617–27.

———. 1992. *Neurofibromatosis: Phenotype, Natural History, and Pathogenesis,* 2nd ed. Baltimore: Johns Hopkins University Press.

———. 1993. Genotype, malleotype, phenotype, and randomness: lessons from neurofibromatosis-I (NF-I). *Am J Hum Genet* 53:301–4.

Riccardi VM, Dobson CE, Chakraborty R, and Bontke C. 1984. The pathophysiology of neurofibromatosis. IX. Paternal age as a factor in the origin of new mutations. *Am J Med Genet* 18:169–76.

Riccardi VM and Eichner JE. 1986. *Neurofibromatosis: Phenotype, Natural History, and Pathogenesis.* Baltimore: Johns Hopkins University Press.

Riccardi VM and Lewis RA. 1988. Penetrance of von Recklinghausen neurofibromatosis: a distinction between predecessors and descendants. *Am J Hum Genet* 42:284–9.

Rodenhiser DI, Andrews JD, Mancini DN, Jung JH, and Singh SM. 1997. Homonucleotide tracts, short repeats and CpG/CpNpG motifs are frequent sites for heterogeneous mutations in the neurofibromatosis type 1 (NF1) tumour-suppressor gene. *Mutat Res* 373:185–95.

Samuelsson B and Åkesson HO. 1989. Neurofibromatosis in Gothenburg, Sweden. IV. Genetic analyses. *Neurofibromatosis* 2:107–15.

Samuelsson B and Samuelsson S. 1989. Neurofibromatosis in Gothenburg, Sweden: I. Background, study design and epidemiology. *Neurofibromatosis* 2:6–22.

Sergeyev AS. 1975. On the mutation rate of neurofibromatosis. *Humangenetik* 28:129–38.

Shen MH, Harper PS, and Upadhyaya M. 1996. Molecular genetics of neurofibromatosis type 1 (NF1). *J Med Genet* 33:2–17.

Spence MA, Bader JL, Parry DM, Field LL, Funderburk SJ, Rubenstein AE, Gilman PA, and Sparkes RS. 1983. Linkage analysis of neurofibromatosis (von Recklinghausen disease). *J Med Genet* 20:334–7.

Spiegel R, Mächler M, Stocker HP, Boltshauser E, and Schmid W. 1991. Neurofibromatose Typ 1: Genetische Untersuchungen mit DNA-Markern bei 38 Familien. *Schweiz Med Wschr* 121:1445–52.

Stephens K, Kayes L, Riccardi VM, Rising M, Sybert VP, and Pagon RA. 1992. Preferential mutation of the neurofibromatosis type 1 gene in paternally derived chromosomes. *Hum Genet* 88:279–82.

Takano T, Kawashima T, Yamanouchi Y, Kitayama K, Baba T, Ueno K, and Hamaguchi H. 1992. Genetics of neurofibromatosis 1 in Japan: mutation rate and paternal age effect. *Hum Genet* 89:281–6.

Tonsgard JH, Yalavarthi KK, Cushner S, Short MP, and Lindgren V. 1997. Do NF1 gene deletions result in a characteristic phenotype? *Am J Med Genet* 73:80–6.

Upadhyaya M, Ruggieri M, Maynard J, Osborn M, Hartog C, Mudd S, Penttinen M, Cordeiro I, Ponder M, Ponder BAJ, Krawczak M, and Cooper DN. 1998. Gross deletions of the neurofibromatosis type 1 (*NF1*) gene are predominantly of maternal origin and commonly associated with a learning disability, dysmorphic features and developmental delay. *Hum Genet* 102:591–7.

Upadhyaya M, Shaw DJ, and Harper PS. 1994. Molecular basis of neurofibromatosis type 1 (NF1): mutation analysis and polymorphisms in the NF1 gene. *Hum Mutat* 4:83–101.

Valero MC, Pascual-Castroviejo I, Velasco E, Moreno F, and Hernádez-Chico C. 1997. Identification of de novo deletions at the NF1 gene: no preferential paternal origin and phenotypic analysis of patients. *Hum Genet* 99:720–6.

Vance JM, Pericak-Vance MA, Yamaoka LH, Speer MC, Rosenwasser GOD, Small K, Gaskell PC, Hung W-Y, Alberts MJ, Haynes CS, Gilbert JR, Aylsworth AS, and Roses AD. 1989. Genetic linkage mapping of chromosome 17 markers and neurofibromatosis type 1. *Am J Hum Genet* 44:25–9.

Viskochil D, Buchberg AM, Xu G, Cawthon RM, Stevens J, Wolff RK, Culver M, Carey JC, Copeland NG, Jenkins NA, White R, and O'Connell P. 1990. Deletions and a translocation interrupt a cloned gene at the neurofibromatosis type 1 locus. *Cell* 62:187–92.

Wallace MR, Marchuk DA, Andersen LB, Letcher R, Odeh HM, Saulino AM, Fountain JW, Brereton A, Nicholson J, Mitchell AL, Brownstein BH, and Collins FS. 1990. Type 1 neurofibromatosis gene: identification of a large transcript disrupted in three NF1 patients. *Science* 249:181–6.

Ward K, O'Connell PO, Carey JC, Leppert M, Jolley S, Plaetke R, Ogden B, and White R. 1990. Diagnosis of neurofibromatosis I by using tightly-linked flanking DNA markers. *Am J Hum Genet* 46:943–9.

Wirth B, Schmidt T, Hahnen E, Rudnik-Schöneborn S, Krawczak M, Müller-Myhsok B, Schönling J, and Zerres K. 1997. De novo rearrangements found in 2% of index patients with spinal muscular atrophy: mutational mechanisms, parental origin, mutation rate, and implications for genetic counseling. *Am J Hum Genet* 61:1102–11.

Wu B-L, Austin MA, Schneider GH, Boles RG, and Korf BR. 1995. Deletion of the entire *NF1* gene detected by FISH: four deletion patients associated with severe manifestations. *Am J Med Genet* 59:528–35.

Wu B-L, Schneider GH, and Korf BR. 1997. Deletion of the entire *NF1* gene causing distinct manifestations in a family. *Am J Med Genet* 69:98–101.

Zöller M, Rembeck B, Åkesson HO, and Angervall L. 1995. Life expectancy, mortality, and prognostic factors in neurofibromatosis type 1. *Acta Derm Venerol (Stockh)* 75:136–40.

5

The Structure and Function of the *NF1* Gene: Molecular Pathophysiology

David H. Viskochil, M.D., Ph.D.

The development of effective therapy for the various features of NF1 requires understanding its pathophysiology—the derangement of function distinct from structural defects. In general, understanding the pathophysiology of a genetic condition is contingent on knowledge of normal biologic processes attributed to the disease gene. This chapter reviews the molecular aspects of the *NF1* gene and its encoded product, neurofibromin, in an attempt to provide insight about the pathophysiology of this complex genetic disorder.

GENE IDENTIFICATION AND STRUCTURE

Initial work on the localization of the *NF1* gene used linkage analysis of a large number of independent families collected by an international consortium to place the locus close to the centromere on the long arm of chromosome 17 (Barker et al. 1987). Subsequently, a detailed genetic marker map of the area was created (O'Connell et al. 1989). There was no evidence of genetic heterogeneity. In 1989, the identification of balanced translocations (Ledbetter et al. 1989; Schmidt et al. 1987) in two unrelated individuals with NF1 led to the transition from genetic mapping to physical mapping of the *NF1* locus (reviewed in Viskochil et al. 1993). By establishing somatic cell hybrids that harbored the derivative translocation chromosomes in rodent cell lines, the human DNA extracted from these respective lines could be used as part of a panel in Southern-blot analysis to map candidate probes derived from chromosome 17. One probe, which was developed as the human homolog to a murine genomic DNA region involved in leukemia-causing ecotropic viral insertions *(evi2)* (Buchburg et al. 1988), mapped between the translocation breakpoints (O'Connell et al. 1990). This genomic segment was used to characterize the locus harboring the *NF1* gene (Cawthon et al. 1990a, 1990b, 1991; Viskochil et al. 1990, 1991; Wallace et al. 1990).

The *NF1* gene is complex, as revealed by the details of its primary structure and organization. It has an open reading frame of 8454 nucleotides (Bernards et al. 1992; Marchuk et al. 1991) and spans approximately 335 kb of genomic DNA (Li et al. 1995). It is transcribed in a centromere-to-telomere direction. The intron–exon structure of the gene has been determined, as detailed in Figure 5-1. Sixty *NF1* exons have been identified. Even though numbered from 1 through 49, further analysis required many *NF1* exons to be split. Both the time at which exons were identified and the initial lack of intronic sequence from genomic clones led to a numbering system that requires the use of letters to designate split exons. The exon lengths are fairly consistent, and two thirds of the NF1 exons are in-frame. There are three known alternatively spliced exons, 9a (30 bp; Danglot et al. 1995), 23a (63 bp; for example, Andersen et al. 1993) and 48a (54 bp; Guttman et al. 1993), although the primary function of their respective encoded domains remains elusive. All but a large section of intron 1 has been sequenced from two sets of overlapping clones, and the intron–exon sequence is available in the GenBank database (accession number AC004526).

Numerous *NF1* homologous loci are scattered throughout the human genome, as detected by both fluorescence in situ hybridization (FISH) analysis and genomic sequence homology of amplified polymerase-chain-reaction (PCR) products (for example, see Purandare et al. 1995). *NF1*-related loci have been mapped to 2q21, 2q33, 14q11.2, 15q11.2, 18p11.2, 21q11.2, and 22q11.2, and there may be two loci on chromosome 15 and two on chromosome 22. Genomic sequence analysis for open reading frames of PCR products derived from various loci and the lack of cDNA harboring non-*NF1* sequence both suggest that the *NF1*-related loci represent unprocessed pseudogenes due to repeated duplications of the *NF1* locus (Bernards 1998). Various types of chromosomal rearrangements are likely explanations for this dispersion of the *NF1* gene sequence in hominid evolution (Regnier et al. 1997). It is intriguing to speculate that these loci may represent reservoirs of mutations that could be crossed into the bona fide *NF1* gene by interchromosomal gene conversion (Cummings et al. 1993). However, review of the NF1 Mutation Database for mutations incorporating genomic sequence derived from *NF1*-related loci failed to identify such an event (Purandare et al. 1995).

NF1 GENE EXPRESSION

The regulation of *NF1* gene expression is also complex. Within the *NF1* gene there are two introns > 45 kb, one of which (27b) contains three embedded genes (*OMGP, EVI2B,* and *EVI2A*) that are transcribed in an orientation opposite to *NF1*. Each of the three embedded genes is comprised of two exons. *EVI2A* is a small gene that encodes a 232 amino acid peptide (Cawthon et al. 1991). It is expressed in the brain and bone marrow, and sequence analysis suggests that it is a short-lived peptide that has a transmembrane domain. *EVI2B* is also a small gene that encodes a 448-amino-acid peptide of unknown function (Cawthon et al. 1990). It is expressed exclusively in the bone marrow. *OMGP* encodes a 416-amino-acid peptide and is expressed primarily in oligodendrocytes (Mikol et al. 1990). The peptide is expressed on the cell surface, and its amino acid sequence predicts an intercellular adhesion function. A phenotype for inactivation of any of these three genes, separate from a mutation in *NF1*, has not been demonstrated in vivo, and functional in vitro model systems have not yet been developed to evaluate the regulatory processes in cells that co-express *NF1* and any of these other genes.

The *NF1* promoter region has been cloned and there is cross-species conservation of sequence upstream of exon 1 (Hajra et al. 1994). The promoter lies in a CpG island (Fountain et al. 1989; Rodenheiser et al. 1993), and, as is typical with low-expression genes, there is not a TATA or CCAAT box to delineate a strong transcriptional start site. The major transcriptional start site is based on identification of cDNA clones showing initiation of transcription 484 bp upstream of the translational start site (Marchuk et al. 1991). By sequence analysis, a number of potential *cis*-acting elements can be identified (Viskochil 1998), and in vitro expression studies of deletion constructs have demonstrated potential transcription regulatory regions within the promoter (Feigenbaum et al. 1996; Purandare et al. 1996). The lack of outstanding *cis*-regulatory determinants for *NF1* transcription suggests that the promoter is likely quite weak and that minor perturbations in gene expression could play a significant role in stochastic changes in intracellular neurofibromin levels.

The 3′ end of the *NF1* gene extends approximately 3.5 kb downstream of the translation stop signal in exon 49 (Li et al. 1995). The high homology within the 3′ untranslated region between mouse and human gene sequences suggests that there are important sequences for mRNA stability in this region. Only a few cDNAs that are polyadenylated have been isolated from the *NF1* mRNA, whereas a number of cDNA clones extend beyond the stop site and randomly terminate within 500 bp downstream, well upstream of the purported polyadenylation signal.

As would be expected from the disorder's diverse clinical manifestations, *NF1* mRNA is ubiquitously expressed (Sherman et al. 1998). The mRNA transcript size is about 12 to 14 kb (Buchberg et al. 1990). The application of sensitive RT-PCR (reverse transcriptase–polymerase chain reaction) has identified *NF1* mRNA in almost all tissues, albeit at low levels. Lymphocytes express enough *NF1* mRNA to provide a ready source of RNA for mutational analysis using in vitro transcription and translation assays. Cells in tissue culture also express *NF1* mRNA and serve as potential model systems for research of the *NF1* gene.

Three major alternatively spliced isoforms have been identified that show significantly different expression patterns with respect to RNA and protein levels. The most widely expressed alternative splice form (type 2 neurofibromin) is that which includes exon 23a (Marchuk et al. 1991). Exon 23a lies within the only known functional domain of the *NF1* gene product (GTPase-activating domain, see below). The isoform that includes exon 23a exhibits decreased catalytic activity of this enzymatic function (Andersen et al. 1993). The type 2 isoform is found in many animal species and appears to be associated with differentiated cells. The alternative splice form containing exon 48a is preferentially expressed

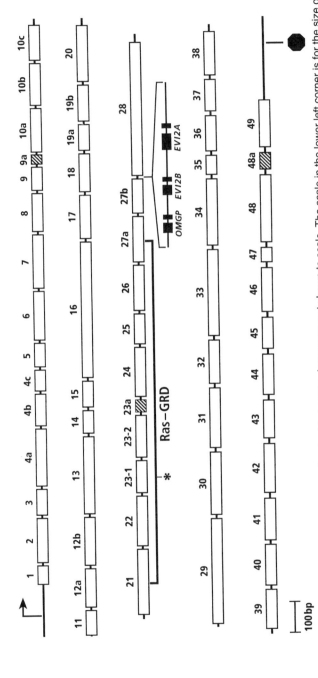

Figure 5-1. Schematic drawing of *NF1* exons and embedded genes. Introns are not shown to scale. The scale in the lower left corner is for the size of exons. The transcription start site is depicted as a horizontal arrow upstream of exon 1. The stop transcription stop site and polyadenylation site are marked with an octagon. The GAP-related domain, *ras*–GRD, is shown spanning exons 21 to 27a (Scheffzek et al., 1998). The alternative splice forms are in-frame insertions of exons 9a, 23a, and 48a, and they are hatched. The embedded genes are shown in bold in intron 27b and are transcribed in the opposite direction (telomere-to-centromere). The t(1;17) and t(17;22) translocation breakpoints lie in intron 27b, upstream of *OMGP*, and in intron 31, respectively. The asterisk in exon 23-1 represents a site of mRNA processing, C3916U, that leads to premature truncation at codon 1303 (Skuse et al., 1996).

in muscle derivatives (Gutmann et al. 1993). A third alternative splice form, involving exon 9a, is found exclusively in the brain during embryogenesis (Danglot et al. 1995; Geist and Gutmann 1996), suggesting potential functions of this encoded domain in central nervous system development. A number of other minor molecular species involving alternative splicing have been identified in various tissues; however, their significance has not been determined.

In addition to the stable alternative splice forms, a potential posttranscriptional regulatory process for *NF1* is RNA editing. Base 3916 in exon 23-1 (Fig. 5-1) is edited from a C to a U by deamination, which leads to premature truncation of translation at codon 1303 (Skuse and Cappione 1997). This phenomenon has been observed in other mRNAs, such as apolipoprotein B (Bass 1993; Driscoll et al. 1989). The finding of different levels of edited *NF1* mRNA in malignant peripheral nerve sheath tumors, benign neurofibromas, and astrocytomas has led to speculation that inactivation of the normal *NF1* allele by editing could lead to abnormal cellular proliferation (Cappione et al. 1997).

Neurofibromin is a relatively large peptide—> 220 kD (DeClue et al. 1991; Golubic et al. 1992; Gutmann et al. 1991). It is expressed in a variety of cell types in adults, including neurons, Schwann cells, oligodendrocytes, keratinocytes, astrocytes, adrenal medulla, and white blood cells (Daston et al. 1992). In animal models, neurofibromin is ubiquitously expressed during embryonic development, with adult tissue expression patterns being established after the first week of postnatal life (Huynh et al. 1994; Gutmann et al. 1995). Subcellular localization studies suggest that neurofibromin may associate with microtubules (see below), smooth endoplasmic reticulum, mitochondria, or nuclear and perinuclear staining, depending on the cell type examined (Bollag et al. 1993; Gregory et al. 1993; Nordlund et al. 1993; Roudebush et al. 1997). As a *ras*-GAP protein, neurofibromin would be expected to localize near *ras* (see below). However, studies have not specifically shown that neurofibromin colocalizes exclusively with membrane-bound *ras*.

THE FUNCTION OF NEUROFIBROMIN

Much of the work on the function of neurofibromin, the protein product of the *NF1* gene, has focused on the small portion of the protein that contains a region of homology to the GTPase-Activating Protein (GAP) family (Buchberg et al. 1990; Xu et al. 1990). There are many GAPs that regulate cellular function by acting on proteins with GTPase activity (G proteins) (reviewed in Boguski and McCormick 1993). The closest relatives of neurofibromin are p120GAP (Trahey and McCormick 1987) and GAPIII (Baba et al. 1995), which share approximately 30% amino acid homology with neurofibromin in the catalytic domain, but no homology outside of it (Kim and Tamanoi 1998). Functional studies have confirmed that both full-length neurofibromin and constructs containing only the GAP-related domain (GRD) stimulate the intrinsic GTPase of p21 *ras* (Fig. 5.2; Ahmadian et al. 1996; Bollag and McCormick 1991).

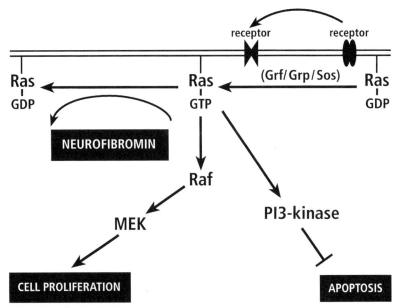

Figure 5-2. Schematic drawing of the role of neurofibromin in *ras* activation and signaling. Growth signals from the cell surface activate guanine nucleotide exchange factors (Sos, Grp, Grf) to dissociate GDP from membrane-bound *ras*. The enables *ras* to bind to free GTP and become activated. Activated *ras*–GTP sends intracellular signals through the phospho-inositol 3' kinase (P13-kinase) pathway to inhibit apoptosis and the *raf*-MAK (mitogen-acti-vated kinase) pathway to stimulate cell proliferation. Neurofibromin inactivates *ras*–GTP by stimulating the intrinsic *ras*–GTPase to hydrolyze GTP to GDP. Inadequate levels of neu-rofibromin (haploinsufficiency) lead to increased signaling through *raf* and P13-kinase. Thus, inactivating *NF1* mutations lead to both increased cell proliferation and increased cell survival.

The *ras* gene is a member of a superfamily of G proteins that are active in a GTP-bound form and inactive when bound to GDP (Lowy and Willumsen 1993; Marshall 1996). Activating *ras* mutations in either amino acid position 12, 13, or 61 prevent conversion of GTP to GDP and result in continuous transduction of signals through downstream pathways. These mutant peptides are functional, and their association with specific malignancies (Bos 1989) has led to the identi-fication of *ras* as a true proto-oncogene. The *ras* protein is anchored to the cell membrane through isoprenylation of its carboxyl end, mediated by farnesyl transferase (Casey et al. 1989). It functions as part of a signal transduction path-way involving receptor tyrosine kinases, such as epidermal growth factor, nerve growth factor, and platelet-derived growth factors (Bernards 1995). Even though *ras* GTPase can be activated in vitro, little, if any, downstream signaling is propagated in vivo through nonanchored *ras* (James et al. 1993; Hancock et al. 1989). The best characterized *ras*-mediated signal transduction pathway in mammalian cells is one that works through another small guanine-binding protein, *raf*, and downstream phosphorylation events, which together are loosely termed the *raf*-MAP kinase pathway (Sternberg and Alberola-Ila 1998). This biochemical cascade ultimately modifies cellular proliferation (see Fig. 5-2).

The role of activated *ras* in various cell systems is complex, including signaling systems such as the *ras*-MAP kinase signaling system, the PI3 kinase and PKB/Akt complexes (Khwaja et al. 1997), and NF-κB (Mayo et al. 1997) to induce antiapoptotic effects (reviewed in Downward 1998) and regulation of the cell cycle. *ras*-mediated induction of cyclin-dependent kinase inhibitors explains some contradictory responses to *ras* signaling found in different cell types; primary cells respond by cell-cycle arrest, whereas activated *ras* in immortalized cell lines induces progression of cell cycling (reviewed in Lloyd 1998). It seems that the accumulation of somatic genetic changes in different cell types could enable the cells to respond to activation of the *ras* signal transduction pathway quite differently.

A number of studies have demonstrated the connection between neurofibromin, *ras* signal transduction, and cell proliferation. Because no direct measurement of the neurofibromin-specific GAP activity has been developed, indirect assays have been substituted. The most commonly used is the intracellular Ras-GTP to Ras-GDP ratio (Basu et al. 1992; DeClue et al. 1992). This ratio has been standardized for a number of tissues, and higher ratios have been found in NF1-related tumors such as neurofibromas and malignant peripheral nerve sheath tumors (Guha et al. 1996). The specificity of the phenotype of the *NF1* gene is difficult to reconcile with the cancer phenotypes associated with activating *ras* mutations. The tumors of NF1 are generally not the same tumors that have somatic mutations involving activated *ras* (Bos 1989; Mulvihill 1994). Only the malignancies of juvenile chronic myeloid leukemia (JCML) overlap, whereby either double inactivation of *NF1* or activating *ras* mutations result in the same tumor phenotype (Kalra et al. 1994; Side et al. 1997). The role of *ras* in downstream signaling in JCML has been demonstrated by assays of MEK phosporylation in NF1-associated JCML tumor cells, which show increased activation of the MAPK pathway (Bollag et al. 1996). The lack of correlation with other tumors suggests that the neurofibromin–*ras* interaction may involve other biochemical pathways, not simply MAP kinase downstream signaling.

Biochemical evaluations of the neurofibromin-ras complex have provided insight into differences between the cellular phenotypes resulting from mutations of *NF1* and *RAS*. First, mutation analysis of the NF1-GRD has led to dissection of the contributions of specific amino acids toward both affinity and catalytic properties of neurofibroma (reviewed in Kim and Tamanoi 1998). Second, the recent crystallization of an NF1-GRD construct, NF1-333, has enabled investigators to determine the structure of the catalytic domain in neurofibromin (Scheffzek et al. 1998). This in comparison with a model for p120GAP (Scheffzek et al. 1996) and its interaction with Ras (Scheffzek et al. 1997) provides some understanding of important molecular interactions between neurofibromin and Ras.

In addition to its interaction with *ras*, neurofibromin has other biochemical properties that are noteworthy. These include other G-protein GAP function, interaction with microtubules, and an inhibitory effect of lipids on NF1-GRD activity. The NF1-GRD interacts with other *ras*-related proteins and catalyzes the intrinsic GTPases of R-*ras* (Rey et al. 1994) and TC21 (Graham et al. 1996). Given that the *ras* superfamily of GTPases consists of more than 50 proteins, it will be important to determine which ones interact with neurofibromin, for both binding and catalysis, in order to understand the complex biochemical role neurofibromin may have as an intracellular GAP.

Neurofibromin has been shown to interact with tubulin (Bollag et al. 1993), and antibody studies demonstrate colocalization of neurofibromin with microtubules in rat kangaroo fibroblasts (Gregory et al. 1993). The structure of tubulin (Nogales et al. 1998) harbors a G-domain fold similar to *ras* (Pai et al. 1990), and the proximity of the N- and C-terminals in the structure of NF1-GRD suggests a possible conformation that is critical in tubulin binding (Scheffzek et al. 1998). This could account for both the tubulin-binding determinants mapping to the N-terminal of the NF1-GRD (Bollag et al. 1993) and the lack of microtubule association of the NF1-GRD mutant constructs (Xu and Gutmann 1997) in vitro. The interaction between neurofibromin and microtubules may reflect a novel function for neurofibromin in regulating microtubule-mediated processes or it could represent one mechanism by which neurofibromin *ras*-GAP activity is controlled in the cell.

The role of lipids in regulating cellular *ras* activity may involve inhibition of GAP activity. Arachidonic acid, phosphatidic acid, and phosphatidylinositol 4,5-bisphosphate (PIP$_2$) inhibit NF1-GRD activity (Golubic et al. 1991) and differential inhibition of NF1-GRD versus P120GAP by phosphatidic acid (Bollag and McCormick 1991) suggests a regulatory function for lipids in *ras* signal transduction. In addition, prostaglandins and prostacyclin (PGI$_2$) also demonstrate differential effects on P120GAP and NF1-GRD activities (Han et al. 1991). This variable responsiveness of *ras*-GAP activities through lipids, prostaglandins, tubulin, and other G proteins may discriminate between the multiple pathways involved in *ras* signal transduction (Downward 1998).

MUTATIONAL ANALYSIS OF THE *NF1* GENE

Mutational analysis of persons with NF1 has proven to be a difficult task because of the large size of the gene and the lack of mutational hot spots. Most reports describe mutation screening by heteroduplex analysis and/or single-strand conformation polymorphism analysis (for example, Abernathy et al. 1997; Upadhyaya et al. 1995). Others have used Southern-blot analysis, fluorescence in situ hybridization (FISH) for large deletions, denaturing gradient-gel electrophoresis, or chemical cleavage of mismatch. The various DNA-based tests have generally identified mutations in no more than 20% of patients with NF1. However, many studies have not screened the entire gene, instead focusing on the domain that has catalytic activity, the NF1-GRD. The most effective single method for *NF1* mutation analysis described to date is the protein truncation test, which has detected mutations confirmed by sequencing in over two thirds of patients in two small studies (Heim et al. 1995; Park and Pivnick 1998). Unfortunately, the sensitivity and specificity of this test in clinical practice have not been reported.

The majority of mutations reported in patients with NF1 are predicted to cause gross truncation of the protein product (Upadhyaya and Cooper 1998; Upadhyaya et al. 1995). Presumably, this results in inactivation of neurofibromin and supports the model that NF1 is caused by decreased amounts of intracellular neurofibromin. Small deletions and insertions are especially common, accounting for about one-third of mutations (Table 5-1). Several polymorphisms have been reported, with heterozygosity frequencies ranging from 0.09 to 0.82 (Shen et al. 1996). The use of these polymorphisms in prenatal diagnosis is discussed in Chapter 3.

Family studies have shown that approximately 95% of all sporadic cases of NF1 result from mutation of the paternal chromosome (Jadayel et al. 1990; Stephens et al. 1992), with the outstanding exception being intragenic deletions, which tend to be derived from the maternal chromosome (Ainsworth et al. 1997; Lazaro et al. 1996).

Identical mutations at the *NF1* gene locus are uncommon. The most common "hotspot" identified to date is a C5839T substitution in exon 31, and it encodes a

Table 5-1. The spectrum of *NF1* mutations reported in patients with NF1

Type of Mutation	Number of Reported Independent Occurrences
Chromosome abnormality	4
Deletion of the entire gene	18
Multi-exon deletion (not whole gene)	38
Small intragenic deletion	55
Large insertion	3
Small insertion	27
Nonsense mutation (premature translation stop)	43
Missense mutation (amino acid substitution)	29
Intronic alteration	25
Alteration of the 3′ untranslated region	4
Total	246

Source: Adapted from the National Neurofibromatosis Foundation International NF1 Genetic Analysis Consortium Database accessed at http://www.nf.org/nf1gene/nf1gene.mutdata.summary.html. Contributing members to this consortium are listed at the site.

premature truncation downstream of the sequences encoding the GAP-related domain (for example, Abernathy et al. 1997). It has been found in 10 unrelated individuals from different ethnic backgrounds, and, in general, the NF1 phenotype associated with this genotype is not unusual. Another recurrent mutation site in exon 37, between nucleotides 6789 and 6792, has been identified in approximately 2% of screened patients with NF1. However, a genotype–phenotype correlation has not been identified (Boddrich et al. 1997; Messiaen et al. 1997). A smattering of recurrent mutations have also been identified associated with repetitive sequences in the gene (Heim et al. 1995; Robinson et al. 1996; Shen and Upadhyaya 1993; Side et al. 1997). The variety of mutations observed probably reflects the fact that several different mechanisms can cause pathogenic changes in the *NF1* gene. In general, different mutations do not appear to be associated with distinctive phenotypic expression of the condition.

A lack of effect of the underlying *NF1* mutation on the resulting phenotype is suggested by the clinical observation that there is little correlation between the clinical features found among relatives with NF1, including affected monozygotic twins (Chapter 2). An exception to the lack of genotype–phenotype correlation is suggested by the clinical findings associated with large deletions in patients who have earlier onset of neurofibromas, more profound developmental delays, distinctive facial features, and other minor anomalies (for example, Wu et al. 1995; see Chapter 3). This finding of a large-deletion phenotype in NF1 suggests that genes contiguous with the *NF1* gene could play some role in the phenotype. Although large gene deletions remove the three embedded genes discussed above, two individuals who have smaller intragenic deletions involving *EVI2A, EVI2B,* or *OMGP* do not have the same phenotype as the whole-gene deletion patients (Viskochil et al. 1990).

The finding of somatic mutations, or "second hits," is key in supporting the hypothesis that the *NF1* gene functions as a true tumor-suppressor gene. The tumor-suppressor gene model was first formulated to explain the occurrence of familial versus sporadic retinoblastoma (Knudson et al. 1975). This hypothesis proposes that "braking" genes exist. Their function is to prevent uncontrolled cellular growth (Fig. 5-3). Genetic changes, either inherited or accumulated during life, may inactivate these genes, leading to tumorigenesis. In the general population, cancers occur singularly and relatively late in life, as both copies of the gene must be inactivated independently. For individuals born with one inactivated copy of a tumor-suppressor gene, each susceptible cell is at a grave disadvantage. With only one remaining copy of the tumor suppressor to be inactivated, multiple tumors of specific cellular types develop relatively early in life. The demonstration of either loss of heterozygosity or homozygous inactivation of *NF1* in a number of tissue samples and cell lines, such as dermal neurofibromas (Colman et al. 1995; Sawada et al. 1996; Serra et al. 1997), malignant peripheral nerve sheath tumors (Glover et al. 1991; Legius et al. 1993; Lothe et al. 1996; Menon et al. 1990; Skuse et al. 1990), pheochromocytomas (Xu et al. 1992), neuroblastomas (Martinsson et al. 1997), and myelogenous leukemias (Side et al. 1997), supports *NF1* as a tumor-suppressor gene.

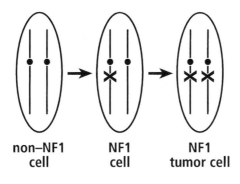

A

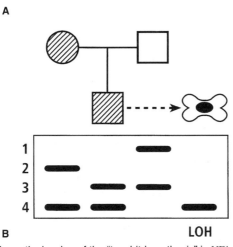

B　　　　　　　　　　　　　　**LOH**

Figure 5-3. (A) Schematic drawing of the "two-hit-hypothesis" in NF1. An NF1 tumor (i.e., juvenile chronic myelogenous leukemia, or JCML) arises as a result of mutations leading to double inactivation of the *NF1* gene on chromosome 17. A normal cell that undergoes somatic *NF1* inactivation retains normal growth properties because the other *NF1* allele provides the necessary function. The same is true of an uninvolved cell in a person with NF1 who has a constitutional mutation of one *NF1* allele. A somatic mutation that inactivates the remaining normal allele in such a cell produces complete loss of *NF1* "tumor-suppressor" activity, leading to cell proliferation. This model holds true for JCML, but somatic mutations involving other loci are likely required for other malignancies in patients with NF1. (B) Schematic drawing of "loss of heterozygosity" (LOH). In a hypothetical example, the pedigree shows an affected mother, an unaffected father, and an affected son with leukemia (bone symbol). Each has a specific genotype at a specific genetic marker locus that is closely linked to *NF1*: mother (2,4), father (1,3), child (3,4), and tumor (–,4). The bands in the box represent alleles of this locus separated by size. The mutant allele is carried on the same chromosome as allele 4 at the marker locus. The DNA from leukemic blasts shows complete loss of the normal allele from the father and retention of the mutant allele from the mother. This represents inactivation of both *NF1* alleles in the tumor; the constitutionally mutant *NF1* allele carried on the same chromosome as the marker allele 4 was inherited from the affected mother. The normal *NF1* allele inherited from the father, along with the marker 3 allele, has presumably been deleted in the tumor cells.

MOSAICISM

A number of individuals have been reported who manifest NF1 features in a localized pattern, termed "segmental NF1." The molecular basis of this phenomenon is likely to be due to a somatic mutation of the *NF1* gene in an early stage of fetal development; however, no molecular confirmation of a mosaic *NF1* mutation in a patient with segmental NF1 has yet been made. In a single case, two patients with NF1 who had unaffected parents were shown to have an identical intragenic deletion of the paternal chromosome, and the father's sperm showed approximately 10% constitution of this mutation (Lazaro et al. 1994, 1995). Mosaicism of large deletions, as demonstrated by lymphocyte FISH analysis, has been reported in several individuals with otherwise typical NF1 (Ainsworth et al. 1997; Colman et al. 1995; Tonsgard et al. 1997; Wu et al. 1997).

HETEROGENEITY

To date, there has been little molecular analysis of persons with other phenotypes that are related to NF1 (Viskochil and Carey 1995). Linkage analysis of families with Watson syndrome (Allanson et al. 1991; Tassabehji et al. 1993), familial café-au-lait spots (Abeliovich et al. 1995; Brunner et al. 1993; Charrow et al. 1993), and NF–Noonan syndrome (Carey et al. 1998; Colley et al. 1991) have shown mixed results (reviewed in Chapter 2). There is a single report of a child with encephalocraniocutaneous lipomatosis who has a germline *NF1* mutation (Legius et al. 1995). Other patients with this rare syndrome have not been studied. A patient with multiple lentigines as part of LEOPARD syndrome was shown to have an *NF1* mutation (Wu et al. 1996); however, this individual may simply have had an atypical presentation of NF1. The rare individuals who have NF1-related features but either do not fulfill the diagnostic criteria or have extensive features not typically seen in NF1 tend to be sporadic cases. Referral of such individuals to a NF clinic with staff who are knowledgeable about the overlap of NF1 features with other genetic conditions is appropriate in order to establish a diagnosis.

MODEL SYSTEMS

The importance of the *NF1*-encoded protein is emphasized by its conservation at the amino acid sequence level in many organisms, including yeast. The yeast neurofibromin homologs, Ira1p and Ira2p, inhibit *ras* activation of the adenylate cyclase pathway and decrease cAMP levels (Tanaka et al. 1990). Ira-deficient mutant strains of yeast have increased levels of cAMP, which leads to a phenotype that can be rescued by NF1-GRD constructs (Ballester et al. 1990; Martin et al. 1990; Xu et al. 1990). There is approximately 20% homology between human neurofibromin (amino acids 900 to 2350) and the GRD-extended sequences in Ira1p and Ira2p. The lack of an Ira phenotype that cannot be rescued by the *NF1*-GRD suggests that the only role for the neurofibromin homolog in yeast is to inhibit *ras*-mediated activation of adenylate cyclase.

The *Drosophila NF1* gene product is approximately 60% homologous with human neurofibromin, and it extends through the full length of the 2803-amino acid peptide. The *Drosophila* model provides a well-characterized *ras* signal transduction system that propagates both cellular proliferation and antiapoptotic signals through the *raf*-MAPK pathway. However, even though *Drosophila NF1* has *ras*-GAP activity, its primary role is the regulation of an adenylate cyclase pathway (Bernards 1998). Homozygous *NF1* null mutants are 20 to 25% smaller with otherwise normal patterning of development, and they demonstrate a reduced escape response that appears to be a behavioral abnormality rather than a physical impediment (The et al. 1997). This phenotype is different from the overexpression-of-*ras* phenotype, and inhibition of *ras* signaling could not rescue the *NF1* null mutants. This was a clue to the identification of the major biochemical pathway of neurofibromin in the fruitfly—regulation of the *rutabaga*-encoded adenylate cyclase. As identified by response to pituitary adenylyl cyclase–activating polypeptide (PACAP38), the NF1 protein is required in the cAMP-induced enhancement of potassium currents specified through an adenylate cyclase (Guo et al. 1997). By virtue of rescue of the *NF1*-deficient growth and behavioral phenotypes through stimulation of the cAMP-dependent protein kinase (PKA) pathway, it is clear that the predominant role for the *Drosophila NF1* gene product is its regulation of cAMP signaling, not the classic *ras*-mediated signal transduction pathway (Bernards 1998).

The development of a transgenic *Nf1* mouse has allowed the examination of this protein in a biologic system that is more similar to humans. This mouse has been engineered with an interruption of the gene segment that corresponds to a premature truncation *NF1* mutation in exon 31 initially identified in an individual with NF1 (Cawthon et al. 1990). The corresponding mouse mutation was constructed by inserting a *neo* gene in exon 31, which causes a similar truncating mutation (Brannan et al. 1994; Jacks et al. 1994). The *Nf1*+/− heterozygous mice do not have an obvious phenotype except late-onset tumors involving the bone marrow and peripheral nervous system. Low-grade gliomas have not been identified, although in a number of mice adrenal tumors developed similar to pheochromocytomas (Jacks et al. 1994). Even though other manifestations of human NF1 such as neurofibromas, skin pigmentation abnormalities, Lisch nodules, or skeletal dysplasias have not been documented, heterozygous mice appear to have learning problems, including poor performance in tests of spatial learning and memory, that can be overcome by extended training (Silva et al. 1997). The *Nf1*+/− heterozygous mice do not show abnormalities in simple associative learning as measured by cued fear conditioning. The brains of these mice have not been shown to have anatomical differences from their wild-type littermates.

Mice homozygous for this construct die in utero at approximately 12 to 14 days of gestation and all have a specific cardiac malformation, double-outlet right ventricle (Brannan et al. 1994; Jacks et al. 1994). This heart defect is not seen in human NF1. There are no other grossly apparent developmental defects at the time of fetal death. To study the most pronounced effects of loss of neurofibromin function, various cell types have been harvested before this embryologic death. Neurons harvested from the peripheral nervous system of these animals show an ability to survive in culture without growth factor stimulation, suggesting a role for neurofibromin in normal programmed cell death, apoptosis, within the nervous system (Vogel et al. 1995). Hematopoietic stem cells show increased cell proliferation, and are more sensitive to GM-CSF stimulation than either heterozygous or wild-type cells (Bollag et al. 1996; Largaespeda et al. 1996). This observation not only supports the tumor-suppressor model for NF1, but also is strong evidence that the neurofibromin-regulated *ras-raf*-MAPK pathway plays a major role in tumorigenesis in individuals with NF1.

SUMMARY

An understanding of the molecular biology of the *NF1* gene and its peptide, neurofibromin, provides an opportunity to develop new therapeutic strategies that were inconceivable only a few years ago. Clearly, targeting the *ras* signal transduction pathway is fertile ground for innovative research. One approach is the application of farnesyl transferase inhibitors to decrease the number of *ras* molecules bound to the inner membrane (Yan et al. 1995). Work along these lines is ongoing, and pharmaceuticals may be available for human trials in the near future, not just for NF1 tumors, but for cancers as well. Another approach is the development of a human reovirus that depends on an activated *ras* signaling pathway for infectivity (Coffey et al. 1998). It is conceivable that tumors could be injected with virus that would infect only cells with activated *ras* and cause direct cell lysis of only those cells with double inactivation of NF1. Finally, knowledge that the GRD of neurofibromin has the same *ras*-GAP activity as the full-length peptide indicates that development of vectors to deliver functional NF1-GRD to affected cells that signal through *ras* is a reasonable approach to future therapy. Cytoplasmic expression of NF1-GRD rescues yeast Ira-mutants; therefore transfection with a gene-therapy vector carrying the NF1-GRD is a reasonable undertaking.

REFERENCES

Abeliovich D, Gelman-Kohan Z, Silverstien S, Lerer I, Chemke J, Merin S, and Zlotogora J. 1995. Familial café au lait spots: a variant of neurofibromatosis type 1. *J Med Genet* 32:985–6.

Abernathy C, Rasmussen S, Stalker H, Zori R, Driscoll DJ, Williams CA Kousseff BG, and Wallace MR. 1997. NF1 mutation analysis using a combined heteroduplex/SSCP approach. *Hum Mutat* 9548–54.

Ahmadian M, Wiesmuller L, Lautwein A, Bischoff F, and Wittinghofer A. 1996. Structural differences in the minimal catalytic domains of the GTPase-activating proteins p120GAP and neurofibromin. *J Biol Chem* 271:16409–15.

Ainsworth P, Chakraborty P, and Weksberg R. 1997. Example of somatic mosaicism in a series of *de novo* neurofibromatosis type 1 cases due to a maternally derived deletion. *Hum Mutat* 9:452–7.

Allanson JE, Upadhyaya M, Watson G, et al. 1991. Watson syndrome: is it a subtype of type 1 neurofibromatosis? *J Med Genet* 28:752–6.

Andersen L, Ballester R, Marchuk D, Chang E, Gutmann D, Saulino A, Camonis J, Wigler M, and Collins F. 1993. A conserved alternative splice in the von Reckling-hausen neurofibromatosis (*NF1*) gene produces two neurofibromin isoforms, both of which have GTPase activating protein activity. *Mol Cell Biol* 13:487–95.

Baba H, Fuss B, Urano J, Poullet P, Watson J, Tamanoi F, and Macklin W. 1995. GapIII, a new brain-enriched member of the GTPase-activating protein family. *J Neurosci* 41:846–58.

Ballester R, Marchuk D, Boguski M, et al. 1990. The *NF1* locus encodes a protein func-tionally related to mammalian GAP and yeast *IRA* proteins. *Cell* 63:851–9.

Barker D, Wright E, Nguyen K, et al. 1987. Gene for von Recklinghausen neurofibro-matosis is in the pericentric region of chromosome 17. *Science* 236:1100–2.

Bass B. 1993. *The RNA World*. Cold Spring Harbor, NY: Cold Spring Harbor Laboratory Press, pp. 383–418.

Basu T, Gutmann D, Fletcher J, et al. 1992. Aberrant regulation of ras proteins in malig-nant tumour cells from type 1 neurofibromatosis patients. *Nature* 356:713–5.

Bernards A. 1995. Neurofibromatosis type 1 and Ras-mediated signaling: filling in the GAPs. *Biochim Biophys Acta* 1242:43–59.

———. 1998. Evolutionary Comparisons. In: Upadhyaya M and Cooper DN, eds. *Neu-rofibromatosis Type 1: From Genotype to Phenotype*. Oxford: Bios Scientific.

Bernards A, Haase V, and Murthy A. 1992. Complete human NF1 cDNA sequence: two alternatively spliced mRNAs and absence of expression in a neuroblastoma line. *DNA Cell Biol* 11:727–34.

Boddrich A, Robinson PN, Schulke M, Buske A, Tinschert S, and Nurnberg P. 1997. New evidence for a mutation hotspot in exon 37 of the *NF1* gene. *Hum Mutat* 9:374–7.

Boguski M and McCormick F. 1993. Proteins regulating ras and its relatives. *Nature* 366:643–54.

Bollag G and McCormick F. 1991. Differential regulation of rasGAP and neurofibro-matosis gene product activities. *Nature* 351:576–9.

Bollag G, Clapp DW, Shih S, Adler F, Zhang YY, Thompson P, Lange BJ, Freedman MH, McCormick F, Jacks T, and Shannon K. 1996. Loss of NF1 results in activation of the Ras signaling pathway and leads to aberrant growth in haematopoietic cells. *Nat Genet* 12:144–8.

Bollag G, McCormick F, and Clark R. 1993. Characterization of full-length neurofi-bromin: tubulin inhibits Ras GAP activity. *EMBO J* 12:1923–7.

Bos JL. 1989. Ras oncogenes in human cancer: a review. *Cancer Res* 49:4682–9.

Brannan C, Perkins A, Vogel K, Ratner N, Nordlund M, Reid S, Buchberg A, Jenkins N, Parada L, and Copeland N. 1994. Targeted disruption of the neurofibromatosis type-1 gene leads to developmental abnormalities in heart and various neural crest-derived tissues. *Genes Dev* 8:1019–29.

Brunner HG, Hulsebos T, Stiejlen PM, der Kinderen DJ, Steen A, and Hamel BCJ. 1993. Exclusion of the neurofibromatosis 1 locus in a family with inherited café au lait spots. *Am J Med Genet* 46:472–4.

Buchberg A, Bedigan G, Taylor B, Brownell E, Ihle J, et al. 1988. Localization of *Evi-2* to chromosome 11: linkage to other proto-oncogene and growth factor loci using inter-specific backcross mice. *Oncogene Res* 2:149–65.

Buchberg A, Cleveland L, and Jenkins N. 1990. Sequence homology shared by neurofi-bromatosis type-1 gene and *IRA-1* and *IRA-2* negative regulators of the *RAS* cyclic AMP pathway. *Nature* 347:291–4.

Cappione A, French B, and Skuse G. 1997. A potential role for NF1 mRNA editing in the pathogenesis of NF1 tumors. *Am J Hum Genet* 60:305–12.

Carey J, Stevenson D, Ota M, Nei1 S, and Viskochil D. 1998. Is there an NF/Noonan syn-drome? Part 2: Documentation of the clinical and molecular aspects of an important family. *Proc Greenwood Genet Cent* 17:52–3.

Casey PJ, Solski PA, Der CJ, and Buss JE. 1989. p21ras is modified by a farnesyl isoprenoid. *Proc Natl Acad Sci USA* 86:8323–7.

Cawthon R, Andersen L, Buchberg A, et al. 1991. cDNA sequence and genomic structure of *EVI2B*, a gene lying within an intron of the neurofibromatosis type 1 gene. *Genomics* 9:446–60.

Cawthon R, O'Connell P, Buchberg A, et al. 1990a. Identification and characterization of transcripts from the neurofibromatosis 1 region: the sequence and genomic structure of *EVI2* and mapping of other transcripts. *Genomics* 7:555–65.

Cawthon R, Weiss R, Xu G, et al. 1990b. A major segment of the neurofibromatosis type 1 gene: cDNA sequence, genomic structure, and point mutations. *Cell* 62:193–201.

Charrow J, Listernick R, and Ward K. 1993. Autosomal dominant multiple café au lait spots and neurofibromatosis-1: evidence of non-linkage. *Am J Med Genet* 45:606–8.

Coffey M, Strong J, Forsyth P, and Lee W. 1998. Reovirus therapy of tumors with activated ras pathway. *Science* 282:1332–4.

Colley P, Colley A, Donnai D, et al. 1991. Large scale mutations at the NF1 locus in Noonan-NF1 and NF1 patients. *Am J Hum Genet* 49(4):21A.

Colman S, Williams C, and Wallace M. 1995. Benign neurofibromas in type 1 neurofibromatosis (NF1) show somatic deletions of the *NF1* gene. *Nat Genet* 11:90–2.

Colman S, Rasmussen S, Ho V, Abernathy C, Wallace M. 1996. Somatic mosaicism in a patient with neurofibromatosis type 1. *Am J Hum Genet* 58:484–90.

Cummings L, Glatfelder A, and Marchuk D. 1993. *NF1*-related loci on chromosomes 2, 12, 14, 15, 21, and 22: a potential role for gene conversion in the high spontaneous mutation rate in NF1? *Am J Hum Genet* 53:672A.

Danglot G, Regnier V, Fauvet D, et al. 1995. Neurofibromatosis 1 (*NF1*) mRNAs expressed in the central nervous system are differentially spliced in the 5′ part of the gene. *Hum Mol Genet* 4:915–20.

Daston M, Scrable H, Nordlund M, et al. 1992. The protein product of the neurofibromatosis type 1 gene is expressed at highest abundance in neurons, Schwann cells, and oligodendrocytes. *Neuron* 8:415–28.

DeClue J, Cohen B, and Lowy D. 1991. Identification and characterization of the neurofibromatosis type 1 protein product. *Proc Natl Acad Sci USA* 88: 9914–8.

DeClue J, Papageorge AG, Fletcher JA, Diehl SR, Ratner N, Vass WC, and Lowy DR. 1992. Abnormal regulation of mammalian p21ras contributes to malignant tumor growth in von Recklilnghausen (type 1) neurofibromatosis. *Cell* 69:265–73.

Downward J. 1998. Ras signaling and apoptosis. *Curr Opin Genet Dev* 8:49–54.

Driscoll DM, Wynne JK, Wallis SC, and Scott J. 1989. An in vitro system for the editing of apolipoprotein B mRNA. *Cell* 58:519–25.

Feigenbaum L, Fujita K, and Collins F. 1996. Repression of the *NF1* gene by tax may explain the development of neurofibromas in human T-lymphotropic virus type 1 transgenic mice. *J Virology* 70:3280–5.

Fountain J, Wallace M, and Bruce M. 1989. Physical mapping of a translocation breakpoint in neurofibromatosis. *Science* 244:1085–7.

Geist R and Gutmann D. 1996. Expression of a developmentally-regulated neuron-specific isoform of the neurofibromatosis 1 (*NF1*) gene. *Neurosci Lett* 211:85–8.

Glover T, Stein C, Legius E, Andersen L, Brereton A, and Johnson S. 1991. Molecular and cytogenetic analysis of tumors in von Recklinghausen neurofibromatosis. *Genes Chromosomes Cancer* 3:62.

Golubic M, Roudebush M, Dobrowolski S, et al. 1992. Catalytic properties, tissue and intracellular distribution of neurofibromin. *Oncogene* 7:2151–9.

Golubic M, Tanaka K, Dobrowolski S, Wood D, Tsai M, Marshall M, Tamanoi F, and Stacey D. 1991. The GTPase stimulatory activities of the neurofibromatosis type 1 and the yeast IRA2 proteins are inhibited by arachadonic acid. *EMBO J* 10:2897–2903.

Graham S, Vojtek A, Huff S, Cox A, Clark G, Cooper J, and Der C. 1996. TC21 causes transformation by Raf-independent signaling pathways. *Mol Cell Biol* 16:6132–40.

Gregory P, Gutmann D, Mitchell A, Park S, Boguski M, Jacks T, Wood D, Jove R, and Collins F. 1993. Neurofibromatosis type 1 gene product (neurofibromin) associates with microtubules. *Somat Cell Mol Genet* 19:265–74.

Guha A, Lau N, Huvar I, Gutmann D, Provias J, Pawson T, and Boss G. 1996. Ras-GTP levels are elevated in human NF1 peripheral nerve tumors. *Oncogene* 12:507–13.

Guo HF, The I, Hannan F, Bernards A, and Zhong Y. 1997. Requirement of Drosophila NF 1 for activation of adenylyl cyclase by PACAP38-like neuropeptide. *Science* 276:795–8.

Gutmann D, Anderson L, and Cole J. 1993. An alternatively spliced mRNA in the carboxy terminus of the neurofibromatosis type 1 (*NF1*) gene is expressed in muscle. *Hum Mol Genet* 2:989–92.

Gutmann D, Cole L, and Collins F. 1995a. Expression of the neurofibromatosis type 1 (NF1) gene during mouse embryonic development. *Prog Brain Res* 105:327–35.

Gutmann D, Geist R, Wright D, et al. 1995b. Expression of the neurofibromatosis 1 (*NF1*) insoforms in developing and adult rat tissues. *Cell Growth Differ* 6:315–23.

Gutmann D, Wood D, and Collins F. 1991. Identification of the neurofibromatosis type 1 gene product. *Proc Natl Acad Sci USA* 88:9658–62.

Hajra A, Martin-Gallardo A, Tarle S, et al. 1994. DNA sequences in the promoter region of the NF1 gene are highly conserved between human and mouse. *Genomics* 21:649–52.

Hancock J, Magee A, Childs J, Marshall C. 1989. All *ras* proteins are polyisoprenylated but only some are palmitoylated. *Cell* 57:1167–77.

Han J, McCormick F, and Macara I. 1991. Regulation of Ras-GAP and the neurofibromatosis-1 gene product by eicosanoids. *Science* 252:576–9.

Heim RA, Kam-Morgan LNW, Binnie CG, Corns DD, Cayouette MC, Farber RA, Aylsworth AS, Silverman LM, and Luce MC. 1995. Distribution of 13 truncating mutations in the neurofibromatosis 1 gene. *Hum Mol Genet* 4:975–81.

Huynh D, Nechiporuk T, and Pulst S. 1994. Differential expression and tissue distribution of type I and type II neurofibromins during mouse fetal development. *Dev Biol* 161:538–51.

Jacks T, Shih TS, Schmitt EM, Bronson RT, Bernards A, and Weinberg RA. 1994. Tumour predisposition in mice heterozygous for a targeted mutation in *Nf1*. *Nat Genet* 17:353–61.

Jadayel D, Fain P, Upadhyaya M, Ponder M, Huson S, Carey J, Fryer A, et al. 1990. Paternal origin of new mutations in Von Recklinghausen neurofibromatosis. *Nature* 343:558–9.

James G, Goldstein J, Brown M, et al. 1993. Benozodiazapine peptidomimetics: potent inhibitors of ras farnesylation in animal cells. *Science* 260:19374–42.

Kalra R, Padernga D, Olson K, and Shannon K. 1994. Genetic analysis is consistent with the hypothesis that *NF1* limits myeloid cell growth through p21Ras. *Blood* 84:3435–9.

Khwaga A, Rodriguez V, Wennstrom S, Warne P, and Downward J. 1997. Matrix adhesion and Ras transformation both activate a phosphoinositide 3-OH kinase and protein kinase B/Akt cellular survival pathway. *EMBO J* 16:2783–93.

Kim MR and Tamanoi F. 1998. Neurofibromatosis 1 GTPase activating protein-related domain and its functional signficance. In: Upadhyaya M and Cooper DN, eds. *Neurofibromatosis Type 1: From Genotype to Phenotype*. Oxford: Bios Scientific.

Knudson AG Jr, Hethcote HW, and Brown BW. 1975. Mutation and childhood cancer: a probabilistic model for the incidence of retinoblastoma. *Proc Natl Acad Sci USA* 72:5116–20.

Largaespada D, Brannan C, Jenkins N, and Copeland N. 1996. Nf1 deficiency causes Ras-mediated granulocyte-macrophage colony stimulating factor hypersensitivity and chronic myeloid leukemia. *Nat Genet* 12:137–43.

Lazaro C, Gaona A, Lynch M, Kruyer H, Ravella A, and Estivill X. 1995. Molecular characterization of the breakpoints of a 12-kb deletion in the *NF1* gene in a family showing germ-line mosaicisim. *Am J Hum Genet* 57:1044–9.

Lazaro C, Ravella A, Gaona A, Volpini V, and Estivill X. 1994. Neurofibromatosis type 1 due to germline mosaicism in a clinically normal father. *N Engl J Med* 331:1403–7.

Lazaro C, Gaona A, Ainsworth P, Tenconi R, Vidaud D, Kruyer H, Ars E, et al. 1996. Sex differences in mutational rate and mutational mechanism in the NF1 gene in neurofibromatosis type 1 patients. *Hum Genet* 98:696–9.

Ledbetter D, Rich D, O'Connell P, et al. 1989. Precise localization of NF1 to 17q11.2 by balanced translocation. *Am J Hum Genet* 44:20–5.

Legius E, Marchuk D, Collins F, and Glover T. 1993. Somatic deletion of the neurofibromatosis type 1 gene in a neurofibrosarcoma supports a tumour suppressor gene hypothesis. *Nat Genet* 3:122–6.

Legius E, Wu R, Eyssen M, Marynen P, Fryns JP, Cassiman JJ. 1995. Encephalocraniocutaneous lipomatosis with a mutation in the *NF1* gene. *J Med Genet* 32:316–9.

Li Y, O'Connell P, Huntsman Breidenbach H, et al. 1995. Genomic organization of the neurofibromatosis 1 gene *(NF1)*. *Genomics* 25:9–18.

Lloyd A. 1998. Ras versus cyclin-dependent kinase inhibitors. *Cur Opin Genet Dev* 8:43–8.

Lothe R, Karhu R, Mandahl N, Mertens F, Saeter G, Heim S, Borresen-Dale A, and Kallioniemi O. 1996. Gain of 17q24 to 17qter detected by comparative genomic hybridization in malignant tumors from pateints with von Recklinghausen's neurofibromatosis. *Cancer Res* 56:4778–81.

Lowy DR and Willumsen BM. 1993. Function and regulation of RAS. *Annu Rev Biochem* 62:851–91.

Marchuk D, Saulino A, Tavakkol R, et al. 1991. cDNA cloning of the type 1 neurofibromatosis gene: complete sequence of the NF1 gene product. *Genomics* 11:931–40.

Marshall CJ. 1996. Ras effectors. *Curr Opin Cell Biol* 8:197–204.

Martin G, Viskochil D, Bollag G, et al. 1990. The GAP-related domain of the NF1 gene product interacts with ras p21. *Cell* 63:843–9.

Martinsson T, Sjoberg R, Gedborg F, and Kogner P. 1997. Homozygous deletion of the neurofibromatosis-1 gene in the tumor of a patient with neuroblastoma. *Cancer Genet Cytogenet* 95:183–9.

Mayo M, Wang C-Y, Cogswell P, Rogers-Graham K, Lowe S, Der C, and Baldwin A. 1997. Requirement of NF-kappaBeta activation to suppress p53-independent apoptosis induced by oncogenic Ras. *Science* 278:1812–5.

Menon AG, Anderson KM, Riccardi VM, Chung RY, Whaley JM, et al. 1990. Chromosome 17p deletions and p53 gene mutations associated with the formation of malignant neurofibrosarcomas in von Recklinghausen neurofibromatosis. *Proc Natl Acad Sci USA* 87:5435–9.

Messiaen L, Callens T, De Paepe A, Craen M, and Mortier G. 1997. Characterization of two different nonsense mutations, C6792A and C6792G, causing skipping of exon 37 in the NF1 gene. *Hum Genet* 101:75–80.

Mikol D, Gulcher J, and Stefansson K. 1990. The oligodendrocyte myelin glycoprotein belongs to a distinct family of proteins and contains the HNK-1 carbohydrate. *J Cell Biol* 110:471–80.

Mulvihill JJ. 1994. Malignancy: epidemiologically associated cancers. In: Huson SM and Hughes RAC, eds. *The Neurofibromatoses: A Pathogenetic and Clinical Overview.* London: Chapman & Hall.

Nogales E, Wolf S, and Downing K. 1998. Structure of the alphabeta tubulin dimer by electron crystallography. *Nature* 391:199–203.

Nordlund, M, Gu X, Shipley M, and Ratner N. 1993. Neurofibromin is enriched in the endoplasmic reticulum of CNS neurons. *J Neurosci* 13:1588–1600.

O'Connell P, Leach R, Ledbetter D, et al. 1989. Fine structure mapping studies of the chromosomal region harboring the genetic defect in neurofibromatosis type1. *Am J Hum Genet* 44:51–7.

O'Connell P, Viskochil D, Buchberg A, et al. 1990. The human homologue of murine *evi-2* lies between two translocation breakpoints associated with von Recklinghausen neurofibromatosis. *Genomics* 7:547–54.

Pai E, Krengel U, Petsko G, Goody R, Kabsch W, and Wittinghofer A. 1990. Refined crystal structure of the triphosphate conformation of H-ras p21 at 1.35 A resolution: implications for the mechanism of GTP hydrolysis. *EMBO J* 9:2351–9.

Park VM and Pivnick EK. 1998. Neurofibromatosis type 1 (NF1): a protein truncation assay yielding identification of mutations in 73% of patients. *J Med Genet* 10:813–20.

Purandare S, Huntsman-Breidenbach H, Li Y, et al. 1995. Identification of neurofibromatosis 1 (*NF1*) homologous loci by direct sequencing, fluorescence in situ hybridization and PCR amplification of somatic cell hybrids. *Genomics* 30:476–85.

Purandare S, Ota A, Neil S, et al. 1996. Identification of *cis*-regulatory elements in the neurofibromatosis 1 gene. *Am J Hum Genet* 59:A157.

Regnier V, Meddeb M, Lecointre G, Richard F, Duverger A, Nguyen V, Dutrillaux B, Bernheim A, and Danglot G. 1997. Emergence and scattering of multiple neurofibromatosis (NF1)-related sequences during hominoid evolution suggest a process of pericentromeric interchromosomal transposition. *Hum Mol Genet* 6:9–16.

Rey I, Taylor-Harris P, van Erp H, and Hall A. 1994. R-ras interacts with rasGAP, neurofibromin and c-raf but does not regulate cell growth or differentiation. *Oncogene* 9:685–92.

Robinson PN, Buske A, Neumann R, Tinschert S, and Nurnberg P. 1996. Recurrent 2-bp deletion in exon 10c of the *NF1* gene in two cases of von Recklinghausen neurofibromatosis. *Hum Mutation* 7:85–8.

Rodenhiser D, Coulter-Mackie M, and Singh S. 1993. Evidence of DNA methylation in the neurofibromatosis type 1 (*NF1*) gene region of 17q11.2. *Hum Mol Genet* 2:439–44.

Roudebush M, Slabe T, Sundaram V, Hoppel C, Golubic M, and Stacey D. 1997. Neurofibromin colocalizes with mitochondria in cultured cells. *Exp Cell Res* 236:161–72.

Sawada S, Florell S, Purandare S, Ota M, Stephens K, and Viskochil D. 1996. Identification of NF1 mutations in both alleles of a dermal neurofibroma. *Nat Genet* 14:110–2.

Scheffzek K, Lautwein A, Kabsch W, Ahmadian M, and Wittinghofer A. 1996. Crystal structure of the GTPase-activating domain of human p120GAP and implications for the interaction with Ras. *Nature* 384:591–6.

Scheffzek K, Ahmadian M, Kabsch W, Wiesmuller L, Lautwein A, Schmitz F, and Wittinghofer A. 1997. The Ras-RasGAP complex: structural basis for GTPase activation and its loss in oncogenic ras mutants. *Science* 277:333–8.

Scheffzek K, Ahmadian M, Biesmuller L, Kabsch W, Stege P, Schmitz F, and Wittinghofer A. 1998. Structural analysis of the GAP-related domain from neurofibromin and its implications. *EMBO J* 17:4313–27.

Schmidt M, Michels V, and Dewald G. 1987. Cases of neurofibromatosis with rearrangements of chromosome 17 involving band 17q11.2. *Am J Med Genet* 28:771–5.

Serra E, Otero D, Gaona A, Kruyer H, Ars E, Estivill X, and Lazaro C. 1997. Confirmation of a double-hit model for the *NF1* gene in benign neurofibromas. *Am J Hum Genet* 61:512–9.

Shen MH and Upadhyaya M. 1993. A *de novo* nonsense mutation in exon 28 of the neurofibromatosis type 1 (*NF1*) gene. *Hum Genet* 92:410–2.

Shen MH, Harper PS, and Upadhyaya M. 1996. Moleuclar genetics of neurofibromatosis type 1 (NF1). *J Med Genet* 33:2–17.

Sherman L, Daston M, and Ratner N. 1998. Neurofibromin: distribution, cell biology, and role in neurofibromatosis type 1. In: Upadhyaya M and Cooper DN, eds. *Neurofibromatosis Type 1: From Genotype to Phenotype*. Oxford: Bios Scientific.

Side L, Taylor B, Cayoutte M, Connor E, Thompson P, Luce M, and Shannon K. 1997. Homozygous inactivation of NF1 in the bone marrows of children with neurofibromatosis type 1 and malignant myeloid disorders. *N Engl J Med* 336:1713–20.

Silva AJ, Frankland PW, Marowitz Z, Friedman E, Lazlo G, Cioffi D, Jacks T, and Bourtchuladze R. 1997. A mouse model for the learning and memory deficits associated with neurofibromatosis type I. *Nat Genet* 15:281–4.

Skuse G and Cappione A. 1997. RNA processing and clinical variability in neurofibromatosis type 1 (NF1). *Hum Mol Genet* 6:1707–12.

Skuse G, Kosciolek B, and Rowley P. 1990. Loss of heterozygosity in malignancies in von Recklinghausen neurofibromatosis: the allele remaining in the tumor is derived from the affected parent. *Am J Hum Genet* 49:600–7.

Stephens K, Kayes L, Riccardi V, Rising M, Sybert V, and Pagon R. 1992. Preferential mutation of the neurofibromatosis type 1 gene in paternally derived chromosomes. *Hum Genet* 88:279–82.

Sternberg PW and Alberola-Ila J. 1998. Conspiracy theory: RAS and RAF do not act alone. *Cell* 95:447–50.

Tanaka K, Nakafuku M, Satoh T, Marshall MS, Gibbs JB, Matsumoto K, Kaziro Y, Tassabehji M, Strachan T, Sharland M, Colley A, Donnai D, Harris R, and Thakker N. 1993. Tandem duplication within a neurofibromatosis type 1 (NF1) gene exon in a family with features of Watson syndrome and Noonan syndrome. *Am J Hum Genet* 53:90–5.

Tassabehji M, Strachan T, Sharland M, Colley A, Donnai D, Harris R, Thakker N. 1993. Tandem duplication within a neurofibromatosis type 1 (NF1) gene exon in a family with features of Watson syndrome and Noonan syndrome. *Am J Hum Genet* 53:90–5.

The I, Hannigan GE, Cowley GS, Reginald S, Zhong Y, Gusella JF, Hariharan IK, and Bernards A. 1997. Rescue of a *Drosophila* NF1 mutant phenotype by protein kinase A. *Science* 276:791–4.

Tonsgard J, Yelvarthi K, Cushner S, Short M, and Lindgren V. 1997. Do NF1 gene deletions result in a characteristic phenotype? *Am J Med Genet* 73:80–6.

Trahey M and McCormick F. 1987. A cytoplasmic protein stimulates normal N-ras p21 GTPase, but does not affect oncogenic mutants. *Science* 238:542–5.

Upadhyaya M and Cooper D. 1998. The mutational spectrum in neurofibromatosis 1 and its underlying mechanisms. In: Upadhyaya M and Cooper DN, eds. *Neurofibromatosis Type 1: From Genotype to Phenotype.* Oxford: Bios Scientific.

Upadhyaya M, Maynard J, Osborn M, Huson S, Ponder M, Ponder B, and Harper P. 1995. Characterization of germline mutations in the neurofibromatosis type 1 (NF1) gene. *J Med Genet* 32:706–10.

Viskochil D. 1998. Gene structure and expression. In: Upadhyaya M and Cooper DN, eds. *Neurofibromatosis Type 1: From Genotype to Phenotype.* Oxford: Bios Scientific.

Viskochil D and Carey J. 1992. Nosological considerations of the neurofibromatoses. *J Dermatol* 19(11):873–80.

Viskochil D, Buchberg A, Xu G, et al. 1990. Deletions and a translocation interrupt a cloned gene at the neurofibromatosis type 1 locus. *Cell* 62:187–92.

Viskochil D, Cawthon R, O'Connell P, et al. 1991. The gene encoding the oligodendrocyte-myelin glycoprotein is embedded within the neurofibromatosis type 1 gene. *Mol Cell Biol* 11:906–12.

Viskochil D, White R, and Cawthon R. 1993. The neurofibromatosis type 1 gene. *Annu Rev Neurosci* 16:183–205.

Vogel K, Brannan C, Jenkins N, Copeland N, and Parada L. 1995. Loss of neurofibromin results in neurotropin-independent survival of embryonic sensory and sympathetic neurons. *Cell* 82:733–42.

Wallace M, Marchuk D, Andersen L, et al. 1990. Type 1 neurofibromatosis gene: identification of a large transcript disrupted in three NF-1 patients. *Science* 249:181–6.

Wu B, Austin M, Schneider G, et al. 1995. Deletion of the entire *NF1* gene detected by FISH: four deletion patients associated with severe manifestations. *Am J Med Genet* 59:528–35.

Wu B-L, Boles R, Yaari H, Weremowicz S, Schneider G, and Korf B. 1997. Somatic mosaicism for deletion of the entire NF1 gene identidfied by FISH. *Hum Genet* 99:209–13.

Wu R, Legius E, Robberecht W, Dumoulin M, Cassiman J-J, and Fryns J-P. 1996. Neurofibromatosis type I gene mutation in a patient with features of LEOPARD syndrome. *Hum Mutat* 8:51–5.

Xu H and Gutmann D. 1997. Mutations in the GAP-related domain impair the ability of neurofibromin to associate with microtubules. *Brain Res* 759:149–52.

Xu G, Lin B, Tanaka K, et al. 1990b. The catalytic domain of the NF1 gene product stimulates ras GTPase and complements IRA mutants of *S. cerevisiae. Cell* 63:835–41.

Xu G, O'Connell P, Viskochil D, et al. 1990b. The neurofibromatosis type 1 gene encodes a protein related to GAP. *Cell* 62:599–608.

Xu W, Mulligan L, Ponder M, Liu L, Smith B, Mathew CGP, et al. 1992. Loss of *NF1* alleles in pheochromocytomas from patients with type 1 neurofibromatosis. *Genes Chromosomes Cancer* 4:337–42.

Yan N, Ricca C, Fletcher J, et al. 1995. Farnesyltransferase inhibitors block the neurofibromatosis type 1 (NF-1) malignant phenotype. *Cancer Res* 55:3569–75.

GLOSSARY

Alternative splicing   A nuclear process whereby the primary transcript is spliced differently from the most prevalent mRNA transcript. Usually, the resultant mRNA contains an open reading frame that encodes a functionally active protein.

CCAAT box   A genomic sequence involved in regulation of transcription that lies upstream of the promoter.

Centromere   The region of a chromosome that serves as a site of attachment for spindle fibers during cell division. Usually centromeres divide the chromosome into a short arm and a long arm.

Chemical mismatch cleavage   A method whereby double-stranded DNA with mismatched "bubbles" are cleaved by exposure to a chemical agent such as hydroxylamine (C or G) or osmium tetroxide (A or T).

***Cis*-acting element**   A genomic sequence that influences the transcription of a gene on the same DNA strand.

Contig   A set of clones containing overlapping DNA inserts that span a specified region of the genome.

Cosmid library   A large group of clones derived from a specific targeted genome or subset of genomic sequences that are contained in phage-plasmid hybrids capable of carrying DNA inserts of 40 to 50 kilobases.

CpG island   Unmethylated cytosine–guanine dinucleotide sequences that are often found near the promoter of genes.

Deletion constructs   Clones that harbor DNA segments that have various amounts of DNA deleted from the normal sequence.

Denaturing gradient-gel electrophoresis   A method of mutation detection in which DNA fragments are electrophoresed through a gel in which there is a changing denaturing factor, such as temperature.

Derivative translocation chromosome   The resultant abnormal chromosome that has been altered by a translocation of material from one chromosome to another.

Exon   Segment of a gene that encodes amino acids in cell translation. Exons are retained in mRNA after the primary transcript has been processed.

Gene conversion   A process whereby one gene is substituted with a homolog by mitotic recombination. Generally the normal allele is replaced by an inactive pseudogene to yield a different phenotype.

Genetic code   The combinations of mRNA codons that specify individual amino acids.

Genetic heterogeneity   Describes diseases in which mutations at distinct loci can produce the same disease phenotype.

Genetic mapping   The ordering of genes on chromosomes according to meiotic recombination frequency.

Heteroduplex analysis   An analysis to detect mismatched hybrid DNA strands between two alleles from a given individual after PCR amplification of target DNA product.

In-frame   An alteration of genomic DNA in a multiple of three resulting in an mRNA that maintains an open reading frame.

Intron   DNA sequence found between two exons. Introns are transcribed into primary mRNA but spliced out in the formation of mature mRNA.

Mosaicism   The existence of two or more genetically different cell lines in an individual.

Mutational "hot spots"   Sites of recurrent mutation in an encoded gene.

NF1-GRD   GAP-related domain of neurofibromin. This domain spans exons 21 through 27a and encodes a pepetide that activates the intrinsic GTPase of *ras.*

Northern blot analysis   A gene expression assay whereby mRNA is transferred from an electrophoresis gel to a membrane and particular mRNA transcripts are identified by size using specific DNA probes for hybridization.

Open reading frame   Stretches of genomic DNA in which the nucleotide sequence predicts possible peptide translation. An open reading frame consists of a series of sequential codons for tRNAs and ends with one or more "stop" codons that terminate translation.

Physical mapping   The determination of physical distances between genome "signposts" using cytogenetic and molecular techniques.

Polyadenylation   The process whereby a tract of adenosine residues is attached to a specified site in the noncoding region of the 3′ end of an mRNA transcript.

Polymerase chain reaction (PCR)   A technique for amplifying a large number of copies of a specific DNA sequence flanked by two oligonucleotide primers. The DNA is alternately heated and cooled in the presence of DNA polymerase and free nucleotides so that the specified DNA segment is denatured, hybridized, and extended by DNA polymerase.

Polymorphisms   A locus in which two or more alleles each have frequencies greater than 0.01 in a population. When this criterion is not fulfilled, the locus is monomorphic. Polymorphisms are usually identified as variations in DNA sequence using PCR or other methods.

Pseudogene   A gene that is highly similar in sequence to a gene at another locus but has been rendered transcriptionally or translationally inactive by mutations.

RT-PCR (reverse transcriptase–polymerase chain reaction)   A procedure in which an mRNA sequence is copied into DNA by reverse transcription and the resulting DNA sequence is amplified by PCR.

Single-strand conformation polymorphism (SSCP) analysis   A laboratory procedure in which an alteration in electrophoretic migration of a DNA strand is used to detect an underlying change in the nucleotide sequence.

Southern blot analysis   A laboratory procedure in which DNA fragments that have been electrophoresed through a gel are transferred to a solid membrane. The DNA blot is then hybridized with a specific labeled probe to detect the fragment sizes for the target DNA.

TATA box   Genomic sequence in the 5′ end of a gene that increases transcription of the gene.

Telomere   The tip of a chromosome, either the long arm or the short arm.

6

Neurofibromas and Malignant Tumors of the Peripheral Nerve Sheath

Bruce R. Korf, M.D., Ph.D.

The neurofibroma is the defining feature of NF1 and the source of much of the morbidity associated with the condition. Neurofibromas are complex tumors that arise from peripheral nerve sheaths. They include multiple cell types and may involve cutaneous, subcutaneous, or deep peripheral or cranial nerves. Sizes may range from a millimeter to tens of centimeters; they may be relatively inconspicuous or can cause major disfigurement. Neurofibromas are benign, but some may undergo transformation to malignant peripheral nerve sheath tumors. Other clinical problems associated with neurofibromas include localized or radicular pain and nerve compression.

von Recklinghausen (1882) first noted that neurofibromas arise from nerve sheaths. His clinical and pathologic description of neurofibromatosis is recognized in the eponym for the disorder, von Recklinghausen neurofibromatosis. In the century since von Recklinghausen's work, much has been added to our knowledge of the natural history of the disorder, now called NF1 (Stumpf et al. 1988). The cloning of the gene responsible for NF1 has resulted in insights into pathogenesis, which in turn has engendered hope that therapeutic agents will be developed to target the pathophysiologic mechanisms that lead to neurofibroma growth. This chapter will review the classification, natural history, and pathogenesis of neurofibromas and malignant peripheral nerve sheath tumors, pointing to areas for further study of natural history and possible opportunities for intervention.

DEFINITIONS AND CLASSIFICATION

Neurofibromas arise from cells in the peripheral nerve sheath and have defining pathologic features that will be described in detail below. Solitary neurofibromas may occur in an individual who does not have a germline NF1 mutation, but multiple neurofibromas tend to develop in persons with such a mutation. In these instances it is helpful to classify neurofibromas in clinical terms. In this chapter I

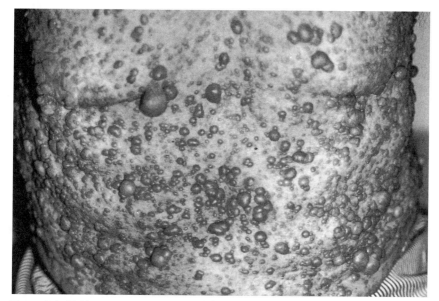

Figure 6-1. Multiple dermal neurofibromas seen on the chest of a patient with NF1.

will refer to two kinds of neurofibromas: discrete and plexiform.* A discrete neurofibroma arises from a single site along a peripheral nerve and presents as a focal mass with well-defined margins. Discrete neurofibromas may arise in or under the skin or may involve deeper peripheral nerves. A plexiform neurofibroma is a peripheral nerve sheath tumor that extends along the length of a nerve. Plexiform neurofibromas may involve multiple nerve fascicles or large branches of a major nerve. These, too, may occur superficially or deeper inside the body. Plexiform neurofibromas often are associated with soft tissue overgrowth and may cause disfigurement.

Both discrete and plexiform neurofibromas are histologically benign lesions. Malignant transformation results in the malignant peripheral nerve sheath tumor (MPNST). In the past these were sometimes referred to as neurofibrosarcomas or malignant schwannomas.

NATURAL HISTORY

DISCRETE NEUROFIBROMAS

Discrete neurofibromas may arise in the superficial dermis, within subcutaneous tissue, and along peripheral nerves that run under the skin or deeper inside the body. Cutaneous neurofibromas may protrude above the surface of the skin (Fig. 6-1), and in some cases may be pedunculated (Fig. 6-2). Alternatively, they may

---

*As discussed in chapter 2, discrete neurofibromas include cutaneous and subcutaneous neurofibromas and plexiform neurofibromas include nodular and diffuse plexiform neurofibromas.

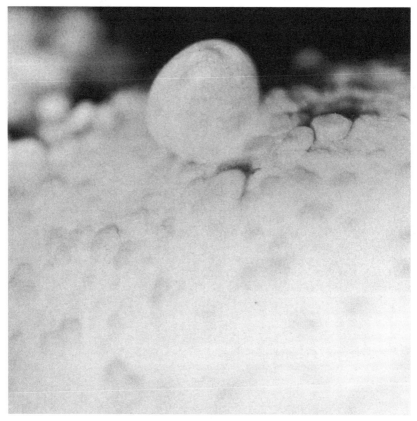

Figure 6-2. Pedunculated dermal neurofibroma.

appear as depressed areas with a violaceous hue in the overlying skin (Fig. 6-3). There may be a defect in the cutaneous connective tissue, so on palpation there is the feeling of placing the finger through a buttonhole ("buttonholing").

Much of the data on the natural history of discrete neurofibromas pertains to cutaneous tumors, which are most accessible to clinical observation. Thus neurofibromas are rarely, if ever, present at birth. Some may be present in early childhood, often seen best with side lighting. The number of dermal neurofibromas tends to increase with age, and varies widely from person to person. Huson et al. (1988) counted cutaneous neurofibromas in 122 individuals with NF1 whose ages ranged from less than 1 year to over 80. Cutaneous neurofibromas were seen in all patients over 16 years of age; the youngest patient found to have cutaneous tumors was 6 years old. Most of the tumors were present on the trunk, and only 17 of 94 patients had tumors on the head and neck. More than half of the subjects older than 30 years had more than 100 dermal tumors.

Neurofibromas often first appear around the time of puberty and may increase in size and number during pregnancy (Dugoff and Sujansky 1996; Huson et al.

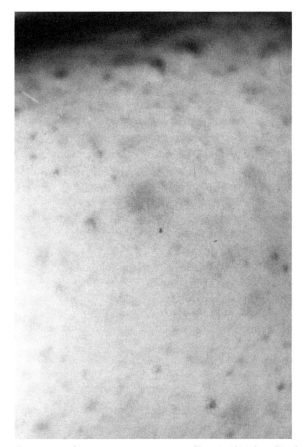

Figure 6-3. Close-up cutaneous neurofibroma showing discoloration of overlying skin.

1988). Cutaneous neurofibromas are usually not painful, although some individuals complain of itching (Riccardi 1981). The major burden imposed by these tumors is cosmetic. In some persons the presence of large numbers of cutaneous tumors can be disfiguring.

Cutaneous neurofibromas are usually soft to the touch and are easily compressible. In contrast, discrete neurofibromas that arise along peripheral nerves under the skin (see Fig. 2-5) tend to be firm to palpation. These subcutaneous neurofibromas may present clinically as beadlike nodules along the length of a nerve. They range in size from pea-sized to several centimeters. Some may be visible with side lighting, but others are only apparent on palpation. Discrete neurofibromas can occur along nerves deeper within the body. Tumors that arise from spinal nerve roots may grow through the neural foramen, assuming a dumb-bell shape (Fig. 6-4). These may cause nerve root compression or compression of the spinal cord. Nerve-root compression will lead to radicular symptoms, including pain, weakness, or sensory loss (Levy et al. 1986).

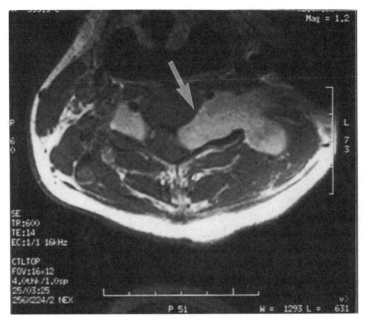

Figure 6-4. Spinal MRI showing neurofibroma of the nerve root that extends through the neural foramen (arrow).

PLEXIFORM NEUROFIBROMA

Plexiform neurofibromas are a major source of morbidity associated with NF1, due mainly to their tendency to grow to large sizes and cause disfigurement. They may extend for some distance along a nerve and can involve multiple nerve branches. Diffuse plexiform neurofibromas have a characteristic "bag of worms" feel on palpation. In classifying plexiform neurofibromas it may be helpful to divide them according to nerve of origin.

The cranial nerves most often involved in plexiform neurofibromas are the fifth, ninth, and tenth nerves. Fifth nerve lesions may extend anteriorly into the orbit (Fig. 6-5A) and may include the cavernous sinus. Orbital tumors are often associated with overgrowth of the upper eyelid and may cause proptosis (Fig. 6-5B) and glaucoma (Boltshauser et al. 1989; Ferguson and Kyle 1993; Jackson et al. 1993; Polito et al. 1993). There may be accompanying dysplasia of the greater wing of the sphenoid (Kjaer et al. 1997) (Fig. 6-5C). Plexiform neurofibromas of the second division of the trigeminal nerve may include the pterygopalatine ganglion, the maxillary region, and the upper gums (Fig. 6-6). Tumors of the third division lead to enlargement of the lower jaw, gums, and anterior two thirds of the tongue. Plexiform neurofibromas of the ninth or tenth nerves present as skull base or cervical masses (Chow et al. 1993; Yumoto et al. 1996). Tumors of the vagus nerve can extend into the mediastinum and even into the abdomen, sometimes following the entire course of this nerve (Fig. 6-7).

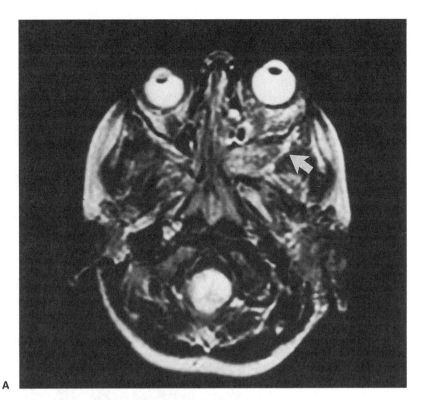

A

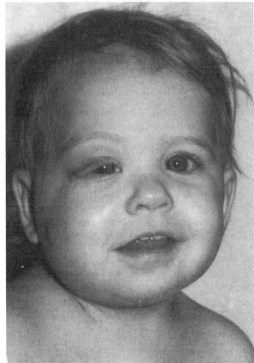

B

Figure 6-5. (A) MRI showing orbital plexiform neurofibroma (arrow); (B) overgrowth of the upper lid due to orbital plexiform neurofibroma.

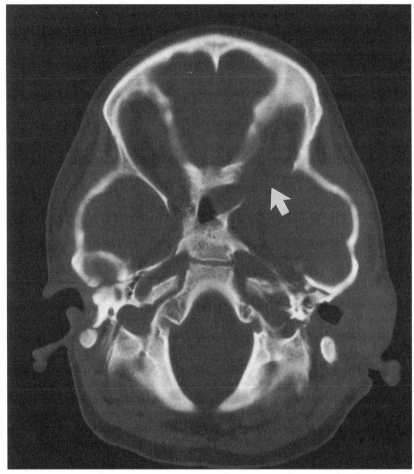

C

Figure 6-5. (C) CT scan showing sphenoid dysplasia (arrow).

Peripheral nerves may give rise to plexiform tumors at any point, from the nerve root to a small distal branch. Multiple root involvement may occur at any point in the spine (Fig. 6-9); individual root tumors may grow through the neural foramen, like discrete neurofibromas. Plexiform tumors can extend along an entire nerve plexus, such as the brachial or lumbar plexus (see Fig. 2-7; Fig. 6-9). These large tumors are often associated with overgrowth of a limb. More superficial plexiform neurofibromas are palpable and associated with thickening and hypertrophy of the skin (Fig. 6-10). Sometimes the skin overlying a plexiform neurofibroma displays hyperpigmentation resembling a large café-au-lait spot (Riccardi 1980, 1981) (see Fig. 2-9). This may be the only clinical sign of a plexiform tumor deep inside the body.

Diffuse plexiform neurofibromas that involve the skin usually become visible within the first 2 years of life. Rapid growth may ensue for the next several years

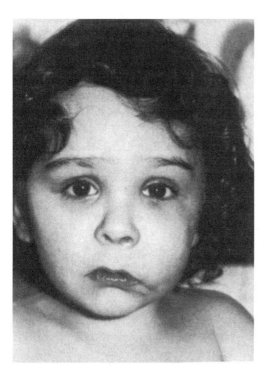

Figure 6-6. Soft-tissue expansion of the upper jaw and nasal region due to plexiform neurofibroma of the second division of the trigeminal nerve.

and then, in many cases, the tumor stabilizes. In some individuals tumor growth continues, or may stop and then resume later in life. Detailed information about the natural history of plexiform neurofibromas at different sites and different ages is much needed.

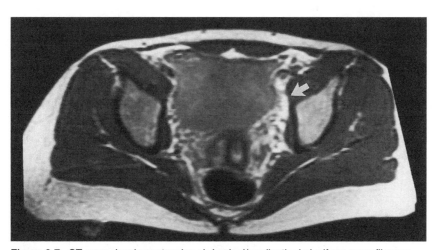

Figure 6-7. CT scan showing extensive abdominal/mediastinal plexiform neurofibroma arising from the vagus nerve.

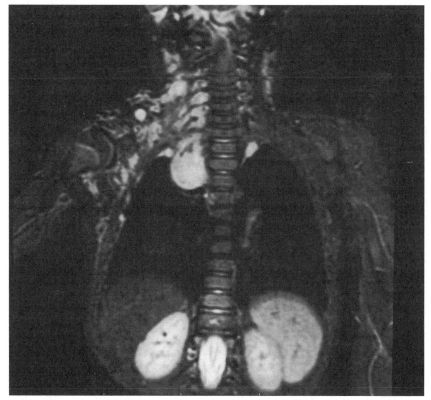

Figure 6-8. MRI showing paraspinal plexiform neurofibroma.

Plexiform neurofibromas occur commonly in individuals with NF1. Huson et al. (1988) identified plexiform neurofibromas on 26.7% of patients with NF1 in a population-based study in Wales. These included tumors on the trunk in 20 of 45 patients, the limbs in 17, and the head or neck in 8. Only 1.2% had significant facial involvement, however. This study identified only clinically apparent plexiform neurofibromas. Studies based on imaging were reported by Tonsgard et al. (1996) and Schorry et al. (1997). The former reported neurofibromas of the chest in 20% of 126 individuals with NF1 aged 16 years or older and tumors of the abdomen or pelvis in 44%. Schorry et al. found nine thoracic tumors in a group of 260 children with NF1. One was a malignant peripheral nerve sheath tumor, but the others were either confirmed (four) or suspected (four) plexiform neurofibromas. Three patients displayed symptoms. These two studies indicate that internal plexiform neurofibromas are common and often are unsuspected clinically. As will be discussed in detail below, this does not imply that routine screening is clinically indicated, however, since many plexiform neurofibromas remain asymptomatic.

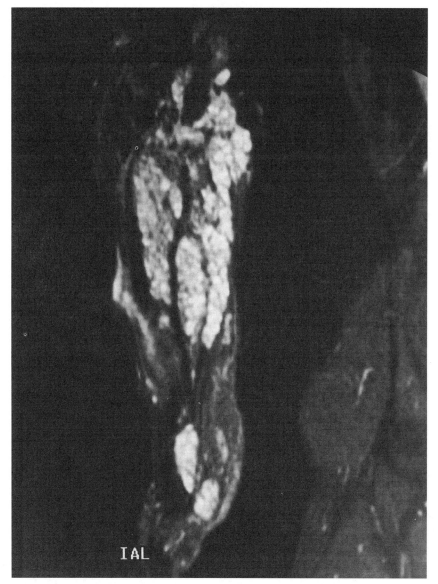

Figure 6-9. MRI showing brachial plexiform neurofibroma extending into arm.

MALIGNANT PERIPHERAL NERVE SHEATH TUMOR

MPNST is a histologically malignant tumor that arises from the peripheral nerve sheath. Like the neurofibroma, this tumor type can occur in the general population but is seen much more commonly in persons with NF1. Dermal tumors, in spite of being present in large numbers, rarely if ever become malignant. Preexisting plex-

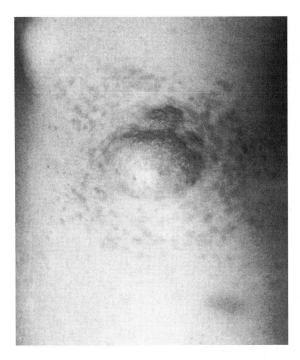

Figure 6-10. Superficial cutaneous plexiform neurofibroma.

iform neurofibromas appear to be the most common precursor to MPNST in persons with NF1. The most important clinical sign of malignant change is the occurrence of unexplained pain. Superficial plexiform neurofibromas may become painful when subjected to minor trauma, but this pain tends to subside within hours to days. Persistent unexplained pain should be investigated as a sign of possible malignant change. Often the pain will be accompanied by growth of a portion of the tumor and a change in consistency from soft to firm. Deeper MPNST can be insidious, however, and may present only with unexplained pain. The clinician should be alert to the possibility of radicular pain, in which the tumor may be located at a nerve root rather than at the apparent site of discomfort. The lifetime risk of MPNST appears to be in the range of 4 to 5% (D'Agostino et al. 1963; Ducatman et al. 1986). The lungs are the most common site of metastasis, although other sites include bone, liver, abdominal cavity, adrenal glands, diaphragm, mediastinum, brain, ovaries, kidneys, and retroperitoneum. Treatment of MPNST will be considered in the section on management below.

PATHOLOGY AND PATHOGENESIS

Neurofibromas are multicellular lesions derived from the nerve sheath. In contrast with schwannomas, in which axons are displaced by the mass of proliferated nerve sheath, in neurofibromas the axons pass through the lesion. There is a proliferation of spindle-shaped cells consisting of Schwann cells and/or perineural fibroblasts (Fisher and Vuzevski 1968; Hirose and Hizawa 1986; Pelto-nen et al. 1988; Stefansson et al. 1982) (Fig. 6-11). Other cellular components are mast cells (Carr and Warren 1993; Nurnberger and Moll 1994; Riccardi 1990) and axons. There is a large amount of extracellular matrix (Penfield 1932) and collagen (Peltonen et al. 1988). Plexiform neurofibromas are usually associ-ated with extensive vascular supplies. MPNST have classical features of anapla-sia (Fig. 6-12), but may also include regions of neurofibroma, suggesting a pre-existing benign lesion as the origin.

The multicellular composition of neurofibromas has presented a major chal-lenge in studies of pathogenesis. Early analysis of clonality gave results indica-tive of a polyclonal composition (Fialkow et al. 1971), but these studies may have been handicapped by admixture of tumor and nontumor cells. Cell admix-ture has also made it difficult to test the possibility that the *NF1* gene functions as a tumor suppressor. No loss of *NF1* heterozygosity was found in benign neu-rofibromas studied by Skuse et al. (1989), Menon et al. (1990), Shimizu et al. (1993), and Lothe et al. (1993). In contrast, Colman et al. (1995) found evidence for loss of heterozygosity of *NF1* in 2 of 5 neurofibromas and Serra et al. (1997) found loss of heterozygosity in 15 of 60 neurofibromas. Direct evidence in sup-port of the tumor-suppressor hypothesis has been provided by Sawada et al. (1996), who identified a point mutation in a dermal neurofibroma from a patient with NF1 whose germline mutation was a complete gene deletion.

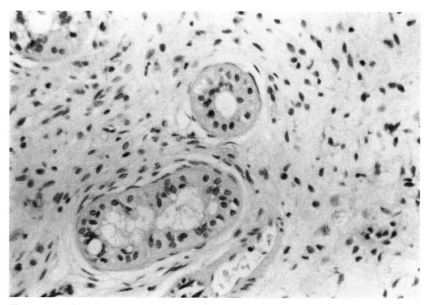

Figure 6-11. Photomicrograph of neurofibroma, showing loosely packed spindle-shaped nuclei and abundant extracellular matrix. Three blood vessels are shown at the center. *Source:* Courtesy of Dr. Antonio Perez-Atayde, Department of Pathology, Children's Hospi-tal, Boston.

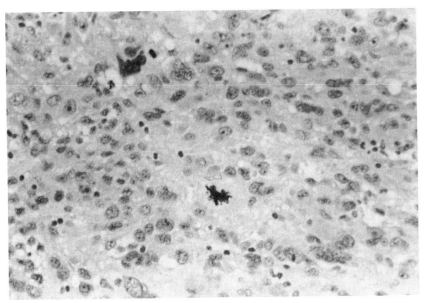

Figure 6-12. Photomicrograph of MPNST, with dense cellularity and a prominent mitotic figure. *Source:* Courtesy of Dr. Antonio Perez-Atayde, Department of Pathology, Children's Hospital, Boston.

Animal studies have also produced data in support of the tumor-suppressor hypothesis for NF1. In mice heterozygous for an *NF1* knockout a neurofibromatosis-like phenotype does not develop, but malignancies do develop, especially leukemias, later in life (Brannan et al. 1994; Jacks et al. 1994). In animals chimeric for homozygous *Nf1 –/–* cells, however, plexiform neurofibromas do develop (Cichowski et al. 1996). This suggests that loss of *NF1* activity is rate limiting for the formation of neurofibromas. The possibility remains, however, that genetic changes at other loci are also required.

The mechanisms whereby loss of *NF1* function leads to formation of neurofibromas remain unknown. The *NF1* gene product is a 2818 amino acid protein with a GTPase-activating protein (GAP) catalytic domain (Ballester et al. 1990; Buchberg et al. 1990; Martin et al. 1990; Xu et al. 1990a, 1990b). Elevated levels of p21 *ras*–GTP have been demonstrated in neurofibromas (Guha et al. 1996, 1998). Studies of fibroblasts and Schwann cells from *Nf1 –/–* mice have revealed phenotypic abnormalities. *Nf1* null fibroblasts proliferate at an increased rate and do not form normal perineurium (Rosenbaum et al. 1995), whereas *Nf1* null Schwann cells reveal abnormalities of proliferation and differentiation (Kim et al. 1995, 1996).

The proliferation of a mixed cell population in neurofibromas suggests the possibility that some of the cell proliferation is due to the presence of mitogens.

HGF (Krasnoselsky et al. 1994), bFGF (Ratner et al. 1990), and IGF-2 (Hansson et al. 1988) have been identified in neurofibromas. Mast cells in neurofibromas have been suggested as one possible source of mitogens (Riccardi 1990). The fact that neurofibroma growth and enlargement occur during puberty and pregnancy may also indicate that hormonal factors play a role. Martuza et al. (1981) found estrogen receptors in one of six neurofibromas, although no evidence for estrogen, progesterone, androgen, or glucocorticoid receptors was seen in any of five neurofibromas in another study (Chaudhuri et al. 1982).

Likewise, the factors that determine the overall number of neurofibromas are unknown. Easton et al. (1993) presented evidence that genetic background may influence numbers of dermal neurofibromas, but not the presence of plexiform neurofibromas. The role of different *NF1* germline mutations has not been explored, with the exception that complete deletion of the *NF1* gene is associated with a distinctive phenotype that includes early onset and the development of large numbers of neurofibromas (Kayes et al. 1994; Leppig et al. 1996; Upadhyaya et al. 1998; Wu et al. 1995). This may be due to complete loss of expression of *NF1* or to loss of expression of one or more contiguous genes.

The factors responsible for malignant transformation to MPNST also remain unknown. MPNSTs have been shown to have loss of heterozygosity for *NF1* and increased levels of p21 *ras*–GTP (Basu et al. 1992; DeClue et al. 1992; Glover et al. 1991; Skuse et al. 1990). It is not clear, however, whether loss of *NF1* activity contributes to the malignant phenotype, or if it is present in the benign neurofibromas prior to malignant transformation. McCarron and Goldblum (1998) found expression of p53 in MPNST but not plexiform neurofibromas. It seems likely that genetic changes of other oncogenes occur in association with the transformation into MPNST and further progression of these malignancies.

MANAGEMENT

No medical treatment is currently available to prevent the growth or reduce the size of neurofibromas. Treatment is currently limited to surgery, although controversy exists about the ideal timing of surgery and about the proper surgical approach.

DISCRETE NEUROFIBROMA

Indications for surgery generally are cosmesis or the presence of discomfort. Dermal neurofibromas are most commonly removed by plastic surgery, but the CO_2 laser has also been used (Becker 1991; Roenigk and Ratz 1987). Laser treatment involves vaporization of the dermal tumor and can be used to remove hundreds of tumors in a single session. There may be a more visible scar than would result from the best outcome of plastic surgery, but surgical treatment of hundreds of tumors at a time may not be practical. So far, however, there have been no large studies of the efficacy and long-term outcome of laser treatments for dermal neurofibromas. Discrete neurofibromas may grow back following surgery, although for individuals with very large tumor burdens it is difficult to distinguish regrowth of an original lesion from the appearance of a new tumor at or near the surgical site.

PLEXIFORM NEUROFIBROMA

Surgery for plexiform neurofibromas is made challenging by the fact that tumors may be large, irregular in shape, highly vascular, and difficult to dissect free from surrounding tissues. These factors make it essentially impossible to completely resect most plexiform neurofibromas. The variable natural history further complicates matters. Small lesions might be most amenable to surgery, but it is difficult to justify surgery if one cannot be sure whether a small tumor will grow. Early and aggressive treatment of orbital plexiform neurofibromas has been advocated (Jackson et al. 1993), but no systematic study of outcomes has been performed. Needle et al. (1997) reviewed outcomes in 121 individuals with NF1 who had plexiform neurofibromas treated surgically. After a median follow-up period of 6.8 years (range, 2 months to 24.5 years), 94 of 168 (56%) tumors did not progress after surgery. Risk factors for progression included age at surgery of less than 10 years and the presence of residual tumor after surgery. Seppala et al. (1995) reported outcomes after surgery in 32 patients with spinal neurofibromas, of whom 22 had NF1. Recurrence of spinal tumors was noted in three patients, two of whom were children. Artico et al. (1997) reported that subtotal resection of plexiform neurofibromas resulted in improvement in 20% of cases. The use of preoperative embolization of feeding vessels has been suggested (Littlewood and Stilwell 1983), but there are few published data on the efficacy of this approach.

MPNST

MPNSTs are lethal if left untreated. Diagnosis, however, may pose a major challenge in persons with NF1. Delay in diagnosis may lead to widespread metastatic disease that is untreatable, but early diagnosis is hampered by the fact that an affected individual may have multiple benign tumors in which some degree of growth occurs commonly. This can make it difficult to detect malignant change in a single tumor. Moreover, only a small portion of a large plexiform neurofibroma may undergo malignant change, making it difficult to diagnosis the malignancy even if a biopsy is performed.

Persons with NF1 should be educated to be alert to unexplained pain or changes in growth patterns of their tumors, particularly large plexiform neurofibromas. Such signs or symptoms are usually investigated by MRI, looking for regions displaying signs of necrosis or unusual appearance. Suspicious areas may be biopsied, but there is a possibility of false negative results due to the large size of some plexiform tumors. Therefore, if a biopsy fails to reveal malignancy but pain or tumor growth continues, close clinical and radiographic monitoring should ensue, and a repeat biopsy should be considered.

The mainstay of treatment is surgical resection, but both radiation and chemotherapy have been used in efforts to improve survival, especially if metastatic disease is present. Numerous studies performed over the years have compared outcomes of treatment of MPNSTs in individuals with or without NF1

(Aguiar Vitacca et al. 1992; Doorn et al. 1995; Ghosh et al. 1973; Hruban et al. 1990; Raney et al. 1987; Sordillo et al. 1981; Storm et al. 1980; Wanebo et al. 1993; White 1971). There is no solid evidence that outcomes in individuals with NF1 are consistently different from those without NF1. Survival is best for those patients whose tumors can be completely resected, with little demonstrated benefit of radiation or chemotherapy over surgery. Adjuvant radiation or chemotherapy tend to be given if the tumor cannot be completely removed (Brennan et al. 1991; Williard et al. 1992). Diagnosis and management of MPNSTs present some of the most significant clinical challenges in the care of persons with NF1 and are best done at a tertiary medical center where medical personnel have experience with this problem.

FUTURE PROSPECTS

The long-term hope is that medical treatment will be developed for neurofibromas. Riccardi (1993) conducted a trial of the mast-cell inhibitor ketotifen, including an open-label trial with 25 patients and a double-blind protocol with 27 patients. This drug was chosen based on the hypothesis that mast cells present in neurofibromas might contribute to the growth of the tumors, perhaps via secretion of growth factors. Both groups treated with ketotifen reported a decrease in itching, pain, and tenderness of neurofibromas. Although a decrease in tumor size was reported by some patients, objective data in support of tumor regression have not been presented.

A new generation of chemotherapeutic agents is now in developn.ent. These include drugs that inhibit growth of blood vessels (Folkman 1995) a. well as agents that target intracellular pathways involving dominant or recessiv. oncogenes. The association of neurofibromin with p21-ras make inhibitors of tι.∍ enzyme farnesyl protein transferase (Yan et al. 1995) particularly attractive ca.٦didates for chemotherapy trials. Although these drugs are being developed ι ٦r treatment of malignant tumors, it is likely that opportunities will arise to tesι their effectiveness on benign or malignant tumors in NF1 as well. Treatment trials will require a new approach to measurement of the size of neurofibromas, such as can be obtained with volumetric MRI (Nelson et al. 1997). Additional data will also be required about the natural history of neurofibromas, including rates of growth and frequency of spontaneous remission of growth, so the efficacy of treatment can be judged objectively. Despite these challenges, however, there is optimism for the first time since the description of neurofibromas by von Recklinghausen that rationally designed drug regimens may supplant the era of symptomatic treatment.

REFERENCES

Aguiar Vitacca S, Sarrazin D, Henry-Amar M, et al. 1992. Neurosarcome associe a une maladie de Von Recklinghausen: a propos de 25 cas observes a l'Institue Gustave-Roussy de 1967 a 1990. *Bull Cancer* 79:101–12.

Artico M, Cervoni L, Wierzbicki V, D'Andrea V, and Nuci F. 1997. Benign neural sheath tumours of major nerves: characteristics in 119 surgical cases. *Acta Neurochir (Wien)* 139:1108–16.

Ballester R, Marchuk D, Boguski M, et al. 1990. The *NF1* locus encodes a protein functionally related to mammalian GAP and yeast *IRA* proteins. *Cell* 63:851–9.

Basu TN, Gutmann DH, Fletcher JA, Glover TW, Collins FS, and Downward J. 1992. Aberrant regulation of *ras* proteins in malignant tumour cells from type 1 neurofibromatosis patients. *Nature* 356:713–5.

Becker DW. 1991. Use of the carbon dioxide laser in treating multiple cutaneous neurofibromas. *Ann Plast Surg* 26:582–6.

Boltshauser E, Stocker H, Sailer H, and Valavanis A. 1989. Intracranial abnormalities associated with facial plexiform neurofibromas in neurofibromatosis type 1. *Neurofibromatosis* 2:274–7.

Brannan CI, Perkins AS, Vogel KS, et al. 1994. Targeted disruption of the neurofibromatosis type-1 gene leads to developmental abnormalities in heart and various neural crest-derived tissues. *Genes Dev* 8:1019–29.

Brennan MF, Casper ES, Harrison LB, Shiu MH, Gaynor J, and Hajdu SI. 1991. The role of multimodality therapy in soft-tissue sarcoma. *Ann Surg* 214:328–36.

Buchberg AM, Cleveland LS, Jenkins NA, and Copeland NG. 1990. Sequence homology shared by neurofibromatosis type-1 gene and *IRA-1* and *IRA-2* negative regulators of the *RAS* cyclic AMP pathway. *Nature* 347:291–4.

Carr NJ and Warren AY. 1993. Mast cell numbers in melanocytic naevi and cutaneous neurofibromas. *J Clin Pathol* 46:86–7.

Chaudhuri PK, Walker MJ, Das Gupta TK, and Beattie CW. 1982. Steroid receptors in tumors of nerve sheath origin. *J Surg Oncol* 20:205–6.

Chow LT, Shum BS, and Chow WH. 1993. Intrathoracic vagus nerve neurofibroma and sudden death in a patient with neurofibromatosis. *Thorax* 48:298–9.

Cichowski K, Shih TS, and Jacks T. 1996. Nf1 gene targeting: toward models and mechanisms. *Semin Cancer Biol* 7:291–8.

Colman SD, Williams CA, and Wallace MR. 1995. Benign neurofibromas in type 1 neurofibromatosis (NF1) show somatic deletions of the *NF1* gene. *Nat Genet* 11:90–2.

D'Agostino AN, Soule EH, and Miller RH. 1963. Sarcomas of the peripheral nerves and somatic soft tissues associated with multiple neurofibromatosis (von Recklinghausen's disease). *Cancer* 16:1015–27.

DeClue JE, Papageorge AG, Fletcher JA, et al. 1992. Abnormal regulation of mammalian $p21^{ras}$ contributes to malignant tumor growth in von Recklinghausen (type 1) neurofibromatosis. *Cell* 69:265–73.

Doorn PF, Molenaar WM, Buter J, and Hoekstra HJ. 1995. Malignant peripheral nerve sheath tumors in patients with and without neurofibromatosis. *Eur J Surg Oncol* 21:78–82.

Ducatman BS, Scheithauer BW, Piepgras DG, Reiman HM, and Ilstrup DM. 1986. Malignant peripheral nerve sheath tumors. *Cancer* 57:2006–21.

Dugoff L and Sujansky E. 1996. Neurofibromatosis type 1 and pregnancy. *Am J Med Genet* 66:7–10.

Easton DF, Ponder MA, Huson SM, and Ponder BAJ. 1993. An analysis of variation in expression of neurofibromatosis (NF) type 1 (NF1): evidence for modifying genes. *Am J Hum Genet* 53:305–13.

Ferguson VMG and Kyle PM. 1993. Orbital plexiform neurofibroma. *Br J Ophthalmol* 77:527–8.

Fialkow PJ, Sagebiel RW, Gartler SM, and Rimoin DL. 1971. Multiple cell origin of hereditary neurofibromas. *N Engl J Med* 284:298–300.

Fisher ER and Vuzevski VD. 1968. Cytogenesis of schwannoma (neurilemmoma), neurofibroma, dermatofibroma, and dermatofibrosarcoma as revealed by electron microscopy. *Am J Clin Pathol* 49:141–54.

Folkman J. 1995. Angiogenesis in cancer, vascular, rheumatoid and other disease. *Nat Med* 1:27–31.

Ghosh BC, Ghosh L, Huvos AG, and Fortner JG. 1973. Malignant schwannoma: a clinicopathologic study. *Cancer* 31:184–90.

Glover TW, Stein CK, Legius E, Andersen LB, Brereton A, and Johnson S. 1991. Molecular and cytogenetic analysis of tumors in von Recklinghausen neurofibromatosis. *Genes Chromosomes Cancer* 3:62.

Guha A. 1998. Ras activation in astrocytomas and neurofibromas. *Can J Neurol Sci* 25:267–81.

Guha A, Lau N, Huvar I, et al. 1996. Ras-GTP levels are elevated in human NF1 peripheral nerve tumors. *Oncogene* 12:507–13.

Hansson HA, Lauritzen C, Lossing C, and Petruson K. 1988. Somatomedin C as a tentative pathogenic factor in neurofibromatosis. *Scand J Plast Reconstr Surg* 22:7–13.

Hirose T and Hizawa K. 1986. Ultrastructural localization of S-100 protein in neurofibroma. *Acta Neuropathol (Berl)* 69:103–10.

Hruban RH, Shiu MH, Senie RT, and Woodruff JM. 1990. Malignant peripheral nerve sheath tumors of the buttock and lower extremity. *Cancer* 66:1253–65.

Huson SM, Harper PS, and Compston DAS. 1988. von Recklinghausen neurofibromatosis. A clinical and population study in south-east Wales. *Brain* 111:1355–81.

Jacks T, Shih TS, Schmitt EM, Bronson RT, Bernards A, and Weinberg RA. 1994. Tumour predisposition in mice heterozygous for a targeted mutation in NF1. *Nat Genet* 7:353–61.

Jackson IT, Carbonnel A, Potparic Z, and Shaw K. 1993. Orbitotemporal neurofibromatosis: classification and treatment. *Plast Reconstr Surg* 92:1–11.

Kayes LM, Burke W, Riccardi VM, Bennett R, Ehrlich P, and Rubenstein AS. 1994. Deletions spanning the neurofibromatosis 1 gene: identification and phenotype of five patients. *Am J Hum Genet* 54:424–36.

Kim H, Ling B, and Ratner N. 1997. NF1-deficient mouse Schwann cells are angiogenic, invasive and can be induced to hyperproliferate: reversion of some phenotypes by an inhibitor of farnesyl protein transferase. *Mol Cell Biol* 17:862–72.

Kim HA, Rosenbaum T, Marchionni MA, Ratner N, and DeClue JE. 1995. Schwann cells from neurofibromin deficient mice exhibit activation of $p21^{ras}$, inhibition of cell proliferation and morphological changes. *Oncogene* 11:325–35.

Kjaer I, Keeling JW, and Fischer H. 1997. Pattern of malformations in the axial skeleton in human trisomy 13 fetuses. *Am J Med Genet* 70:421–6.

Krasnoselsky A, Massay MJ, DeFrances MC, Michalopoulos G, Zarnegar R, and Ratner N. 1994. Hepatocyte growth factor is a mitogen for Schwann cells and is present in neurofibromas. *J Neurosci* 14:7284–90.

Leppig KA, Viskochil D, Neil S, et al. 1996. The detection of contiguous gene deletions at the neurofibromatosis 1 locus with fluorescence in situ hybridization. *Cytogenet Cell Genet* 72:95–8.

Levy WJ, Latchaw J, Hahn JF, Sawhny B, Bay J, and Dohn DF. 1986. Spinal neurofibromas: A report of 66 cases and a comparison with meningiomas. *Neurosurgery* 18:331–4.

Littlewood AH and Stilwell JH. 1983. The vascular features of plexiform neurofibroma with some observations on the importance of pre-operative angiography and the value of pre-operative intra-arterial embolisation. *Br J Plast Surg* 36:501–6.

Lothe RA, Saeter G, Danielsen HE, Stenwig AE, Hoyheim B, and O'Connell P. 1993. Genetic alterations in a malignant schwannoma from a patient with neurofibromatosis (NF1). *Pathol Res Pract* 189:465–71.

McCarron KF and Goldblum JR. 1998. Plexiform neurofibroma with and without associated malignant peripheral nerve sheath tumor: a clinicopathological and immunohistochemical analysis of 54 cases. *Mod Pathol* 11:612–7.

Martin GA, Viskochil D, Bollag G, et al. 1990. The GAP-related domain of the neurofi-bromatosis type 1 gene product interacts with ras p21. *Cell* 63:843–9.

Martuza RL, Maclaughlin DT, and Ojemann RG. 1981. Specific estradiol binding in schwannomas, meningiomas, and neurofibromas. *Neurosurgery* 9:665–71.

Menon AG, Anderson KM, Riccardi VM, et al. 1990. Chromosome 17p deletions and p53 gene mutations associated with the formation of malignant neurofibrosarcomas in von Recklinghausen neurofibromatosis. *Proc Natl Acad Sci USA* 87:5435–9.

Needle MN, Cnaan A, Dattilo J, et al. 1997. Prognostic signs in the surgical management of plexiform neurofibroma: the Children's Hospital of Philadelphia experience, 1974–1994. *J Pediatrics* 131:678–82.

Nelson SJ, Huhn S, Vigneron DB, et al. 1997. Volume MRI and MRSI techniques for the quantitation of treatment response in brain tumors: presentation of a detailed case study. *J Magn Reson Imaging* 7:1146–52.

Nurnberger M and Moll I. 1994. Semiquantitative aspects of mast cells in normal skin and in neurofibromas of neurofibromatosis types 1 and 5. *Dermatology* 188:296–9.

Peltonen J, Jaakkola S, Lebwohl M, et al. 1988. Cellular differentiation and expression of matrix genes in type 1 neurofibromatosis. *Lab Invest* 59:760–71.

Penfield W. 1932. Tumors of the sheaths of the nervous system. *Arch Neurol* 27:1298–1309.

Polito E, Leccisotti A, and Frezzotti R. 1993. Cosmetic possibilities and problems in eye-lid neurofibromas. *Ophthalmic Paediatr Genet* 14:43–50.

Raney B, Schnaufer L, Ziegler M, Chatten J, Littman P, and Jarrett P. 1987. Treatment of children with neurogenic sarcoma. *Cancer* 59:1–5.

Ratner N, Lieberman MA, Riccardi VM, and Hong D. 1990. Mitogen accumulation in von Recklinghausen neurofibromatosis. *Ann Neurol* 27:298–303.

Riccardi VM. 1980. Pathophysiology of neurofibromatosis. V. Dermatologic insights into heterogeneity and pathogenesis. *J Am Acad Dermatol* 3:157–66.

———. 1981. Cutaneous manifestation of neurofibromatosis: cellular interaction, pig-mentation, and mast cells. *Birth Defects: Original Article Series,* vol. 17, no. XX. New York: Liss, pp. 29–45.

———. 1990. The potential role of trauma and mast cells in the pathogenesis of neurofi-bromas. In Ishibashi Y and Hori Y, ed. *Tuberous Sclerosis and Neurofibromatosis: Epidemiology, Pathophysiology, Diagnosis, and Management.* Amsterdam Elsevier, pp. 167–90.

———. 1993. A controlled multiphase trial of ketotifen to minimize neurofibroma-associated pain and itching. *Arch Dermatol* 129:577–81.

Roenigk RK and Ratz JL. 1987. CO2 laser treatment of cutaneous neurofibromas. *Dermatol Surg Oncol* 13:187–90.

Rosenbaum T, Boissy YL, Kombrinck K, et al. 1995. Neurofibromin-deficient fibroblasts fail to form perineurium in vitro. *Development* 121:3583–92.

Sawada S, Florell S, Purandare SM, Ota M, Stephens K, and Viskochil D. 1996. Identifi-cation of *NF1* mutations in both alleles of a dermal neurofibroma. *Nat Genet* 14:110–2.

Schorry EK, Crawford AH, Egelhoff JC, Lovell AM, and Saal HM. 1997. Thoracic tu-mors in children with neurofibromatosis-1. *Am J Med Genet* 74:533–37.

Seppala MT, Haltia MJ, Sankila RJ, Jaaskelainen JE, and Heiskanen O. 1995. Long-term outcome after removal of spinal neurofibroma. *J Neurosurg* 82:572–7.

Serra E, Otero D, Gaona A, Kruyer H, Ars E, Estivill X, and Lazaro C. 1997. Confirma-tion of a double-hit model for the NF1 gene in benign neurofibromas. *Am J Hum Genet* 61:512–9.

Shimizu E, Shinohara T, Mori N, et al. 1993. Loss of heterozygosity on chromosome arm 17p in small cell lung carcinomas, but not in neurofibromas, in a patient with von Recklinghausen neurofibromatosis. *Cancer* 71:725–8.

Skuse GR, Kosciolek BA, and Rowley PT. 1989. Molecular genetic analysis of tumors in von Recklinghausen neurofibromatosis: loss of heterozygosity for chromosome 17. *Genes Chromosomes Cancer* 1:36–41.

————. 1990. Loss of heterozygosity in malignancies in von Recklinghausen neurofibromatosis: the allele remaining in the tumor is derived from the affected parent. *Am J Hum Genet* 49:600–7.

Sordillo PP, Helson L, and Kajdus SI. 1981. Malignant schwannoma: clinical characteristics, survival, and response to therapy. *Cancer* 47:2503–9.

Stefansson K, Wollmann R, and Jerkovic M. 1982. S-100 protein in soft tissue tumours derived from Schwann cells and melanocytes. *Am J Pathol* 106:261–8.

Storm FK, Eilber FR, Mirra J, and Morton DL. 1980. Neurofibrosarcoma. *Cancer* 45:126–9.

Stumpf DA, Alksne JF, Annegers JF, et al. 1988. Neurofibromataosis. *Arch Neurol* 45:575–8.

Tonsgard JH, Short MP, Kwak S, and Dachman A. 1996. Computed tomographic imaging in neurofibromatosis. *Ann Neurol* 40:278–8.

Upadhyaya M, Ruggieri M, Maynard J, Osborn M, Hartog C, Mudd S, Penttinen M, Cordeiro I, Ponder M, Krawczak M, and Cooper DN. 1998. Gross deletions of the neurofibromatosis type 1 (NF1) gene are predominantly of maternal origin and commonly associated with a learning disability, dysmorphic features and developmental delay. *Hum Genet* 102:591–7.

von Recklinghausen FD. 1882. *Ueber die multiplen Fibrome der Haut und ihre Beiehung zu den multiplen Neuromen.* Berlin: August Hirschwald.

Wanebo JE, Malik JM, VandenBerg SR, Wanebo HJ, Driesen N, and Persing JA. 1993. Malignant peripheral nerve sheath tumors: a clinicopathologic study of 28 cases. *Cancer* 71:1247–53.

White HR. 1971. Survival in malignant schwannoma: an 18-year study. *Cancer* 27:720–9.

Williard WC, Collin C, Casper EC, Hajdu SI, and Brennan MF. 1992. The changing role of amputation for soft tissue sarcoma of the extremity in adults. *Surg Gynecol Obstet* 175:389–96.

Wu BL, Austin MA, Schneider GH, Boles RG, and Korf BR. 1995. Deletion of the entire *NF1* gene detected by FISH: four deletion patients associated with severe manifestations. *Am J Med Genet* 59:528–35.

Xu G, Lin B, Tanak K, et al. 1990a. The catalytic domain of the neurofibromatosis type 1 gene product stimulates ras GTPase and complements ira mutants of *S. cerevisiae.* *Cell* 63(4):835–41.

Xu G, O'Connell P, Viskochil D, et al. 1990b. The neurofibromatosis type 1 gene encodes a protein related to GAP. *Cell* 62:599–608.

Yan N, Ricca C, Fletcher J, Glover T, Seizinger BR, and Manne V. 1995. Farnesyltransferase inhibitors block the neurofibromatosis type 1 (NF1) malignant phenotype. *Cancer Res* 55:3569–75.

Yumoto E, Nakamura K, Mori T, and Yanagihara N. 1996. Parapharyngeal vagal neurilemmoma extending to the jugular foramen. *J Laryngol and Otol* 10:485–9.

7

Cognitive Function and Academic Performance

Kathryn North, M.D., M.B.B.S., B.Sc(Med)

NF1 is associated with a wide variety of obvious and often disfiguring physical manifestations that capture the attention of clinicians and patients. However, the most common consequence of the disorder in childhood, and often the major concern of the parent of a child with NF1, is cognitive impairment. Although mental retardation is not a common feature of NF1 (see below), a wide range of learning disabilities occurs in 40 to 60% of children with NF1 and can be responsible for significant lifetime morbidity in terms of academic underachievement, behavioral problems, failure to complete higher education, and limitation of career choice. In addition a combination of factors, including altered physical appearance, school failure, difficulties with social interaction, and the stigma of having a "chronic disorder" contribute to low self-esteem and poor self-image in individuals with NF1.

Until the late 1980s there were few systematic studies of the NF1 cognitive phenotype. As noted in 1992, "Relatively few published reports deal with the topic of developmental and intellectual deficits in NF1. Even fewer provide data from specific measurements of the performance of patients with NF1. . . . The pathogenetic mechanism or mechanisms to account for the mental retardation seen in NF1 are totally obscure, and little work on this problem has been performed" (Riccardi 1992). Over the past decade, a number of studies have specifically addressed these concerns. In this chapter we will summarize our current understanding of the frequency and nature of cognitive deficits and learning disability in children with NF1, theories concerning pathogenesis, and the current approach to management.

HOW COMMON ARE COGNITIVE DEFICITS IN NF1?

Mental retardation is defined as an intellectual handicap associated with IQ scores two or more standard deviations below the mean (i.e., full-scale IQ score < 70), along with deficits in adaptive behavior. By definition, 3% of the general population are mentally retarded. Although mental retardation is often associated with school performance problems, it is important to differentiate children with academic underachievement due to low IQ from those with "specific learning disability" because the implications for appropriate intervention will differ. *Specific learning disability* is a controversial term—but commonly used in the literature—and is defined as "significantly impaired achievement that is not explained by sensory deficits, motor deficits, social and emotional problems, with IQ in the normal range" (National Joint Committee on Learning Disabilities 1982). Simply stated, specific learning disability represents a major discrepancy between ability (intellect or aptitude) and achievement (performance).

Early reports of cognitive function in patients with NF1 markedly overestimated the incidence of mental retardation. For example, in the Michigan study (Crowe et al. 1956), a mean IQ of 45 was found in 20 institutionalized patients as compared with a mean IQ of 77 in 15 of 203 noninstitutionalized patients for whom such data were available. In a population-based study in Gothenburg, Sweden, formal IQ testing was not performed, and estimates of intelligence were based on school placement and school performance (Samuelsson and Axelson 1981). Of 71 patients in whom intelligence was so assessed, 45% showed "slight mental retardation," and two of these patients were thought to be "somewhat more retarded than the remainder."

As exemplified by these studies, there are many limitations to the interpretation of data concerning intellectual function in NF1 before the early 1980s. No formal diagnostic criteria were available at that time; there was no clear distinction between NF1, NF2, and other forms of neurofibromatosis (e.g., segmental NF)—all of which may have different implications for cognitive development. Often only patients with severe manifestations of the disease were identified, introducing a significant ascertainment bias. More importantly, in the absence of standardized psychometric assessment, academic achievement was wrongly interpreted as a measure of intelligence. Consequently "learning disability"—a common manifestation of NF1—was equated with "mental retardation." Interestingly, neither of the two original patients described by von Recklinghausen (1882) appeared to have cognitive deficits. About subject 1, he commented, "Apart from a great attraction to the male sex, she exhibited nothing unusual in her mental sphere"; and of subject 2, he noted, "His intelligence did not seem exceptional nor, on the other hand, below average."

Accurate figures for the incidence of mental retardation in NF1 can be based only on population studies (to exclude ascertainment bias), in which standardized objective measures of IQ are performed (the Wechsler Intelligence Scales for Children [WISC] are the most commonly used; Wechsler 1974). In addition, the consequences of clinical variables, such as intracranial tumors and epilepsy, need to be considered. No such study exists and thus the true incidence of mental retardation in NF1 is unknown. In the population-based study of Huson et al. (1988) formal assessment of IQ was not performed, and the incidence of mental retardation was estimated at 3.2% (based on retrospective analysis of educational needs)—only slightly higher than the general population (3%). Despite some ascertainment bias, the results of clinic-based studies, in which objective psychometric testing was performed, are likely to provide a more accurate estimate of the frequency of mental retardation in patients with NF1.

The results of 11 such clinic-based studies are summarized in Table 7-1. The frequency of mental retardation (full-scale IQ > 2 standard deviations below the population mean) ranged between 4.8 percent (North et al. 1994, 1995) and 11 percent (Wadsby et al. 1989). The true incidence likely lies somewhere between these two estimates—and thus the risk for mental retardation in NF1 is approximately two to three times the risk for the general population.

All of the studies summarized in Table 7-1 reported a lowering of IQ scores in children with NF1 compared to normative data for the population (Eliason 1986; Ferner et al. 1996; Legius et al. 1994; Moore et al. 1994; North et al. 1994; Stine and Adams 1989; Varnhagen et al. 1988) or to unaffected sibling controls (Dilts et al. 1996; Hofman et al. 1994). The mean IQ score of patients with NF1 ranges between 89 and 98 (as measured on WISC-R) (i.e., within one standard deviation of the normal population) (mean, 100, SD, 15). Varnhagen et al. (1988), in a study of 16 children, found there was increased cognitive deficit as a function of the severity of physical disease manifestations. The effect was most marked on performance IQ and in tests of sequential and simultaneous processing. However, interpretation of this study is limited by the small number of patients, necessitating the use of nonparametric statistical analysis. No other study has supported this association with clinical severity and the general consensus is that there is no apparent association between the left shift in IQ and any clinical variable (such as socioeconomic status, gender, clinical severity of disease, macrocephaly, or family history of NF1) (Ferner et al. 1996; Hofman et al. 1994; North et al. 1994). The important exception to this rule is the association between intracranial tumors in NF1 and lowering of IQ. Moore et al. (1994) studied 65 children with NF1 (without intracranial pathology on MRI) and compared their intellectual function and academic achievement with children with and

Table 7-1. Results of studies of cognitive function in patients with NF1 on whom quantitative psychometric assessment (WISC-R) was performed

Study	No. of Patients	% with FSIQ <70	Mean FSIQ	Mean VIQ	Mean PIQ
Varnhagen et al. 1988	16	NA	94.5	94.0	93.5
Wadsby et al. 1989	27	11	NA	NA	NA
Stine and Adams 1989	18	NA	91.8	92.1	91.6
Eldridge et al. 1989	13	NA	93.9	91.6	97.8
Riccardi 1992	203	8.4	NA	NA	NA
North et al. 1994, 1995	40	4.8	93.3	92.6	95.4
Legius et al. 1994*	31	6.5	87.7	92.9	83.9
Moore et al. 1994	65	6	92.9	91.4	96.0
Denckla et al. 1996	19	NA	94.8	NA	NA
Ferner et al. 1996	103	8	88.6	90.5	88.1
Dilts et al. 1996	19	5.3	98.3	97.4	100.0

NA = not performed or analysis not appropriate to draw conclusion; FSIQ = full-scale IQ; VIQ = verbal IQ; PIQ = performance IQ; LD = learning disability.
*n = those aged 6–16 years.

without NF1 who had brain tumors. Children with brain tumors alone performed significantly better than patients with NF1 alone, and children with NF1 and brain tumor performed at a lower level than children with NF1 alone. It is thus important to control for the presence or absence of intracranial pathology in any study of cognitive function in NF1; unless stated otherwise, children with intracranial pathology are excluded in all studies cited below.

It is unclear from individual studies whether there is a general lowering of IQ scores in all patients with NF1 or whether only a subset of patients has NF-related cognitive deficits. Preliminary data from two studies would suggest that lowering of IQ in NF1 is an "all-or-nothing" phenomenon—akin to other complications of the disorder (e.g., optic glioma and scoliosis, which occur in a subset of patients). Although the sample size was too small to draw definitive conclusions, North et al. (1994) noted a bimodal distribution of IQ scores in 40 patients studied (with modal values of 85 and 100). In their study of 65 children with NF1, Moore et al. (1994) noted that the distribution of IQ scores in NF1 was skewed to the left, so children with NF1 were "overrepresented in lower ranges of academic performance and underrepresented in the higher ranges." Cluster analysis was conducted to identify subgroups of children with NF1 based on intellectual function and academic achievement (Brewer et al. 1997). This analysis suggested that there were three subsets of children with NF1; those with normal intellectual function and appropriate academic performance for IQ, those with normal intellect and significant specific deficits, and those with mild global deficits and no specificity. Neither of these studies included a control group to account for other socioeconomic, genetic, or environmental factors that may have an impact on cognitive function.

While many of the cutaneous manifestations of NF1 appear to worsen with age (e.g., number of cutaneous neurofibromas, size of plexiform neurofibromas), the natural history of cognitive deficits in NF1 is unclear. Cross-sectional data from Riccardi and Eichner (1986) suggested that IQ scores vary with age in groups of patients with NF1. The average IQ for children aged 6 to 17 years (n = 67) was at or near 90, compared to a mean IQ of 99.3 for patients 17 years or older (n = 89). However, there have been no systematic longitudinal studies to confirm this difference in function with time, and a recent study of 103 patients with NF1 aged 6 to 75 years did not show a correlation between age and neurocognitive deficits in NF1 (Ferner et al. 1996).

LEARNING DISABILITY IN NF1

Despite discrepancies in estimates of intellectual handicap, all studies to date agree on the high incidence of specific learning disability (SLD) in children with NF1. The reported frequency of learning disabilities ranges between 30% and 65% (Table 7-2); the discrepancy between figures is most likely due to differences in definition of SLD. As noted above, the two population studies of NF1 (Samuelsson and Axelsson 1981; Huson et al. 1988) assessed cognitive performance on the basis of school placement. In the Swedish study, 30 of 71 patients

Table 7-2. Frequency of learning disability in children with NF1

Study	n	Study Population	Definition of LD	% with LD
Samuelsson and Axelsson 1981	71	Population-based	School placement	42
Huson et al. 1988	135	Population-based	School placement	27
Wadsby et al. 1989	27	Hospital-based	Teacher questionnaire	59
Stine and Adams 1989	106	NF clinic	Parent questionnaire	41
Riccardi 1992	203	NF clinic	Teacher report Psychometrics	30
North et al. 1995	40	NF clinic	School placement	45
			Psychometrics	65
Legius et al. 1994	38	NF clinic	Psychometric	61
Moore et al. 1994	65	NF clinic	Psychometric	30
Dilts et al. 1996	19	NF clinic Support groups	Psychometric School placement	32

LD = learning disability; psychometric = definition based on psychometric assessment including tests of academic achievement.

(42%) were assessed as functioning at the "remedial class level" and 2 of 71 were at the "special school level." In the Welsh study, 10% of children with NF1 attended special schools and 17% were in remedial classes, as compared with 5% of individuals who had affected parents but did not have NF1. All other studies that provide estimates of the frequency of learning disabilities in children with NF1 have derived study populations from hospital-based NF or genetics clinics, with or without referrals from family support groups. In two studies, the diagnosis of "learning disability" was based on parent or teacher questionnaires. In the study of Wadsby et al. (1989), 47% of the children with NF1 were defined as performing "below normal" as compared with their peers; 36% had behavioral problems such as hyperactivity and poor concentration, 49% had reading or writing problems and 59% required special educational assistance, usually educational support while attending a mainstream school. Stine and Adams (1989) found that 41% of children with NF1 were perceived as learning disabled, as compared with 4% of their unaffected siblings.

In the remaining studies, comprehensive psychometric assessment was performed and specific learning disability objectively defined as a discrepancy between IQ scores and performance in tests of academic achievement. Riccardi and Eichner (1986) noted learning disability in 30% of children with NF1 and estimated that 40 to 50% of children had coordination problems and 50% had speech abnormalities—although coordination and language were not formally assessed. In a study of 40 children aged 8 to 16 years (excluding patients with intracranial pathology or full-scale IQ less than 70), North et al. (1995) found that 26 of 40 children (65%) had impaired performance in at least one test of academic achievement. Forty-five percent of children performed more than 2 years below chronologic age in reading accuracy, and 47.5% had impaired performance on reading comprehension tasks. Thirty-two percent of the group had impaired performance in spelling while 27.5% had math scores more than 1.96 SD below the mean. From parent questionnaires concerning their children's school performance, 18 of 40 children (45%) were receiving some form of special educational assistance (e.g., special class, integration aide, speech therapy). In their study of 65 children, Moore et al. (1994) found that mean scores on tests of academic achievement in reading, spelling, and mathematics were all more than 1 SD below the population mean, and that over 30% of children with NF1 would be classified as learning disabled based on discrepancy between IQ scores and performance on tests of academic achievement. Dilts et al. (1996) found that academic achievement of subjects with NF1 was significantly lower in all areas as compared with their unaffected siblings. Thirty-seven percent of the subjects with NF1 had previously received special education services (compared to 11% of unaffected siblings) and 63% met preliminary criteria for special education (learning disability with or without communication or behavior disorder), as compared with 1 of 19 (5%) unaffected siblings. Thirty-two percent of the subjects with NF1 (6 of 19) had specific learning disabilities in written expression (3), math (2), or reading.

THE NF1 COGNITIVE PHENOTYPE

The nature of SLD in children with NF1 has been addressed in the literature only in the past decade; the conclusions of the major studies to date are summarized in Table 7-3. Early studies of neuropsychological profiles in children with NF1 proposed that nonverbal learning problems (characterized by difficulty with written work, poor organizational skills, impulsivity, and a decreased ability to perceive social cues) were predominant in the population with NF1. The basis for this proposal was a discrepancy between verbal and performance IQ (VIQ > PIQ) found on two studies (Eliason et al. 1986, 1988; Wadsby et al. 1989), poor performance in tests of spatial memory (Varnhagen et al. 1988), and consistent deficits in the Judgement of Line Orientation (JLO) (Benton et al. 1976), a test of visuospatial function (Eliason 1986; Eldridge et al. 1989).

More recent studies, which include evaluation of language and reading, demonstrate that language-based learning problems (e.g., reading and spelling) are at least as common as nonverbal learning deficits in children with NF1 (Dilts et al. 1996; Ferner et al. 1996; Hofman et al. 1994; Legius et al. 1994; Mazzocco et al. 1995; Moore et al. 1994; North et al. 1994, 1995). Specific verbal deficits include poorer performance on measures of word definition, naming, written vocabulary, receptive syntactic language, and verbal reasoning and recall (North et al. 1995; Mazzocco et al. 1995). The discrepancy between VIQ and PIQ is not reproducible between studies and is of questionable significance (see Table 7-3). Interestingly, the JLO is consistently abnormal in all studies to date, with mean scores for the NF1 study population more than 2 SD below the mean. Thus, at some level, the JLO is a robust indicator of NF1-related neuropsychological deficits (Eliason 1986; Eldridge et al. 1989; Hofman et al. 1994; Joy et al. 1995). Poor attentional and organizational skills affect performance in many areas, al-

Table 7-3. Studies of the cognitive phenotype in patients with NF1

Study	n	VIQ and PIQ	Conclusions re Cognitive Phenotype
Eliason 1986, 1988	32	VIQ > PIQ	Predominance of visuoperceptual deficits (VIQ > PIQ, poor performance on JLO). Profile specific for NF1. Note that 25% of children with NF1 had intracranial pathology.
Wadsby et al. 1989	27	VIQ > PIQ	Verbal performance better than nonverbal. High incidence of attention problems and reading difficulties.
Eldridge et al. 1989	13	PIQ > VIQ	Poor performance on JLO, suggesting visuospatial deficits.
Riccardi 1992	203	NA*	Wide-ranging deficits, including easy distractability, poor visual motor coordination, and deficits in language and vocabulary.
Legius et al. 1994	38	VIQ > PIQ	Both verbal and nonverbal learning disabilities noted. Attentional problems in children with IQ > 85.
Moore et al. 1994	65	PIQ > VIQ	Deficits in motor and visuospatial function, as well as language and concentration; poor performance in reading, spelling, and mathematics.
North et al. 1994, 1995	40	VIQ = PIQ	Both verbal and nonverbal deficits. Poor performance in JLO. High incidence of attentional and organizational deficits, which undermine performance in many areas. No deficits in memory tasks.
Hofman et al. 1994 Mazzocco et al. 1995	19	NA	Sibling controls. Specific verbal deficits, visuomotor spatial deficits, mathematics and reading skill deficits, attention problems.
Ferner et al. 1996	103	PIQ = VIQ	Age- and sex-matched controls. Weaknesses in reading skills and short-term memory. Impaired attention, difficulty with complex and unfamiliar tasks. Similarity to patients with frontal lobe dysfunction.
Dilts et al. 1996	19	Mixed*	Sibling controls. Deficits in language, spatial judgment, visuomotor integration. No deficits in memory tasks.

NA = not performed or analysis not appropriate to draw conclusion; VIQ = verbal IQ; PIQ = performance IQ; JLO = Judgement of Line Orientation (a test of visuospatial function).
*8 of 19 patients had VIQ/PIQ discrepancy—PIQ > VIQ in 5 and VIQ > PIQ in 3.

though increased distractability is not usually associated with hyperactivity (Ferner et al. 1996; Hofman et al. 1994; North et al. 1995). Speech (articulation) problems are common (~25%) but rarely severe enough to affect intelligibility. Motor coordination is frequently impaired; up to one third of children demonstrate significant impairment in tests of manual dexterity, balance, and ball skills (North et al. 1995).

In summary, there does not appear to be a profile of learning disabilities specific to NF1. As Mazzocco et al. (1995) concluded, "from this and other research . . . the NF1 cognitive phenotype is characterized by (a) verbal weakness in vocabulary, phonological awareness and additional verbal skills as measured by the WISC-R; (b) motor-free and visual-motor spatial deficits; and (c) mathematics and reading skills deficits." Consequently, academic learning disability may be associated with depressed performance in verbal tasks such as reading and spelling, and/or non-verbal tasks such as mathematics. Nevertheless, learning disability is not thought to be secondary to global intellectual impairment in the majority of children with NF1. Mean IQ scores are well within the average range, performance of memory tasks is not impaired (Dilts et al. 1996; Joy et al. 1995), and there are no group differences (as compared with controls) in neuropsychologic measures typically influenced by overall intellectual impairment (Mazzocco et al. 1995).

Clinical variables, such as disease severity, macrocephaly, and family history of NF1, have not been demonstrated to influence performance in tests of intellect, language, or visuospatial function. However, male gender and lower socioeconomic status are associated with poorer performance in tests of academic achievement. In addition, boys with NF1 demonstrate poorer adaptive functioning and social skills and a higher incidence of behavioral problems than girls (North et al. 1995). This sex difference is consistent with a higher incidence of learning disabilities in males in the general population (Vogel 1990). In one study, a family history of NF1 was strongly associated with lower socioeconomic status based on ratings of employment and education. This result is probably a secondary effect of the high incidence of learning disabilities in the NF population; that is, individuals with NF1 are less likely to complete tertiary education and will fall into lower socioeconomic groups (North et al. 1995).

Two studies attempted to correlate NF1 cognitive deficits with dysfunction of specific regions of the brain. Ferner et al. (1996) noted that, compared to age- and sex-matched controls, patients with NF1 have particular weaknesses in reading skills and short-term memory. In addition, the group with NF1 had slower mean reaction times, impaired attention, and were slow to develop and adapt strategies for complex and unfamiliar tasks. The authors observed that the difficulties experienced by patients with NF1 were similar to those of patients with frontal lobe disorders. Interestingly, MRI studies suggest that lesions in the NF1 brain are more common in the anterior and subcortical areas of the brain (see below). Chapman et al. (1996) addressed this observation specifically in a study of 10 children with NF1. A consistent neurobehavioral profile emerged characterized by verbal and motor disinhibition, compromised social discourse, poorly regulated attention, and awkward motor output. It was concluded that deficits referable to dysfunction of frontal/subcortical areas were overrepresented in the NF1 group as compared with NF1/LD controls who did not have NF1 or learning disabilities. Surprisingly, this outcome was manifest only in females, and macrocephaly was also observed only in females. Although the numbers are too small to draw firm conclusions, and cranial MRI was not performed in the study cohort, these initial observations provide an interesting foundation for further neuropsychologic studies in patients with NF1, which aim to correlate anatomical and cognitive deficits.

NF1 COGNITIVE PHENOTYPE IN YOUNG CHILDREN

All of the above studies focused exclusively on school-age children. There are a paucity of data on the neurodevelopmental performance of infants and toddlers with NF1, and yet, better characterization of this group is essential to determine predictors of learning disability which may allow earlier appropriate intervention. Samango-Sprouse et al. (manuscript in preparation) recently completed a study of 90 children with NF1 whose mean age was 34.6 months. Fifty-four children had cranial MRI, and all were assessed in each of the following areas: cognitive capability (to approximate IQ), gross and fine motor function, visual-perceptual skill, and receptive and expressive language. There was a "shift to the left" in mean scores in all developmental domains; 13% of children were "mentally retarded." A family history of NF1 also appeared to correlate with poorer performance in tests of cognitive and language ability. This may be due to a pervasive influence of the NF1 gene, but is more likely to be due to a synergistic effect of a less-optimal environment with a predisposition for developmental disabilities. Children in higher socioeconomic groups also appeared to perform better in all areas except gross motor development. The presence of asymptomatic prechiasmatic optic nerve gliomas (in 12 of 54 cases [22%]) did not have an impact on developmental performance. Boys were significantly more hypotonic than girls, but there was no gender difference in the other domains of development. While early presentation with diminished truncal tone and depressed scores on the developmental scales may be precursors to, or predictors of, the cognitive and motor deficits seen in school-age children with NF1, only longitudinal studies will determine the predictive value of early assessment and therapeutic value of early intervention.

BEHAVIORAL PHENOTYPE AND SELF-IMAGE

Despite the psychosocial implications of a diagnosis of NF1, there has been very little research into the impact of NF1 on the functioning of the individual. One retrospective study (Benjamin et al. 1993) found that almost 50% of individuals with NF1 were distressed by the presence of neurofibromas and had changed their dressing and social behavior to hide them. Many individuals experienced anxiety about physical aspects of NF1, had been teased at school about the skin manifestations of the disorder, and felt that NF1 had hindered them in forming new friendships. Porter Counterman et al. (1995) found that children with NF1 were often unhappy with their own behavioral conduct and that those with more severe disease manifestations had a lower sense of self-worth.

The behavioral phenotype of children with NF1 has been indirectly assessed in two additional studies that administered the Child Behavior Checklist (Achenbach and Edelbrock 1979) to parents and teachers (Dilts et al. 1996; North et al. 1995). Findings were similar in both studies. Children with NF1 were reported to have difficulties with social interaction and, as a group, had more difficulty getting on with friends and family members than would be expected for their peer group. Neither the parent nor teacher reports suggested any externalizing behaviors (e.g., aggression, delinquency, poor conduct, hyperactivity) or other behavior traits that were disruptive or attention-seeking. There was a high frequency of internalizing features, which are often associated with anxiety and depression, and higher rates of inattention and impulsivity. Subjects with NF1 were less functionally independent than expected for age and were less involved or less skilled in sports and in non-sport activities. On the social problems subscale, common items identified included "frequently teased," "not liked by peers," "acts young," "prefers younger children," and "clumsy." A combination of factors including altered physical appearance, school failure, difficulties with social interactions, and the stigma of having a chronic illness potentially contribute to the psychosocial burden of NF1.

SUMMARY: WHAT DO WE KNOW ABOUT COGNITIVE FUNCTION AND ACADEMIC PERFORMANCE IN NF1?

1. NF1 is associated with a lowering of IQ in a subset of patients. There is a slight increase in the incidence of mental retardation over and above the incidence for the general population (4 to 8%).
2. There is a high incidence of academic learning disability in the NF1 population (40 to 60%).
3. There is no consistent discrepancy between verbal and performance IQ.
4. There is no specific or characteristic profile of learning disability in children with NF1. Both language-based learning problems and nonverbal deficits occur.
5. The Judgment of Line Orientation (a test of visuospatial function) is consistently abnormal in all studies of NF1 to date and thus, at some level, is a robust indicator of NF1-related neuropsychologic deficits.
6. Attentional and organizational deficits undermine performance in many areas. Attentional deficits are not usually associated with hyperactivity.
7. Although all aspects of school performance may be affected, reading and spelling tend to be more affected than mathematics.
8. Speech (articulation) problems are common but rarely severe enough to affect intelligibility.
9. Motor coordination is frequently impaired and clumsiness usually manifests at an early age.
10. Cognitive and physical manifestations of NF1 may have a negative effect on self-esteem and self-image. Children with NF1 may have difficulties interacting with their peers and appear withdrawn or anxious.
11. Macrocephaly and other clinical variables are not specifically associated with cognitive deficits.

IMPLICATIONS FOR ASSESSMENT AND MANAGEMENT

There have been no systematic studies to date to determine the best way to manage cognitive deficits and learning disability in children with NF1. Nevertheless, we can draw certain conclusions from studies of the cognitive phenotype to provide guidelines for assessment and intervention. Since children with NF1 are at high risk of learning disability, this risk should be discussed with parents in the same way that the other manifestations of the disorder are explained during medical assessment and counseling. The diagnostic label of NF1 should alert clinicians, parents, and teachers to the need to monitor for learning disability. A developmental history and review of school progress should be incorporated in the yearly review of all children with NF1. If any areas of concern are identified, then a formal educational assessment should be performed, including measures of language and motor performance, attention, and academic achievement. Children should be followed throughout their school career, as the vulnerabilities identified persist and may manifest at a later age when demands on performance increase.

Individual total scores on formal tests of intellectual, language, and motor function rarely fall below 2 SD from the mean. If this cutoff point is used to define "impaired performance," then standard assessment tools will underestimate the incidence of learning disabilities in this population. Performance across a range of subtests and a qualitative assessment of the child's approach to problem solving or more detailed neuropsychologic assessment are necessary to define the functional problems of the individual child.

Since no specific profile of learning disability has been identified in this group, management of problems need not differ from that of other learning-disabled populations, although the underlying medical "diagnosis" may assist in obtaining special services. In younger children, hypotonia and motor incoordination may be the predominant problems, and referral to an occupational therapist would be beneficial. Remediation in school-age children should focus on providing the child with skills aimed at compensating for areas of weakness. Self-esteem is often poor in children with NF1 due to both the physical and cognitive manifestations of the disorder. Therefore, these children will benefit from a modified teaching approach, which also focuses on their relative strengths and allows them to achieve optimal results on a day-to-day basis. The preservation of intellect and the ability to learn rules presented in an appropriate way, and to apply them, provides the most important base for appropriate and successful remediation of children with NF1. They will benefit from a structured learning environment and individualized teaching, such as provided in smaller remedial classes.

The predominance of attentional and organizational problems, the difficulties, with social interaction, the high incidence of speech and language difficulties and the preservation of learning and memory in this population suggests the possibility of attention deficit disorder without hyperactivity (ADDWO) as a diagnostic label for some of these children. Hyperactivity, disruptive or oppositional behavior, or conduct disorder, as encountered in attention deficit disorder with hyperactivity (ADDH; DSM III-R 1987) are not frequently present in children with NF1. ADDWO is characterized by more-subtle deficits in cognitive processing, attention span, language problems, and social withdrawal in the absence of obvious disruptive behavior (Cantwell and Baker 1992). Later presentation of these subtle learning deficits may result in anxiety, depression, and poor peer relationships, such as those that are identified in many children with NF1. Attentional and organizational deficits in these children also suggested an indication for the use of stimulant medication. Several children in the study of North et al. (1995) were treated with dexamphetamine or methylphenidate, with good response reported by parents and teachers. Similar beneficial response to stimulant medication has been noted by others North et al. (1997).

Early identification of learning disability reflects the current best practice in educational and clinical management. If the school experience can become less than the overwhelming frustration that it tends to be for children with NF1, the long-term outlook in terms of later occupational and social performance will be greatly improved.

THE PATHOGENESIS OF COGNITIVE DEFICITS IN PATIENTS WITH NF1

The high incidence of cognitive deficits in children with NF1 raises a number of important questions concerning the role of the NF1 gene product, neurofibromin, in the brain. It is intriguing to hypothesize that abnormal expression of the NF1 gene results in cognitive deficits through a direct effect on neuronal or glial development and function. While histopathologic studies and cranial imaging provide an insight into the role of neurofibromin in the brain, molecular studies and the analysis of animal models for NF1 are more likely to provide us with a better understanding of the pathogenesis of cognitive deficits in NF1.

PATHOLOGIC STUDIES OF THE CENTRAL NERVOUS SYSTEM IN NF1

Surprisingly, there are a paucity of data on the neuropathology of NF1. The much-quoted study of Rosman and Pearce (1967) examined autopsy specimens to determine if mental retardation and epilepsy observed in patients with NF1 was due to a primary brain dysplasia. Assessment of intellectual function in the 10 deceased adult subjects relied on obtaining their occupational and social history from medical records. On histopathology, disordered cortical architecture with random orientation of neurons, disarray of cortical lamination, and heterotopic neurones within the cortical molecular layer were found in the majority of patients. Three of five "mentally deficient" patients had additional heterotopias in the deep cerebral white matter as compared with none of five "normal" patients, who also had less disorder of their cortical architecture. On this basis, an association between cortical heterotopias and intellectual handicap was postulated. Rubinstein (1986) reviewed 11 postmortem cases of NF1 as part of a larger study of the neuropathology of NF1 and NF2. No correlation was made with intellectual function in the patients studied. Three of the eleven patients in this study showed focal proliferation of glial cells in subependymal regions to form well-defined gliofibrillary nodules. One of the eleven patients had hyperplastic gliosis, and one patient had a micro-nodular, hyperplastic focus of blood vessels.

Nordlund and colleagues (1995) demonstrated that GFAP (gliofibrillary acidic protein), a marker for astrocytes, was up-regulated in three brains from patients with NF1 studied by immunohistochemistry; there was a 4- to 18-fold increase in GFAP levels in the NF1 brains as compared with controls. Such an increase reflects reactive astrocytic gliosis—a phenomenon that has been reported in many neurodegenerative diseases, including Down syndrome, Alzheimer disease, and Parkinson disease. Histologic examination of these brains demonstrated some consistent abnormalities. There were foci of gliosis, with hypertrophic astrocytes in two cases, and an increase in the perivascular spaces was present in all cases. In one case, focal heterotopias and focal cellular disorganization in the thalamus and neocortex were also evident (D. Anthony K. North, unpublished observations). These data, while sparse, suggest that astrogliosis and other white matter abnormalities could be related to cognitive deficits in patients with NF1.

MRI T_2 SIGNAL ABNORMALITIES IN NF1

In recent years the use of magnetic resonance imaging (MRI) has allowed more precise definition of intracranial lesions as well as an insight into their pathogenesis. Cranial MRI signal abnormalities in patients with NF1 are well described. Focal areas of high signal intensity on T_2 weighted images are considered characteristic of NF1 (Fig. 7-1). These lesions have been variously called hamartomas, heterotopias, unidentified bright objects (T_2), and unidentified neurofibromatosis objects (Pont and Elster 1992). These areas are characterized by increased T_2 signal intensity and isointensity on T_1-weighted images; they exert no mass effect, there is no surrounding edema, they do not enhance with contrast, and are not visible on CT scan. They most commonly occur in the basal ganglia, cerebellum, brain stem, and subcortical white matter (Bognanno et al. 1988; Dunn and Roos 1989; Pont and Elster 1992; Sevick et al. 1992; Van Es et al. 1996). They are not associated with focal neurologic deficits (Duffner et al. 1989; North et al. 1994). The reported incidence of areas of increased T_2 signal intensity on MRI examination varies between 43% (Bognanno 1988, in a study including patients with NF2), 52% (Dunn and Roos 1989), 53% (DiMario et al. 1993), 53.5% (Zimmerman 1992), 60% (Aoki et al. 1989), 62% (Duffner et al. 1989), 64% (Van Es et al. 1996), 77% (Itoh et al. 1994), and 79% (Sevick et al. 1992). Aoki et al. (1989) found an age effect in that increased T_2 signals were rare over the age of 20 years. Sevick et al. (1992) followed 18 patients with an increased T_2 signal on serial MRI examinations and found that in all patients over the age of 10 years, the lesions remained static or decreased with time. Similarly, Itoh et al. (1994) found that T_2 lesions were much more common in young patients with NF1 and occurred in up to 93% of patients less than 15 years old (compared to 29% of patients over 31 years). Thus, the variation in the reported frequency of areas of increased T_2 signal is probably secondary to the variation in the age range of patients in individual studies.

ANATOMIC CORRELATES

There has been much speculation about the nature of areas of increased T_2 signal intensity on MRI. They have been considered as regions of dysplasia or heterotopia (Bognanno 1988; Duffner et al. 1989; Dunn and Roos 1989). This assump-

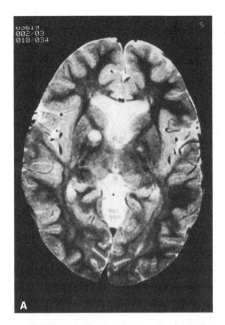
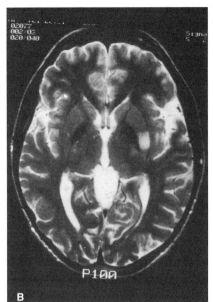

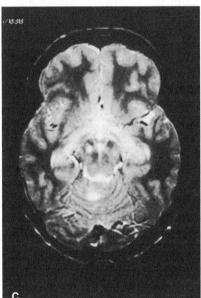

Figure 7-1. Areas of increased T_2 signal intensity on cranial MRI: (A, B) discrete lesions involving the basal ganglia; (C) diffuse involvement of the optic tracts bilaterally.

tion is based on the studies of Rosman and Pearce (1967) and of Rubinstein (1986). There are many limitations in relating these pathologic studies to the areas of increased T_2 signal on MRI examination seen in children and young adults with NF1. Neither of the studies correlated pathologic findings with neuroimaging. The majority of patients in the pathologic studies were adults and the lesions described occurred in different parts of the brain to areas of increased T_2 signal on MRI examination. In addition, developmental anomalies such as hamartomas, heterotopias, or benign or malignant proliferations of glial cells would not be expected to have reversible signal abnormalities such as have been observed on MRI (Aoki et al. 1989). Sevick et al. (1992) proposed that areas of increased T_2 signal intensity represent the formation of chemically abnormal myelin that was subsequently broken down by normal metabolic processes to be replaced by myelin with a more stable conformation.

Only one study has correlated pathologic studies with MRI findings. Zimmerman et al. (1992) (subsequently published in detail by DiPaolo et al. 1995) performed autopsies on two pediatric patients with NF1 and studied histologically five areas of brain tissue (two globus pallidus and three midbrain peduncle specimens) that correlated with areas of high T_2 signal intensity on MRI examinations performed before death. The five areas examined had similar histologic appearances. These consisted of atypical glial infiltrate with "bizarre" hyperchromatic nuclei, foci of microcalcification associated with perivascular gliosis, areas of dymyelination on specific staining, and spongy change in the white matter (spongiform myelinopathy) at the periphery of the lesions. The latter was thought to be due to intramyelinic edema. It was concluded that the high signal intensity lesions on MRI represented increased fluid within the myelin associated with hyperplastic or dysplastic glial proliferation. These areas were not malignant or premalignant. The MRI changes and associated pathologic changes were thought to be unique to NF1 and it was postulated that the abnormal MRI signals may disappear with time with resolution of the intramyelinic edema and replacement of abnormal myelin.

DEVELOPMENTAL CORRELATES

The high frequency of these MRI lesions has led to the hypothesis that these lesions are associated with the occurrence of cognitive deficits in children with NF1. Several studies have been performed to test this hypothesis, with mixed results (summarized in Table 7-4). The general consensus is that MRI T_2 hyperintensities may represent a marker for developmental abnormalities in the brain parenchyma, which result in cognitive deficits, and that they may provide an insight into the pathogenesis of cognitive deficits in NF1. However, additional studies need to be performed before the nature of the association, and the influence of variables such as the anatomic location and number of lesions, can be determined.

Three initial studies (Duffner et al. 1989; Dunn and Roos 1989; Ferner et al. 1993) found no association between the presence of MRI T_2 hyperintensities and cognitive deficits in patients with NF1. These three studies were based on small populations and covered a wide age range, quantitative IQ assessment was not performed in all patients, and there was no comparison between the distribution of test scores in the T_2+ and T_2- groups. It is not surprising that estimates of learning disability based on reports of school performance problems, IQ scores below 70, or academic skills more than two years below grade level, with

Table 7-4. Studies of the relationship between MRI T_2<-> hyperintensities and cognitive function in NF1

Study	n (range of ages, in years)	Methodology	Conclusions
Dunn and Roos 1989	31 (6–20)	IQ testing not performed in all patients. LD defined as performance two or more grade levels below IQ.	No significant difference in the incidence of LD, MR, or incoordination in T_2+ vs T_2-.
Duffner et al. 1989	46 (1–18)	IQ testing performed in 30% children. 30% had seizures, 25% had structural lesions on head CT. LD defined as placement in special class.	No association between placement in special class and increased T_2 signal on MRI.
Ferner et al. 1993	38 (3–63)	36% patients with intracranial pathology. IQ testing not performed in 25% of patients. Patients divided into 3 groups based on IQ.	No association between T_2+ and group with more severe intellectual impairment.
North et al. 1994	40 (8–16)	Patients with intracranial pathology excluded. Quantitative assessment of IQ, language, and visuospatial function.	Significantly lower IQ, language, and visuospatial function and academic achievement in T_2+ group.
Hofman et al. 1994	12 (8–16)	Unaffected sibling controls. Quantitative assessment of IQ, neuropsychological and language performance.	Number of T_2 hyperintensities correlate with pairwise deficits in IQ.
Legius et al. 1995	20 (4–16)	Patients with intracranial pathology excluded. Quantitative assessment of IQ.	No significant difference in IQ between T_2+ and T_2- group.
Moore et al. 1996	64 (8–16)	Patients with intracranial pathology excluded. Quantitative assessment of IQ.	No significant difference in IQ between T_2+ and T_2- group. Significant association between deficits in IQ and T_2 lesions in thalamus and hypothalamus.
Samango-Sprouse et al. 1997b	94 (1–6)	Quantitative assessment of IQ.	Presence of T_2 hyperintensities significantly related to decrease in neuromotor outcome.

LD = learning disability; MR = mental retardation.

analysis based on the arbitrarily defined presence or absence of cognitive deficit, did not reveal any association with MRI abnormalities. In addition, these studies included a large number of patients with CNS pathology (such as epilepsy and intracranial tumors), which could have an additional effect on cognitive function (Moore et al. 1994).

Three independent studies using clinic-based study samples and quantitative neuropsychological assessment have found a significant association between lowering of IQ and T_2-weighted hyperintensities in children with NF1. North et al. (1994) studied 40 children with NF1 and no intracranial pathology to determine whether those with areas of increased T_2 signal intensity on MRI examination differed significantly in intellectual, language, motor, or academic performance from those without abnormal findings. Areas of T_2 hyperintensity (T_2+) were present in 62.5% of the study population and there was no significant association with other clinical disease manifestations, age, socioeconomic status, gender, macrocephaly, or family history of NF1.

The distribution of full-scale IQ scores for the entire study population was bimodal, suggesting that there are two populations of patients with NF1: those with and those without cognitive impairment. There was no significant association between lower IQ scores and any clinical variable. However, children with T_2 hyperintensities on MRI (T_2+) had significantly lower IQ scores than children without these lesions, suggesting that the areas of increased T_2 signal are associated with the presence of a cognitive deficit (Fig. 7-2). Scores in tests of language function, visuomotor integration, and coordination were also significantly lower in the T_2+ group.

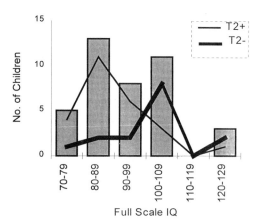

Figure 7-2. Full-scale IQ scores for the study population and association with areas of increased T_2 signal (T_2+) on MRI examination. The presence or absence of abnormal signal (T_2+/T_2-) divides the study population into two distinct groups. The T_2- group has a mean IQ score of 103.7, which does not differ significantly from normative values for the general population. The T_2+ group has a mean IQ score of 87.0 and significantly lower performance in tests of cognitive function.

The 15 children without areas of abnormal T_2 signal on MRI scan (T_2–) did not differ significantly from the general population in any parameter measured. In contrast, the T_2+ group had mean scores on all test parameters that differed significantly from the T_2– group. Although there was a general lowering of mean IQ scores in association with NF1, most of this left shift was accounted for by the results of the T_2+ group. Similar results were found for tests of language and motor function. The majority of children with impaired performance in tests of academic achievement were in the T_2+ group. Behavioral problems such as anxiety, depression, and poor peer relationships were predominant in this group, either as a primary manifestation or secondary to their learning disability. Seventeen children in the T_2+ group were already receiving some form of special educational assistance (as compared with one child in the T_2– group). The association between T_2 signal lesions and impaired academic achievement was independent of other clinical variables, including gender and socioeconomic status, but may be a secondary effect of the lower mean IQ scores in the T_2+ group.

On analysis of subtests of the WISC-R and neuropsychologic assessment (Joy et al. 1995), the presence of T_2-hyperintensities was associated with specific cognitive deficits. The T_2+ group performed significantly lower on all verbal subtests of the WISC-R, in two performance subtests, and in neuropsychologic tests of attention, visuospatial, and organizational function. Although the deficits were widespread, these results emphasized that the learning disabilities in this population were specific rather than a manifestation of global cognitive impairment.

A number of studies by Denckla and colleagues also found a significant association between T_2 hyperintensities and cognitive dysfunction (Denckla et al. 1994, 1996; Hofman et al. 1994; Mott et al. 1994). The study design used rigorous exclusion criteria, unaffected sibling controls, quantitative assessment of neuropsychological and language performance, and volumetric MRI analysis. The only limitations to the validity of this study are the small size of the study population (20 sibling pairs in the study by Denckla et al. 1996) and the higher proportion of patients with T_2 hyperintensities on MRI compared to other studies (93%—the same series reported by Itoh et al. 1994). Thus, no comparison of T_2+ and T_2– groups was possible in this study. Denckla and colleagues concluded that the number and volume of T_2 hyperintensities were highly correlated with pairwise deficits in IQ scores (compared to unaffected siblings), and pilot data suggested an association between impaired visuospatial function (as demonstrated in the Judgement of Line Orientation) and the volume of T_2 hyperintensities in the most commonly involved site, the basal ganglia. They suggested that many of cognitive deficits in NF1 are attributable largely to involvement of subcortical structures.

Samango-Sprouse and colleagues (1997) confirmed an association between intellectual development and the T_2 hyperintensities in a study of 94 preschool children (age range, 18 to 72 months). The mean IQ for the entire study group was 95.3, and the presence of T_2 foci was significantly related to a decrease in neuromotor outcome ($p < .01$) and intellectual developmental income ($p < .008$). Interestingly, in the presence of T_2 hyperintensities, males were found to be more impaired than females in spatial cognition.

Despite the convergent results among these three studies, the association between T_2 hyperintensities and learning disabilities remains controversial. Legius
et al. (1995) performed cognitive assessment and cranial MRI in 28 children
with NF1 between 4 and 16 years old. The cohort included eight children with
intercurrent neurologic disease (epilepsy, hydrocephalus, intracranial tumors).
As a group, these eight children had significantly lower mean IQ scores than
children without other neurologic problems (74.5 v. 95). Eighteen of twenty-
eight children (including all eight children with other neurologic problems) had
T_2 hyperintensities on MRI. No significant difference in full-scale IQ score was
noted between the T_2+ and T_2- group, even when the eight children with other
neurologic lesions were excluded from the analysis. Although the total study
numbers were small, this study questioned the association between T_2 hyperintensities in NF1 and lowering of IQ.

Moore and colleagues (Moore 1995; Moore et al. 1996) studied 84 patients
from a Houston NF clinic, performing neuropsychologic evaluations and MRI
examinations. When patients with brain tumors were excluded (n = 20, or 23.8%
of the study sample), the final sample size was 64. The study sample was comparable to the Sydney cohort (North et al. 1994), since patients were ascertained se-
quentially from an NF clinic, age and socioeconomic status were comparably
distributed, sex incidence was equal, and 55% of patients had areas of increased
T_2 signal on MRI. The study population appeared to differ only in their ethnic
makeup (for n = 84; 55 white, 15 black, and 14 Hispanic) and the fact that patients with asymptomatic optic gliomas were not included (compared to three
such patients in the Sydney cohort).

Mean full-scale IQ for the full study group demonstrated a left shift as compared with the general population (mean full-scale IQ was 94, as compared with
93.3 in the Sydney study), yet there was no statistical difference in overall IQ
scores between the T_2+ and T_2- groups. However, when the results were analyzed according to the site of increased T_2 lesions, there was a significant association between deficits in IQ, memory, motor function, and attention span and T_2
signal lesions in the thalamus and hypothalamus (but not the basal ganglia, brain
stem, or cerebellum).

It is not immediately clear why these ostensibly similar studies yield different
results. Apart from the difference in the ethnic backgrounds of the study populations from Sydney, Australia, and Houston, Texas, the subjects were otherwise
very similar. It is possible that there is some difference in the definition of T_2 hyperintensities. There is no disagreement concerning the definition of T_2 hyperintensities in the basal ganglia, cerebellum, and brain stem—where the areas of increased T_2 signal appear as discrete rounded lesion (see Fig. 7-1A, B). However,
in the Sydney study, many patients also had diffuse areas of increased T_2 signal
involving the optic tracts (e.g., Fig. 7-1C). Apart from the three patients with
asymptomatic optic gliomas, these areas were not associated with abnormalities
of the optic nerve, chiasm, or hypothalamus, did not exert a mass effect, were not
evident on CT scan or T_1-weighted images, did not enhance with gadolinium,

and tended to disppear with age. Hence, these lesions were considered to fulfill the definition of T_2 hyperintensities. In the Houston study, these lesions may have been classified as optic pathway tumors (Moore et al. 1996). The question is thus raised, "Are all T_2 hyperintensities the same?" Unfortunately, there are no neuropathologic or functional imaging data to answer this question. When data from the Sydney study were reanalyzed, excluding the three patients with asymptomatic optic pathway gliomas, the statistical association between cognitive deficits and MRI lesions remained highly significant (North 1995).

In the absence of adequate neuropathologic studies, functional brain imaging may provide additional information concerning MRI T_2 lesions and cortical function; however, preliminary studies have been confusing and contradictory. Kaplan et al. (1994) studied 10 patients with NF1 and increased T_2 signal intensities on MRI with PET (positron emission tomography) using fluoro-2-deoxy-D-glucose and found that all large T_2 lesions were metabolically inactive. Balestri et al. (1994) used PET to study subcortical T_2 lesions in four patients with NF1 and found the lesions to have a normal metabolic level. Proton MR spectroscopy of areas of increased T_2 signal intensity showed patterns similar to those in the normal brain (Castillo et al. 1995). Despite conflicting results concerning the metabolic activity of T_2 signal lesions, both Kaplan et al. (1994) and Balestri et al. (1994) found inhomogeneous and decreased cortical metabolism on PET in the brains of patients with NF1, which may reflect cortical astrocytic gliosis in NF1 brains.

In conclusion, although there appears to be some association between T_2 high-intensity lesions on MRI and cognitive deficits in children with NF1, the exact nature of this association and its relationship to the number, volume, and location of lesions remains to be elucidated. If, indeed, areas of increased T_2 signal on MRI prove to be consistently associated with cognitive deficits in children with NF1, then this observation has theoretical implications for our understanding of underlying pathogenesis. A radiologic marker for risk of cognitive dysfunction has been identified, and children with areas of increased T_2 signal on MRI are at higher risk for cognitive deficits and academic learning disabilities.

It would be too simplistic and naive to view these MRI lesions as a firm predictor of cognitive deficits in children with NF1. Not all children in the T_2+ group had significant school performance problems and several had above average IQs. MRI should not be used as a screening procedure for learning disabilities in NF1, because it would not be appropriate to provide educational intervention on the basis of an MRI result. The most valuable information concerning a child's development can be obtained from developmental evaluation. The possible association between T_2 hyperintensities and cognitive deficits in NF1 is of primary interest in helping to understand the pathogenesis of learning disability in a subset of children with NF1 and hence is of theoretical rather than practical import. In the future, clinical studies of learning disabilities in children with NF1 should consider the T_2+ and T_2- groups separately. Definition of associated neuropathology and the underlying molecular mechanisms may provide us with a better understanding as to why cognitive deficits occur in NF1.

MOLECULAR INSIGHTS INTO THE ROLE OF NEUROFIBROMIN IN THE BRAIN

Part of the protein encoded by the NF1 gene, neurofibromin, shares high sequence homology with the GAP (GTPase Activator Protein) family of proteins that interact with Ras proteins to regulate cell growth and differentiation (Bollag and McCormack 1991; Xu et al. 1990). The GAP activity of neurofibromin and the identification of mutations in both NF1 alleles in malignant tumors associated with NF1 (Legius et al. 1993; Shannon et al. 1994) and in benign neurofibromas (Colman et al. 1995) has led to the classification of the NF1 gene as a tumor-suppressor gene. It is not known whether loss of both NF1 alleles is associated with all NF1 disease manifestations.

A number of studies have implicated a role for neurofibromin in brain function, and hence have provided initial insight into the pathogenesis of cognitive deficits in patients with NF1. The results of these studies can be summarized as follows:

1. Neurofibromin is expressed early during embryonic development with high levels of expression in the brain. These data suggest that neurofibromin plays an important role in regulating the orderly differentiation of central nervous system neurons (Daston and Ratner 1993; Daston et al. 1992; Gutmann et al. 1995; Huynh et al. 1994).
2. In the adult, the expression of the NF1 gene is largely restricted to neuronal tissues. In normal brains, neurofibromin is enriched in large projection neurons of the cortex (especially pyramidal and Purkinje cells) and is also present in oligodendrocytes (Nordlund et al. 1993). Ultrastructural analysis of rat and human brains revealed that neurofibromin is localized to the smooth endoplasmic reticulum in neurons. Microglia, astrocytes, and endothelial cells did not show any staining on immunohistochemistry.
3. The intensity of neurofibromin immunoreactivity was similar in normal human brains and in three brains from adult NF1 patients (aged 30, 31, and 37 years, all with normal MRI scans) (Nordlund et al. 1995). Although the NF1 group may have mutations in their NF1 gene that allow production of nonfunctional forms of neurofibromin, these data demonstrate that gross abnormalities in the levels or distribution of neurofibromin are not necessarily present in NF1 patients. However, as noted above, GFAP was upregulated in the brains of patients with NF1, suggesting that neurofibromin may be a critical growth regulator for astrocytes and that activation of astrocytes may be a pathologic feature of the disorder.
4. Gregory et al. (1993) demonstrated that neurofibromin is expressed predominantly in the cytoplasm and is associated with microtubules in cultured fibroblasts and in mammalian brain. Microtubule-associated proteins are involved in stabilizing microtubules and in actively promoting microtubule movement and microtubule-mediated intracytoplasmic transport. Some populations of microtubules have also been implicated in signal transduction pathways involving surface receptors and neurotransmitters.

5. An alternately spliced exon of neurofibromin, exon 9a, has been identified and shown to be expressed almost exclusively in human and rodent CNS tissues (Danglot et al. 1995). Expression of this exon is enriched in the forebrain, it is present in neurons, not astrocytes, and its expression increases during CNS neuronal differentiation in vivo and in vitro (Geist and Gutmann 1996). The identification of a CNS neuron-specific NF1 isoform supports the hypothesis that neurofibromin has brain-specific functions that may relate to the high incidence of cognitive deficits in NF1 individuals.

6. Vogel et al. (1995) demonstrated that neurons isolated from neurofibromin deficient mouse embryos (*NF1 −/−*) survive in the absence of neurotrophic factors, suggesting that neurofibromin may act as a negative regulator of neurotrophin-mediated signaling, and that abnormal expression of neurofibromin may affect signal transduction within the nervous system.

Further studies of the role of neurofibromin in the central nervous system are required before we can determine whether any of these early observations have functional implications for the pathophysiology of cognitive deficits in NF1.

ANIMAL MODELS FOR COGNITIVE DEFICITS IN NF1

Jacks and colleagues (1994) successfully generated a mouse *Nf1* knockout by homologous recombination. Mice heterozygous for a mutation in the *Nf1* gene (*Nf1 +/−*) show hyperplasia of some neuronal populations (Brannan et al. 1994), as well as behavioral abnormalities that bear striking similarity to the learning disability observed in humans with NF1 (Silva et al. 1997). Adult mice do not have focal neurologic deficits, but a subset of mice (50 to 60%) have impaired performance in the spatial version of the Morris water maze test. They have deficits in spatial learning, as compared with unaffected littermates, but are able to learn tasks with extended training. Other cognitive functions such as associative learning are unaffected. The mouse brains also demonstrate astrogliosis similar to that observed in humans (Rizvi et al. 1999). Silva et al. (1997) hypothesized that the "learning deficits" in mice heterozygous for a mutation in the *Nf1* gene may be due to (1) an effect on the ras signaling during hippocampal-dependent learning, (2) an effect on modulation of neurotrophin signaling, (3) an effect on modulation of potassium currents, (4) pathologic changes in the brain such as glial proliferation, or (5) mutations at a modifying genetic locus. Obviously, this animal model will be invaluable in determining the pathologic and molecular processes involved in cognitive deficits in NF1.

Drosophila (fruit flies) homozygous for null mutations of an NF1 homolog have also been generated and are small in size and behaviorally "sluggish" compared to wild type (The et al. 1997). Studies in the *Drosophila* NF1 mutant have demonstrated that NF1 is necessary for activation of adenylyl cyclase in response to certain neuropeptides (PACAP38) at the neuromuscular junction. Moreover, the NF1 defect was rescued by exposure to pharmacologic treatment that increased concentrations of cAMP (Guo et al. 1997). While it would be overzealous to analyze these findings with respect to the pathophysiology of NF1 in humans, the fly model of NF1 provides further evidence for the role of neurofibromin in *ras*-mediated pathways. In addition, it raises the possibility that depletion of cAMP within the CNS may contribute to occurrence of cognitive deficits in NF1 individuals.

A MODEL FOR THE PATHOGENESIS OF COGNITIVE DEFICITS IN NF1

Current understanding of the function of the *NF1* gene, the nature of cognitive deficits in this disorder, and early correlations between neuroradiologic, pathologic, and neuropsychologic findings allow us to develop a possible model for the pathogenesis of cognitive deficits in NF1 (North et al. 1997). If mutations in the NF1 gene result in aberrant control of cell growth and differentiation in the central nervous system (i.e., through loss of GAP-related or other potential functions of neurofibromin), then this may result in areas of dysplastic gliosis and aberrant myelination within the brain parenchyma which, in turn, appear as areas of increased T_2 signal intensity on MRI. These lesions disrupt important neuronal circuits involved in higher cognitive processing and manifest as specific cognitive deficits rather than focal neurologic signs. For example, the basal ganglia have been demonstrated to have a role in the preparation for, and execution of, cognitive, limbic, oculomotor, and motor functions (Afifi 1994; Alexander et al. 1986). A lesion in the basal ganglia may disrupt feedback loops to and from the cerebral cortex and affect performance of many complex tasks. Whether the disruption of "information flow" has a secondary effect on the level of cortical metabolism (as suggested by PET findings) remains to be elucidated.

The *NF1* gene is classified as a tumor-suppressor gene, but it is not known how *NF1* gene mutations cause many of the nontumor manifestations of the disorder, such as cognitive deficits. At the molecular level there are two possibilities; heterozygous mutations in the *NF1* gene may, in themselves, affect orderly differentiation of neurons and glial cells and result in both focal (T_2 hyperintensities, heterotopias) and generalized (astrocytic gliosis) lesions seen in NF1 brains. Alternatively, a "second hit," with loss of heterozygosity for the NF1 gene in a subpopulation of cells, may be necessary for the development of CNS lesions. The latter possibility is of interest considering the focal nature of many MRI lesions. A third possibility is that a combination of mechanisms are operating at a molecular level to explain the concurrence of focal and more generalized abnormalities.

To date no phenotype–genotype correlation has been possible concerning cognitive deficits in NF1. The exception to the rule is the occurrence of mental retardation in association with dysmorphism and an increased cutaneous tumor load in patients with large deletions of the whole NF1 gene and surrounding DNA (Kayes et al. 1992, 1994). It is not known whether the cognitive deficits in these cases are due to absence of one NF1 allele or are the result of a contiguous gene syndrome involving deletion of a gene or genes adjacent to the NF1 locus.

FUTURE DIRECTIONS

Although there has been much progress toward gaining a better understanding of the cognitive deficits that occur in children with NF1, many important questions remain to be answered. For example, it is still unclear whether the distribution of IQ scores in patients with NF1 is unimodal or bimodal; that is, is there a general "shift to the left" in IQ scores in all patients with NF1? Or are only a subset of patients affected? What is the natural history of the cognitive dysfunction in patients with NF1? Is there an improvement over time, and is this related to the disappearance of T_2 hyperintensities on MRI with age? In addition, a consistent relationship between MRI T_2 signal lesions and cognitive deficits needs to be established.

In terms of pathogenesis, it is not known if the neuropathology of NF1 is due to a GAP-related function of neurofibromin or possible other functions of the protein (e.g., microtubular association, aberrant response to neurotrophic factors). How does mutation in the *NF1* gene result in aberrant myelination and astrocytic proliferation? Are abnormalities due to altered phenotypes of neurons and/or glial cells? Are the CNS abnormalities in NF1 a static/ "developmental" problem or an ongoing process; that is, is there potential for intervention?

NF1 provides a unique opportunity to begin to uncover a molecular basis for cognitive impairment. If we can determine the mechanism by which abnormalities in neurofibromin affect the function of the brain and neuronal pathways, it will provide an insight into the pathogenesis of cognitive impairment and learning disabilities in the general population. By understanding the etiology of cognitive deficits in NF1, we can then strive to develop therapies that go beyond "symptomatic" educational intervention.

REFERENCES

Achenbach TM and Edelbrock CS. 1979. Achenbach child behaviour checklist. *J Consult Clin Psychol* 47:223–33.

Afifi AK. 1994. Basal ganglia: functional anatomy and physiology. *J Child Neurol* 9:352–61.

Alexander GE, Delong MR, and Strick PL. 1986. Parallel organisation of functionally segregated circuits linking basal ganglia and cortex. *Annu Rev Neurosci* 9:357–81.

Aoki S, Barkovich AJ, Nishimura K, Kjos BO, Machida T, Cogen P, Edwards M, and Norman D. 1989. Neurofibromatosis types 1 & 2: cranial MR findings. *Radiology* 172:527–34.

Balestri P, Lucignani G, Fois A, Magliani L, Calistri L, Grana C, DiBartolo RM, Perani D, and Fazio F. 1994. Cerebral glucose metabolism in neurofibromatosis type 1 assessed with [18F]-2-fluoro-2-deoxy-D-glucose and PET. *J Neurol Neurosurg Psychiatry* 57:1479–83.

Benjamin CM, Colley A, Donnai D, Kingston H, Harris R, and Kerzin-Storrar L. 1993. Neurofibromatosis type 1 (NF1): knowledge, experience, and reproductive decisions of affected patients and families. *J Med Genet* 30:567–74.

Benton A, Varney N, and Hamsher K. 1976. *Judgement of Line Orientation.* Iowa City Department of Neurology, University of Iowa.

Bognanno JR, Edwards MK, Lee TA, Dunn DW, Roos KL, and Klatte EC. 1988. Cranial MR imaging in neurofibromatosis. *AJNR Am J Neuroradiol* 9:461–8.

Bollag G and McCormack F. 1991. Regulators and effectors of ras proteins. *Annu Rev Cell Biol* 7:601–32.

Brannan CI, Perkins AS, Vogel KS, Ratner N, Nordlund ML, Reid SW, Buchberg AM, Jenkins NA, Parada LF, and Copeland NG. 1994. Targeted disruption of the neurofibromatosis type 1 gene leads to developmental abnormalities in heart and various neural crestderived tissues. *Genes Dev* 8:1019–29.

Brewer VR, Moore BD, and Hiscock M. 1997. Learning disability subtypes in children with neurofibromatosis. *J Learn Disabil* 30:521–33.

Cantwell DP and Baker L. 1992. Attention deficit disorder with and without hyperactivity: a review and comparison of matched groups. *J Am Acad Child Adolesc Psychiatry* 31:432–8.

Castillo M, Green C, Kwock L, Smith K, Wilson D, Schiro S, and Greenwood R. 1995. Proton MR spectroscopy in patients with neurofibromatosis type 1: evolution of hamartomas and clinical correlation. *AJNR Am J Neuroradiol* 16:141–7.

Chapman CA, Waber DP, Bassett N, Urion DK, and Kork BR. 1996. Neurobehavioral profiles of children with Neurofibromatosis 1 referred for learning disabilities are sex-specific. *Am J Med Genet* 67:127–32.

Colman SD, Williams CA, and Wallace MR. 1995. Benign neurofibromas in type 1 neurofibromatosis (NF1) show somatic deletions of the NF1 gene. *Nat Genet* 11:9092.

Crowe FW, Schull WJ, and Neel JV. 1956. *A Clinical, Pathological and Genetic Study of Multiple Neurofibromatosis.* Springfield, Ill.: Charles C Thomas, pp. 1–181.

Danglot G, Regnier V, Fauvet D, Vassal G, Kujas M, and Bernheim A. 1995. Neurofibromatosis 1 (NF1) mRNAs expressed in the central nervous system are differentially spliced in the 5′ part of the gene. *Human Mol Gen* 4:915–20.

Daston MM and Ratner N. 1993. Neurofibromin, a predominantly neuronal GTPase activating protein in the adult, is ubiquitously expressed during development. *Dev Dynam* 195:216–26.

Daston MM, Scrable H, Norlund M, Sturbaum AK, Nissen LM, and Ratner N. 1992. The protein product of the neurofibromatosis type 1 gene is expressed at highest abundance in neurons, Schwann cells and oligodendrocytes. *Neuron* 8:415–28.

Denckla MB, Hofman K, Bryan N, Reiss A, Harris E, Melhem E, Lee J, Cox C, and Schuerholz L. 1994. Evidence that cognitive deficits in NF-1 are related to T2-weighted hyperintensities on MRI. *Neurology* (Suppl 2):A381–2.

Denckla MD, Hofman K, Mazzocco MMM, Melhem E, Reiss AL, Bryan RN, Harris EL, Lee J, Cox CS, and Schuerholz LJ. 1996. Relationship between T_2-weighted hyperintensities (unidentified bright objects) and lower IQs in children with neurofibromatosis-1. *Am J Med Genet* 67:98–102.

Dilts CV, Carey JC, Kircher JC, Hoffman RO, Creel D, Ward K, Clark E, and Leonard CO. 1996. Children and adolescents with neurofibromatosis 1: a behavioral phenotype. *Dev Behav Pediatr* 17:229–39.

DSM III-R. 1987. *Diagnostic and Statistical Manual of Mental Disorders,* 3rd edition, rev. Washington, D.C.: American Psychiatric Association, pp. 50–3.

DiMario FJ, Ramsby G, Greenstein R, Langshur S, and Dunham B. 1993. Neurofibromatosis type 1: magnetic resonance imaging findings. *J Child Neurol* 8:32–9.

DiPaolo DP, Zimmerman RA, Rorke LB, Zackai EH, Bilaniuk LT, and Yachnis AT. 1995. Neurofibromatosis type 1: pathologic substrate of high-signal intensity foci in the brain. *Radiology* 195:721–4.

Duffner PK, Cohen ME, Seidel FG, and Shucard DW. 1989. The significance of MRI abnormalities in children with neurofibromatosis. *Neurology* 39:373–8.

Dunn DW and Roos KL. 1989. MRI evaluation of learning difficulties and incoordination in neurofibromatosis type 1. *Neurofibromatosis* 2:1–5.

Eldridge R, Denckla MB, Bien E, Myers S, Kaiser-Kupfer MI, Pikus A, Schlesinger SL, Parry DM, Dambrosia JM, Zasloff MA, and Mulvihill JJ. 1989. Neurofibromatosis type 1 [Recklinghausen's disease]: neurologic and cognitive assessment with sibling controls. *Am J Dis Child* 143:833–7.

Eliason MJ. 1986. Neurofibromatosis: Implications for learning and behaviour. *J Dev Behav Pediatr* 7:175–9.

———. 1988. Neuropsychological patterns: Neurofibromatosis compared to developmental learning disorders. *Neurofibromatosis* 1:17–25.

Ferner RE, Chaudhuri R, Bingham J, Cox T, and Hughes RAC. 1993. MRI in neurofibromatosis 1: the nature and evolution of increased intensity T_2 weighted lesions and their relationship to intellectual impairment. *J Neurol Neurosurg Psychiatry* 56:492–5.

Ferner RE, Hughes RAC, and Wenman J. 1996. Intellectual impairment in neurofibromatosis 1. *J Neurol Sci* 138:125–33.

Geist RT and Gutmann DH. 1996. Expression of a developmentally regulated neuron specific isoform of the neurofibromatosis 1 (NF1) gene. *Neurosci Lett* 211:85–8.

Gregory PE, Gutmann DH, Boguski M, Mitchell AM, Parks S, Jacks T, Wood DL, Jove R, and Collins FS. 1993. The neurofibromatosis type 1 gene product, neurofibromin, associates with microtubules. *Somat Cell Molec Genet* 19:265–74.

Guo HF, The I, Hannan F, Bernards A, and Zhong Y. 1997. Requirement of Drosophila NF1 for activation of adenylyl cyclase by PACAP38-like neuropeptides. *Science* 276:795–8.

Gutmann DH, Geist RT, Wright DE, and Snider WD. 1995. Expression of the neurofibromatosis 1 (NF1) isoforms in developing and adult rat tissues. *Cell Growth Dev* 6:315–22.

Hofman KJ, Harris EL, Bryan RN, and Denckla MB. 1994. Neurofibromatosis type 1: the cognitive phenotype. *J Pediatr* 124:S1–8.

Huson SM, Harper PS, and Compston DAS. 1988. von Recklinghausen neurofibromatosis: a clinical and population study in south east Wales. *Brain* 111:1355–81.

Huynh DP, Nechiporuk T, and Pulst SM. 1994. Differential expression and tissue distribution of type I and type II neurofibromins during mouse fetal development. *Dev Biol* 161:538–51.

Itoh T, Magnaldi S, White RM, Denckla MB, Hofman K, Naidu S, and Bryan RN. 1994. Neurofibromatosis type 1: the evolution of deep gray and white matter MR abnormalities. *AJNR Am J Neuroradiol* 15:1513–9.

Jacks T, Shih TS, Schmitt EM, Bronson RT, Bernards A, and Weinberg RA. 1994. Tumor predisposition in mice heterozygous for a targeted mutation in NF1. *Nat Genet* 7:353–61.

Joy P, Roberts C, North K, and De Silva M. 1995. Neuropsychological function and MRI abnormalities in neurofibromatosis type 1. *Dev Med Child Neurol* 37:906–14.

Kaplan AM, Lawson MA, Bonstelle CT, and Wodrich DL. 1994. Positron emission tomography (PET) in children with NF1. Paper presented at the International Child Neurology Association Conference, San Francisco. (Abstract 607)

Kayes LM, Burke W, Riccardi VM, et al. 1994. Deletions spanning the Neurofibromatosis 1 gene: identification and phenotype of five patients. *Am J Hum Genet* 54:424–36.

Kayes LM, Riccardi VM, Burke W, Bennett RL, and Stephens K. 1992. Large de novo DNA deletion in a patient with sporadic neurofibromatosis, mental retardation and dysmorphism. *J Med Genet* 29:686.

Legius E, Marchuk DA, Collins FS, and Glover TW. 1993. Somatic deletion of neurofibromatosis type 1 gene in a neurofibrosarcoma supports a tumor suppressor gene hypothesis. *Nat Genet* 3:122–6.

Legius E, Descheemaeker MJ, Spaepen A, Casaer P, and Fryns JP. 1994. Neurofibromatosis type 1 in childhood: a study of the neuropsychological profile in 45 children. *Genet Couns* 5:51–60.

Legius E, Descheemaeker MJ, Steyaert J, Spaepen A, Vlietinck R, Casaer P, Demaeral P, and Fryns JP. 1995. Neurofibromatosis type 1 in childhood: correlation of MRI findings with intelligence. *J Neurol Neurosurg Psychiatr* 59:638–40.

Mazzocco MMM, Turner JE, Denckla MB, Hofman KJ, Scanlon DC, and Vellutino FR. 1995. Language and reading deficits associated with neurofibromatosis type 1: evidence for not-so-nonverbal learning disability. *Dev Neuropsychol* 11:503–22.

Moore BD. 1995. NF1, cognition and MRI. *Neurology* 45:1029.

Moore BD, Ater JL, Needle MN, Slopis J, and Copeland DR. 1994. Neuropsychological profile of children with neurofibromatosis, brain tumor or both. *J Child Neurol* 9:368–77.

Moore BD, Slopis JM, Schomer D, Jackson EF, and Levy B. 1996. Neuropsychological significance of areas of high signal intensity on brain magnetic resonance imaging scans of children with neurofibromatosis. *Neurology* 46:1660–8.

Mott S, Kkryja PB, Baumgardner T, Abrams M, Reiss A, and Denckla M. 1994. Neurofibromatosis type I (NF1): association between volumes of T_2 weighted high intensity signals (UBOs) on magnetic resonance imaging (MRI) and impaired performance on the Judgement of Line Orientation (JLO). Paper presented at the conjoint meeting of the CNS and ICNA. October 2–8, San Francisco, Calif.

National Joint Committee on Learning Disabilites. 1982. Learning Disabilities: issues on definition. *ASHA* 24:945.

Nordlund M, Gu X, Shipley MT, and Ratner N. 1993. Neurofibromin is enriched in the endoplasmic reticulum of CNS neurons. *J Neurosci* 13:1588–1600.

Nordlund ML, Rizvi TA, Brannan CI, and Ratner N. 1995. Neurofibromin expression and astrogliosis in neurofibromatosis (type 1) brains. *J Neuropathol Exp Neurol* 54:588–600.

North K. 1995. Learning difficulties in neurofibromatosis type 1: the significance of MRI abnormalities. *Neurology* 45:1029–30.

North K, Joy P, Yuille D, Cocks N, and Hutchins P. 1995. Cognitive function and academic performance in children with Neurofibromatosis type 1. *Dev Med Child Neurol* 37:427–36.

North K, Joy P, Yuille D, Cocks N, Hutchins P, McHugh K, and de Silva M. 1994. Learning difficulties in neurofibromatosis type 1: the significance of MRI abnormalities. *Neurology* 44:878–83.

North KN, Riccardi V, Samango-Sprouse C, Moore BD, Ferner F, Legius E, Ratner N, and Denckla MB. 1997. Cognitve function and academic performance in neurofibromatosis 1: consensus statement from the NF1 Cognitive Disorders Task Force. *Neurology* 48:1121–7.

Pont MS and Elster AD. 1992. Lesions of skin and brain: modern imaging of the neurocutaneous syndromes. *AJR Am J Roentgenol* 158:1193–1203.

Porter Counterman A, Saylor CF, and Pai S. 1995. Psychological adjustment of children and adolescents with neurofibromatosis. *Child Health Care* 4:223–34.

Riccardi VM. 1992. *Neurofibromatosis: Phenotype, natural history, and pathogenesis,* 2nd ed. Baltimore: Johns Hopkins University Press, pp. 88–95.

Riccardi VM and Eichner JE. 1986. *Neurofibromatosis: Phenotype, Natural History, and Pathogenesis.* Baltimore: Johns Hopkins University Press.

Rizvi TA, Akunuru S, de Courten-Myers G, Switzer RC, Nordlund ML, Ratner N. 1999. Region-specific astrogliosis in brains of mice heterozygous for mutations in the neurofibromatosis type 1 (Nf1) tumor suppressor. *Brain Res* 816:111–23.

Rosman NP and Pearce J. 1967. The brain in multiple neurofibromatosis (von Recklinghausen's disease): a suggested neuropathological basis for the associated mental defect. *Brain* 90:829–38.

Rubinstein LJ. 1986. The malformative central nervous system lesions in the central and peripheral forms of neurofibromatosis: a neuropathological study of 22 cases. *Ann N Y Acad Sci* 486:14–29.

Samango-Sprouse CA, Cohen MS, Mott SH, Brasseux C, Custer DA, Vaught DR, Lutz-Armstrong M, Rosenbaum KN, Stern HJ, and Tifft CJ. 1997a. A comprehensive study of the neurodevelopmental profile in young children with neurofibromatosis type 1 and the influence of the mode of transmission.

Samango-Sprouse C, Vezina LG, Brasseux C, Tillman, and Tifft CJ. 1997b. Cranial magnetic resonance findings and the neurodevelopmental performance in the young child with neurofibromatosis 1. *Am J Hum Genet* 61:A35.

Samuelsson B and Axelsson R. 1981. Neurofibromatosis: a clinical and genetic study of 96 cases in Gothenburg, Sweden. *Acta Derm Venereol* 95:67–71.

Sevick RJ, Barkovich AJ, Edwards MSB, Koch T, Berg B, and Lempert T. 1992. Evolution of white matter lesions in neurofibromatosis type 1: MR findings. *AJR Am J Roentgenol* 159:171–5.

Shannon KM, O'Connell P, Martin GA, Paderanga D, Olson K, Dinndorf P, and McCormick F. 1994. Loss of the normal NF1 allele from the bone marrow of children with type 1 neurofibromatosis and malignant myeloid disorders. *N Engl J Med* 330:597–601.

Silva AJ, Frankland PW, Marowitz Z, Friedman E, Lazlo G, Cioffi D, Jacks T, and Bourtchuladze R. 1997. A mouse model for the learning and memory deficits associated with neurofibromatosis type 1. *Nat Genet* 15:281–4.

Stine SB and Adams WV. 1989. Learning problems in neurofibromatosis patients. *Clin Orthop* 245:43–8.

The I, Hannigan GE, Cowley GS, Reginald S, Zhong Y, Gusella JF, Hariharan IK, and Bernards A. 1997. Rescue of a Drosophila NF1 mutant phenotype by protein kinase A. *Science* 276:791–4.

Van Es S, North K, McHugh K, and de Silva M. 1996. MRI abnormalities in children with NF1. *Paediatr Radiol* 26:478–87.

Varnhagen CK, Lewin S, Das JP, Bowen P, Ma K, and Klimek M. 1988. Neurofibromatosis and psychological processes. *J Dev Behav Pediatr* 9:257–65.

Vogel SA. 1990. Gender differences in intelligence, language, visual-motor abilities and academic achievement in males and females with learning disabilities: a review of the literature. *J Learn Disabil* 23:44–52.

Vogel KS, Brannan CI, Jenkins NA, Copeland NG, and Parada LF. 1995. Loss of neurofibromin results is neurotrophin independent survival of embryonic sensory and sympathetic neurons. *Cell* 82:733–42.

von Recklinghausen F. 1882. *Ueber die multiplen Fibrome der Haut und ihre Beziehung zue den multiplen Neuromen. Berlin: August Hirschwald.*

Wadsby M, Lindenhammer H, and Eeg-Olofsson O. 1989. Neurofibromatosis in childhood: neuropsychological aspects. *Neurofibromatosis* 2:251–60.

Wechsler D. 1974. *Manual for Wechsler Intelligence Scale for Children–Revised (WISC-R).* New York: Psychological Corporation.

Xu G, O'Connell P, Viskochil D, Cawthon R, Robertson M, Culver M, Dunn D, Stevens J, Gesteland R, White R, and Weiss R. 1990. The neurofibromatosis type 1 gene encodes a protein related to GAP. *Cell* 62:599–608.

Zimmerman RA, Yachnis AT, Rorke LB, Rebsamen SL, Bilaniuk LT, and Zackai E. 1992. Pathology of findings of high signal intensity findings in neurofibromatosis type 1. Abstract from 78th Scientific Assembly of the Radiological Society of North America. *Radiology* 186(P):123.

8

Abnormalities of the Nervous System

David H. Gutmann, M.D.,-Ph.D.

Neurofibromatosis type 1 (NF1) affects the nervous system in many ways. Some of the significant CNS manifestations of NF1 include the development of astrocytomas and, in particular, optic pathway/hypothalamic gliomas, learning disabilities, MRI hyperintense lesions on T_2-weighted images, and precocious puberty. These manifestations will be dealt with elsewhere in this book. In this chapter, attention will focus on two common CNS abnormalities (macrocephaly and headaches) as well as several less common manifestations of NF1 (epilepsy, cerebral vascular abnormalities, aqueductal stenosis, and psychiatric illness). The frequencies of these central nervous system abnormalities in NF1 are listed in Table 8-1.

MACROCEPHALY

Macrocephaly in NF1 is defined as a fronto-occipital circumference greater than or equal to 2 SD above the mean for sex and age (DeMeyer 1972; Meredith 1971). Macrocephaly unrelated to CNS pathology (e.g., hydrocephalus) is observed in 29 to 45% of individuals with NF1 (Carey et al. 1979; Huson et al. 1988; North et al. 1993; Riccardi 1992). This enlarged head circumference is not indicative of an underlying calvarial bone defect but rather reflects the size of the

Table 8-1. Other central nervous system abnormalities in NF1

Feature	% of Patients with NF1		
	North (1993)	Huson et al. (1988)	Riccardi (1992)
Macrocephaly (> 2 SD)	43	45	29
Headache	9	—	10
Epilepsy	3.5	7.3	6
Aqueductal stenosis	2.5	1.5	1
Psychiatric disturbances	2.5	—	1
Cerebrovascular abnormalities	—	—	< 1

brain. In studies by Riccardi and coworkers, increased head circumference was observed at every age level as compared with the general population (Riccardi 1981, 1992). This was significant for both males and females and did not vary according to racial, ethnic, or socioeconomic background. In this regard, once macrocephaly became apparent, it continued to be a feature characteristic of an individual with NF1. Studies by Bale and coworkers (1991) demonstrated that NF1 is a true macrocephaly syndrome, again, supporting the notion that macrocephaly is an associated feature of NF1.

NATURAL HISTORY

In the small number of longitudinal studies, macrocephaly, once detected, remains a feature throughout the life of an individual affected with NF1 (Riccardi 1992). The degree of macrocephaly is not dependent on other manifestations of NF1 and does not correlate with the severity of the disease.

PATHOLOGY AND PATHOGENESIS

The pathogenesis underlying the macrocephaly observed in NF1 is unknown. It does not appear to be related to any underlying bony defects but merely reflects the size of the brain. Preliminary studies examining brains from individuals with NF1 have demonstrated an increased number of glial fibrillary acidic protein (GFAP)–immunoreactive astrocytes (Nordlund et al. 1995). Whether this increased number of astrocytes accounts for the relative macrocephaly seen in individuals with NF1 will require further study. Interestingly, morphometric studies have demonstrated increased white matter volumes in children with NF1 (Greenwood et al. 1997; Said et al. 1996). The availability of the heterozygous *Nf1* knockout mouse genetically engineered to harbor one normal and one mutant copy of the *NF1* gene in all cells of the body may provide an experimental model to address this issue.

EVALUATION AND MANAGEMENT

As part of the routine evaluation of an infant, careful fronto-occipital circumference measurements are taken annually and charted as a function of age. In children with NF1, macrocephaly is commonly observed, with the head circumference growing along an isopleth at least 2 SD from the average. Isolated macrocephaly in individuals with NF1 is not an indication for MRI of the brain. However, accelerated head growth deviating from the established isopleth, the presence of an abnormal neurologic examination, papilledema, or persistent/-unusual headaches warrants further evaluation.

HEADACHE

Headaches are commonly associated with NF1 and have been described in 9 to 10% of affected individuals (North 1993; Riccardi 1992). In one study involving 181 patients with NF1, headaches were present in 55 patients (Clementi et al. 1996). Fifty-two of these cases were not associated with CNS pathology. Five individuals had migraine headaches, while 47 suffered from episodic tension-type headaches. In 3 of the 55 cases, obstructive hydrocephalus was related to the presence of a brain tumor. In all three of these cases, the headaches were described as "tension"-type headaches. Thirteen of the 181 patients who underwent routine CT or MRI studies of the brain had abnormal results. In 7 of these 13 patients, there was no associated headache. Abnormal findings included 4 optic pathway gliomas and 1 individual with aqueductal stenosis. In the 6 patients with an abnormal imaging study and headache, 3 were symptomatic, 2 patients harbored optic pathway gliomas, 1 had hydrocephalus, and another had a cerebellar astrocytoma.

NATURAL HISTORY

Although the presentation of headaches in the context of NF1 does not appear to differ from headaches in the general population, population-based studies are required to prove this. The frequency and natural history of headaches in NF1 not associated with CNS pathology also appear indistinguishable from that in the general population. In one study of individuals with NF1, headaches appeared more commonly in the 7- to 14-year-old age group and seemed to decrease with age, such that headaches were less commonly described over the age of 18 (Clementi et al. 1996).

Migraine headaches in children may also manifest as visual abnormalities such as vivid visual hallucinations, scotomata, visual-field deficits, or flashing lights. Paroxysmal disorders such as torticollis of infancy, recurrent abdominal pain, and benign positional vertigo may be an initial manifestation of migraines in children. Complicated migraines in which associated transient neurologic deficits occur may be observed in children with NF1. The appearance of transient neurologic deficits, whether or not in the setting of headache, warrants further investigation to exclude occlusive cerebrovascular etiologies seen in individuals with NF1 (see section on "Cerebrovascular Abnormalities" below).

EVALUATION AND TREATMENT

The evaluation of uncomplicated headache in an individual with NF1 includes a detailed history with attention focused on the frequency, duration, characteristics, and associated symptoms (including visual complaints) that accompany the headaches. Patients should be instructed to maintain a "headache diary" to log detailed information regarding their headaches. Any family history of headaches (migraines) should be explored. Physical examination should include a general physical examination, a careful neurologic examination, and a complete ophthalmologic evaluation for all patients with headaches. Further evaluation should be driven by the clinical history and neurologic examination. Patients with neurologic or neuro-ophthalmologic abnormalities should be studied by brain MRI to exclude hydrocephalus or the presence of an intracranial tumor. When appropriate, cerebral arteriography should be performed to exclude cerebrovascular etiologies.

Complicated migraine headaches are uncommon but have been observed in children with NF1. Affected individuals may present with hemiplegia, aphasia, brain-stem symptoms (ophthalmoplegic migraine), and altered mental status. Often there is a history of vague recurrent headaches or migraines in other first-degree relatives. In addition, the neurologic deficits can manifest even in the absence of headache in some individuals. All individuals with NF1 and complicated migraines should be evaluated by brain MRI and cerebral angiography (in some cases) to exclude the presence of intracranial pathology.

Currently, treatment of headaches in individuals affected with NF1 does not differ from the treatment of individuals without NF1. In general, treatment should be conservative. Standard treatment for tension headaches in children includes acetaminophen, nonsteroidal antiinflammatory medicines (ibuprofen), and amitriptyline. Headaches in adults can be managed similarly. Children and adults should be encouraged to lie down in a quiet darkened room to facilitate the onset of sleep. In addition, migraine headaches can be treated prophylactically either using propranolol or amitriptyline. In adults, abortive therapy can be initiated with ergotamine preparations for severe infrequent migraines. In children, medicines such as cyproheptadine and methysergide may have some utility. Dietary manipulation in individuals with a clear temporal relationship between food ingestion and headache may be helpful. The use of antiseizure medicines such as carbamazepine, phenobarbital, and phenytoin may have benefit in selected cases.

EPILEPSY

Epilepsy is associated with NF1 and has been reported with a frequency of 3.5 to 7.3% (Huson et al. 1988; Kulkantrakorn and Geller 1997; North 1993; Riccardi 1992). The seizures associated with NF1 do not differ from seizures seen in the general population. Epilepsy can occur at any age and include a wide variety of seizure types, such as grand mal tonic–clonic seizures, absence seizures, complex partial seizures, petit mal seizures, and hypsarrhythymia. In the study by Huson and coworkers (1988), 10 of 135 individuals with NF1 had a seizure disorder, with the majority occurring in adulthood. Two were associated with hypsarrhythmia on electroencephalogram (EEG) and were responsive to adrenocorticotrophin hormone (ACTH) treatment. An additional two had an associated intracranial abnormality (aqueductal stenosis). In the remaining six, no known cause could be identified. Three of these were grand mal tonic–clonic seizures, one represented grand mal and absence seizures, and one each were complex partial seizures and petit mal seizures. All were well controlled with routine antiepileptic drugs. Korf and coworkers (1993) reported 22 cases of epilepsy out of 359 individuals with NF1. Eleven of these individuals had seizures that appeared to be unrelated to NF1, including two patients with perinatal/neonatal seizures associated with cerebral atrophy on MRI of the brain, three with primary generalized epilepsy, and six with febrile seizures. Two patients had aqueductal stenosis and the remainder had complex partial seizures with normal MRIs of the brain. Eight of the nine with complex partial seizures had abnormal EEGs. This frequency of individuals with nonfebrile seizures matches that described in the general population. None of the 22 patients in this study who had NFI and epilepsy in this study harbored a structural lesion in the brain. In summary, epilepsy appears to be a less common feature of NF1, but when present, seizures have a natural history similar to that of epilepsy in the general population.

PATHOLOGY AND PATHOGENESIS

The pathogenesis of epilepsy in the context of NF1 is unclear. Although it is tempting to postulate that abnormal CNS development as a result of the defects in *NF1* gene function underlie the development of seizure foci, there is no direct evidence to support this contention. Further studies examining the role of the *NF1* gene in astrocyte and neuronal function within the CNS may provide some clues to the relationship between epilepsy and NF1.

EVALUATION AND TREATMENT

The initial evaluation of seizures in individuals with NF1 should include an MRI scan of the brain as well as an EEG. Laboratory studies to exclude metabolic and infectious etiologies are routine (e.g., complete blood count, urinalysis, serum electrolytes, and blood sugar). Lumbar puncture is indicated if a CNS infection is suspected and there is no evidence of increased intracranial pressure. In the absence of underlying CNS pathology, the treatment of NF1-related seizures does not differ from treatment of seizures in the general population. The same spectrum of antiepileptic drugs is as efficacious in the treatment of seizures in children and adults with NF1 as it is for individuals without this disorder.

PSYCHIATRIC ILLNESS

True psychiatric illness as defined by DSM-IV-R diagnostic criteria is uncommon in NF1 and has been reported in 1 to 2% of individuals (North 1993; Riccardi 1992). There is no evidence to support an excess of "mental illness" in individuals with NF1. Although the psychosocial impact of having NF1 may present excessive stress for a particular individual, there is no evidence for an overrepresentation of dementia, neuroses, psychoses, or personality disorders in individuals with NF1.

AQUEDUCTAL STENOSIS

Both frank hydrocephalus and asymptomatic ventricular dilatation are potentially important complications of NF1 (Davidson 1980; Horwich et al. 1983; Senveli et al. 1989; Spadaro et al. 1986a, 1986b). The anatomic and/or functional bases for these abnormalities are not established except in instances of hydrocephalus that develop as a result of intracranial tumors or surgery. In most instances, the ventricular enlargement spares the fourth ventricle and indicates a stenosis at the level of the aqueduct of Sylvius (Fig. 8-1). Aqueductal stenosis

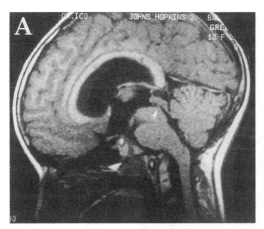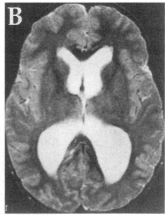

Figure 8-1. Primary aqueductal stenosis in a patient with NF1. Brain MRI shows enlargement of the third and lateral ventricles in sagittal (A) and axial (B) orientations. No enlargement of the fourth ventricle was observed, arguing that the obstruction occurred above the level of the fourth ventricle. The arrow denotes the narrowed Sylvian aqueduct. Typically, enlargement of the third ventricle is also observed. *Source:* Photographs provided by Dr. Bruce Korf (Children's Hospital, Boston).

has been reported in 1 to 2.5% of individuals with NF1 (North 1993; Huson et al. 1988; Riccardi 1992). Individuals with aqueductal stenosis and hydrocephalus may be asymptomatic and may not come to medical attention in the absence of a brain imaging study. For those symptomatic individuals, aqueductal stenosis may manifest as headache, gait disturbance, ocular disturbance, seizures, or speech difficulties. Review of previously reported cases in the literature suggests that children more commonly present with gait disturbances and visual abnormalities whereas adults may manifest with seizures as well as visual abnormalities and gait disturbances (Spadaro et al. 1986a, 1986b). There is no unique profile for children versus adults with NF1 who present with hydrocephalus secondary to aqueductal stenosis. The distribution of aqueductal stenosis in NF1 as a function of age is illustrated in Figure 8-2. The majority of cases reported in individuals affected with NF1 occur between the ages of 6 and 35. Initial presentation before age 5 or after age 50 is unusual.

NATURAL HISTORY

Aqueductal stenosis impairs the normal flow of cerebrospinal fluid through the brain ventricular system and subarachnoid spaces. Constriction of the aqueduct above the level of the fourth ventricle leads to ventricular dilatation, predominantly of the third and lateral ventricles. Expanding hydrocephalus will eventually lead to abnormal CNS function. These abnormalities include headache, gait disturbances, difficulties with speech, seizures, decreased vision, and cranial nerve abnormalities. The finding of papilledema on funduscopic exam should alert the physician to the possibility of increased intracranial pressure and hydrocephalus.

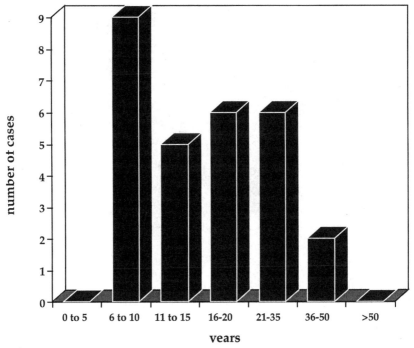

Figure 8-2. Age distribution of aqueductal stenosis in patients with NF1. Review of the reported cases in the literature resulted in the generation of an age histogram for this uncommon feature of NF1. The number of cases are depicted along the y axis, while the age at presentation of symptoms from the aqueductal stenosis is divided according to epoch of life along the x axis. A total of 28 cases were included in which sufficient clinical information was provided.

PATHOLOGY AND PATHOGENESIS

Review of the world literature demonstrates eight cases with proven pathologic correlates (Spadaro et al. 1986a). In these individuals with primary aqueductal stenosis, there were three cases of septal formation, three with forking of the aqueduct and two with surrounding gliosis (Radhakrishnan et al. 1981). MRI evaluation of nine cases of hydrocephalus in NF1 demonstrates periaqueductal gliosis in six patients, while gliomas (two cases) and basiocciput dysplasia (one case) accounted for the remaining three cases (Pou-Serradell and Ugarte-Elola 1989). The contribution of the *NF1* gene to the development of the ventricular outflow system of the brain is unknown. It is tempting to speculate that aqueductal stenosis resulting from surrounding gliosis may be related to locally increased astrocyte proliferation due to inactivation of the *NF1* gene. Further studies are required to determine what role the *NF1* gene plays in regulating astrocyte proliferation in the brain.

EVALUATION AND DIAGNOSIS

Individuals with NF1 who present with an abnormal neurologic or ophthalmologic examination suggestive of intracranial pathology should be evaluated by high-quality enhanced MRI of the brain with thin cuts through the area of the aqueduct to exclude the presence of aqueductal stenosis and hydrocephalus. In particular, abnormalities such as sixth cranial nerve palsy, decreased vision, and severe headaches warrant further investigation. Symptomatic individuals with hydrocephalus resulting from aqueductal stenosis should be surgically treated with placement of a ventricular shunt by an experienced neurosurgeon. Initial follow-up should include MRI of the brain and monitoring for signs of shunt failure.

CEREBROVASCULAR ABNORMALITIES

True cerebrovascular abnormalities are not common in NF1 (Erickson et al. 1980; Rizzo and Lessell 1994; Sobata et al. 1988; Tomsick et al. 1976; Woody et al. 1992). However, 3 to 4% of individuals with cerebrovascular disease have been diagnosed with NF1. Most commonly, the cerebrovascular abnormalities seen in individuals with NF1 result from cerebrovascular stenoses or occlusions involving the carotid, middle cerebral artery, and anterior cerebral arteries (Halpern and Currarino 1965; Lehrnbecher et al. 1994; Levinsohn et al. 1978; Zochodne 1984). The most commonly involved intracranial vessel is the internal carotid artery with obstruction at the level of the siphon. Involvement of the posterior cerebral artery is infrequent. Because of the luminal compromise, small collateral vessels form. On angiography, these small telangiectatic vessels sprouting around the area of the stenosis appear as a puff of smoke (Brooks et al. 1987). This radiographic appearance on cerebral angiography has been termed "moya-moya" (Fig. 8-3).

Guidelines for the diagnosis and treatment of moya-moya disease have been formulated (Fukui 1997). The diagnosis is typically based on cerebral angiography demonstrating stenosis or occlusion at the terminal portion of the internal carotid artery and/or the proximal portion of the anterior or middle cerebral arteries as well as abnormal vascular networks in the vicinity of the occlusion/-stenosis. These findings should be present bilaterally. The diagnosis can also be made by magnetic resonance imaging/angiography (MRI-MRA) demonstrating similar findings. Since moya-moya is idiopathic, other etiologies should be eliminated, including hypertension, autoimmune disease, meningitis, brain neoplasm, head trauma, or irradiation to the head.

Juvenile moya-moya with a peak incidence at 5 years of age typically presents with ischemia in contrast to adult moya-moya (30 to 49 years of age), which presents with hemorrhage due to breakdown of the collateral vessels. Individuals with NF1 and cerebrovascular disease tend to be young, with an equal representation of males and females (Tomsick et al. 1976). Cerebrovascular abnormalities should be suspected in any patient with NF1 who presents with abrupt onset of a neurologic deficit.

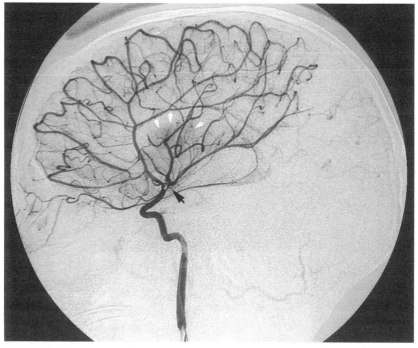

Figure 8-3. Moya-moya radiographic appearance in a patient with NF1. A cerebral arteriogram illustrates the "puff of smoke" appearance in small telangiectatic blood vessels that surround the stenosis at the level of the internal carotid artery (ICA). Telangiectatic blood vessels are denoted by the "blush" of radiographic contrast dye (white arrows) surrounding the ICA occlusion (black arrow). *Source:* Photograph provided by Dr. Bruce Korf (Children's Hospital, Boston).

Clinically, children most commonly present with weakness, involuntary movements, headaches, or seizures. Adults present with similar symptoms, although the sudden onset of neurologic deficits may result from intracranial hemorrhage. Approximately half of all deaths are due to hemorrhage.

NATURAL HISTORY

It is not known whether the cerebrovascular abnormalities in NF1 are evolving or static lesions in which the vascular lumen is narrowed. The formation of small collateral vessels may represent a long-standing adaptation to a large-vessel stenosis. Acute presentation of neurologic deficits can be seen at any age and may reflect the formation of a thrombus and subsequent embolization of a smaller vessel distal to the stenosis.

PATHOLOGY AND PATHOGENESIS

Careful pathologic studies on cerebrovascular disease in NF1 were performed by Salyer and Salyer (1974). They described four different pathologic appearances in NF1-related cerebrovascular disease. These included: (1) pure intimal small vessel thickening and fibrosis, (2) advanced intimal thickening with proliferation, (3) intimal thickening and fibrosis with loss of the smooth muscle layer in the media, and (4) a nodular type with spindle-cell proliferation between the media and adventitial layers. Subsequent analysis of these "spindle cells" revealed cells to be rapidly proliferating vascular smooth muscle cells and not Schwann cells as often reported (Greene et al. 1974; Malecha and Rubin 1992).

Of the 43 cases reported in the literature, three subgroups of individuals with NF1 cerebrovascular disease have been described (Sobata et al. 1988). Group A represents occlusive cerebrovascular disease with an average age of onset of 14 years and a relative female predominance. Group B represents individuals with a cerebral aneurysm with an average of onset of 40 years and a female predominance. Group C represents a combination of occlusive and aneurysmal disease with an average age of onset of 47 years and a female predominance. In individuals with occlusive disease, the majority presented with cerebral ischemia. These individuals tended to be younger as opposed to those with a hemorrhagic presentation. In 10 of these 37 patients with occlusive disease, the cerebrovascular abnormality was an accidental finding. The moya-moya angiographic pattern was detected in 31 of these 37 patients. In individuals with NF1 presenting with cerebral aneurysms, the internal carotid artery was the most common site (four cases), followed by the anterior communicating artery (three cases), and one each in the vertebral posterior-inferior cerebellar artery (PICA) and posterior choroidal artery distributions.

MOLECULAR INSIGHTS

The role of the *NF1* gene as a growth regulator for vascular smooth muscle cells has only recently been investigated (Ahlgren-Beckendorf et al. 1993; Norton et al. 1995). Expression of the *NF1* gene product, neurofibromin, has been detected in vascular endothelial cells as well as vascular smooth muscle cells (Norton et al. 1995). It is plausible that reduced *NF1* gene expression results in increased vascular smooth muscle proliferation and accounts for the vascular hyperplasia that limits the lumen size and results in cerebral ischemia. Likewise, abnormalities in endothelial cell biology as a result of *NF1* gene dysfunction may disrupt the integrity of the blood vessel and lead to aneurysm formation. Formal proof for the role of the *NF1* gene as a negative growth regulator for these cells will require further experiments.

EVALUATION AND TREATMENT

Individuals with NF1 who present with the sudden onset of a neurologic deficit should be promptly evaluated. Initial evaluation includes brain imaging and, in appropriate cases, cerebral angiography. Angiography is appropriate when the history and MRI suggest neurologic and/or structural deficits, respectively, in a vascular distribution. The role of MRA in the evaluation of individuals with NF1 remains to be tested. Because cerebral ischemia without cerebrovascular abnormalities may develop in patients with NF1, appropriate studies should be performed as indicated to exclude cardiac sources (e.g., echocardiogram and Holter monitoring) and other less common etiologies for stroke (e.g., hypercoagulable states). Treatment of cerebrovascular abnormalities in individuals with NF1 is identical to the management of individuals without NF1 and includes both surgical and medical options. Medical treatment typically involves aspirin therapy (at least 80 mg/day), aspirin combined with antiplatelet agents (ticlopidine), or less commonly, systemic anticoagulation (warfarin). None of these treatments has proven efficacy for the prevention of further ischemic events in the setting of NF1 cerebrovascular disease, but experience with cerebrovascular ischemia in adults supports their use.

Surgical approaches include (1) superior temporal artery–middle cerebral artery (STA-MCA) bypass, (2) encephaloduroarteriosynangiosis (EDAS), and encephalomyosynangiosis (EMS). STA-MCA bypass can be effective for revascularization of the brain distal to the occluded vessel but is limited by the difficulty in finding satisfactory donor and recipient arteries of sufficient caliber in patients with moya-moya disease. Surgical experience with this procedure has demonstrated partial normalization of cerebral circulation and good clinical outcomes (Okada et al. 1998). EDAS is an indirect revascularization procedure in which a patent STA is sutured along the dura to approximate the artery to the brain surface. EDAS procedures are often easier and safer to perform in small children and can be combined with an STA-MCA anastomosis (Matsushima et al. 1997). EMS represents another indirect procedure that involves suturing the temporalis muscle to the dura to promote neovascularization on the surface of the brain. This procedure either alone or in combination with STA-MCA bypass has achieved excellent results (reviewed in Ueki et al. 1994).

REFERENCES

Ahlgren-Beckendorf JA, Maggio WW, Chen F, and Kent TA. 1993. Neurofibromatosis 1 mRNA expression in blood vessels. *Biochem Biophys Res Commun* 197:1019–24.
Bale SJ, Amos CI, Parry DM, and Bale AE. 1991. Relationship between head circumference and height in normal adults and in the nevoid basal cell carcinoma syndrome and neurofibromatosis type 1. *Am J Med Genet* 40:206–10.
Brooks BS, Gammal TE, Adams RJ, Hartlage PL, and Smith WB. 1987. MR imaging of moyamoya in neurofibromatosis. *AJNR Am J Neuroradiol* 8:178–9.
Carey JC, Laub JM, and Hall BD. 1979. Penetrance and variability in neurofibromatosis: a genetic study of 60 families. *Birth Defects Original Articles Series*, vol. 15, no. 5B. New York: Liss, pp. 271–81.
Clementi M, Battistella PA, Rizzi L, Boni S, and Tenconi R. 1996. Headache in patients with neurofibromatosis type 1. *Headache* 36:10–3.
Davidson RI. 1980. Primary hydrocephalus in adolescence. *Surg Neurol* 14:137–40.
DeMeyer W. 1972. Megalencephaly in children. *Neurology* 22:634–43.
Erickson RP, Wooliscroft J, and Allen RJ. 1980. Familial occurrence of intracranial arterial occlusive disease (moyamoya) in neurofibromatosis. *Clin Genet* 18:191–6.
Fukui M. 1997. Guidelines for the diagnosis and treatment of spontaneous occlusion of the circle of Willis ("moyamoya" disease). *Clin Neurol Neurosurg* 99:S238–40.
Greene JF, Fitzwater JE, and Burgess J. 1974. Arterial lesions associated with neurofibromatosis. *Am J Clin Pathol* 62:481–7.

Greenwood RS, Said SM, Yeh T-L, El-Fatatry MA, Tupler LA, and Krishnan KRK. 1997. Changes in the brain volume in children with neurofibromatosis 1. *Ann Neurol* 42:500–1.

Halpern M and Currarino G. 1965. Vascular lesions causing hypertension in neurofibromatosis. *N Engl J Med* 273:248–52.

Horwich A, Riccardi WM, and Francke U. 1983. Aqueductal stenosis leading to hydrocephalus—an unusual manifestation of neurofibromatosis. *Am J Med Genet* 14:577–81.

Huson SM, Harper PS, and Compston DAS. 1988. Von Recklinghausen neurofibromatosis: a clinical and population study in South East Wales. *Brain* 111:1355–81.

Korf BR, Carrazana E, and Holmes GL. 1993. Patterns of seizures observed in association with neurofibromatosis 1. *Epilepsia* 34:616–20.

Kulkantrakorn K and Geller TJ. 1997. Seizures in neurofibromatosis type 1. *Neurology* 48:A402.

Lehrnbecher T, Gassel AM, Rauh V, Kirchner T, and Huppertz H-I. 1994. Neurofibromatosis presenting as a severe systemic vasculopathy. *Eur J Pediatr* 153:107–9.

Levisohn PM, Mikhael MA, and Rothman SM. 1978. Cerebrovascular changes in neurofibromatosis. *Dev Med Child Neurol* 20:789–92.

Malecha MJ and Rubi R. 1992. Aneurysms of the carotid arteries associated with von Recklinghausen's neurofibromatosis. *Pathol Res Pract* 188:145–7.

Matsushima T, Inoue TK, Suzuki SO, Inoue T, Ikezaki K, Fukui M, and Hasuo K. 1997. Surgical techniques and the results of a fronto-temporo-parietal combined indirect bypass procedure for children with moyamoya disease: a comparison with the results of encephalo-duro-arterio-synangiosis alone. *Clin Neurol Neurosurg* 99:S123–7.

Meredith H. 1971. Human head circumference from birth to early adulthood: racial, regional and sex comparisons. *Growth* 35:233–51.

Nordlund ML, Rizvi TA, Brannan CI, and Ratner N. 1995. Neurofibromin expression and astrogliosis in neurofibromatosis (type 1) brains. *J Neuropathol Exp Neurol* 54:588–600.

North K. 1993. Neurofibromatosis type 1: review of the first 200 patients in an Australian clinic. *J Child Neurology* 8:395–402.

Norton KK, Xu J, and Gutmann DH. 1995. Expression of the neurofibromatosis 1 gene product, neurofibromin, in blood vessel endothelial cells and smooth muscle. *Neurobiol of Dis* 2:13–21.

Okada Y, Shima T, Nishida M, Yamane K, Yamada T, and Yamanaka C. 1998. Effectiveness of superficial temporal artery-middle cerebral artery anastamosis in adult moyamoya disease. *Stroke* 29:625–30.

Pou-Serradell A and Ugarte-Elola AC. 1989. Hydrocephalus in neurofibromatosis. *Neurofibromatosis* 2:218–26.

Radhakrishnan K, Kak VK, Sridharan R, and Chopra JS. 1981. Adult aqueductal stenosis with Recklinghausen's neurofibromatosis. *Surg Neurol* 16:262–5.

Riccardi VM. 1981. von Recklinghausen neurofibromatosis. *N Engl J Med* 305:1617–26.

———. 1992. *Neurofibromatosis: Phenotype, Natural History and Pathogenesis,* 2nd ed. Baltimore: Johns Hopkins University Press.

Rizzo JF and Lessell S. 1994. Cerebrovascular abnormalities in neurofibromatosis type 1. *Neurology* 44:1000–2.

Said SMA, Yeh T-L, Greenwood RS, Whitt JK, Tupler LA, and Krishnan KRR. 1996. MRI morphometric analysis and neuropsychological function in patients with neurofibromatosis. *Neuroreport* 7:1941–4.

Salyer WR and Salyer DC. 1974. The vascular lesions of neurofibromatosis. *Angiology* 25:510–9.

Senveli E, Altinors N, Kars Z, Arda N, Turker A, Cinar N, et al. 1989. Association of von Recklinghausen's neurofibromatosis and aqueductal stenosis. *Neurosurgery* 24:99–101.

Sobata E, Ohkuma H, and Suzuki S. 1988. Cerebrovascular disorders associated with von Recklinghausen's neurofibromatosis: a case report. *Neurosurgery* 22:544–9.

Spadaro A, Ambrosio D, Moraci A, and Albanese V. 1986a. Nontumoral aqueductal stenosis in children affected by von Recklinghausen's disease. *Surg Neurol* 26:487–95.

Spadaro A, Ambrosio D, Moraci A, Conforti R, and Albanese V. 1986b. Aqueductal stenosis as isolated localization involving the central nervous system in children affected by von Recklinghausen disease. *J Neurosurg Sci* 30:87–93.

Tomsick TA, Lukin RR, Chambers AA, and Benton C. 1976. Neurofibromatosis and intracranial arterial occlusive disease. *Neuroradiology* 11:229–34.

Ueki K, Meyer FB, and Mellinger JF. 1994. Moya-moya disease: the disorder and surgical treatment. *Mayo Clinic Proc* 69:749–57.

Woody RC, Perrot LJ, and Beck SA. 1992. Neurofibromatosis cerebral vasculopathy in an infant: clinical, neuroradiographic and neuropathologic studies. *Pediatr Pathol* 12:613–9.

Zochodne D. 1984. von Recklinghausen vasculopathy. *Am J Med Sci* 287:64–5.

9

Tumors of the Optic Pathway

Robert Listernick, M.D., and David H. Gutmann, M.D.,-Ph.D.

One of the most common tumors in patients with NF1 is the optic pathway glioma. Although tumors of the optic pathway account for only 2 to 5% of all brain tumors in childhood, as many as 70% are associated with NF1. While these tumors generally are benign, optic pathway gliomas may lead to signs as diverse as visual loss and precocious puberty. Before the past 15 years, studies of optic pathway gliomas in NF1 were hampered by the inaccurate diagnosis of NF1, the unavailability of noninvasive neuroimaging techniques, and the frequent rendering of what would now be considered unnecessary, overaggressive therapy. Recognition of the various forms of neurofibromatosis, as well as insights into its pathogenesis, has enabled us to more accurately identify optic pathway gliomas and to elucidate their natural history.

HISTORY

The first recorded case of an optic pathway glioma in association with NF1 was in 1873. Michael reported an autopsy finding of "glial hyperplasia" of the right optic nerve and chiasm in a boy who had "elephantiasis" of one leg. In 1902, Emmanuel noted that these tumors may involve both optic nerves in children with von Recklinghausen disease and that the tumors did not behave in a "malignant" fashion. Both observations, the multicentric nature of optic pathway gliomas in NF1 and their often indolent growth pattern, are central to our understanding of these tumors today. Despite isolated case reports, this association was not widely accepted until Davis (1940) reviewed the literature and reported on five cases (three children, two adults) of optic pathway gliomas in von Recklinghausen disease. He recognized that these tumors often occurred in young children in whom the other manifestations of von Recklinghausen disease, such as café-au-lait spots and neurofibromas, may be minimal or absent, obscuring the true diagnosis. In addition, he clearly pointed out that these lesions were histologically distinct from neurofibromas and should be classified as gliomas.

The next advance in our understanding of optic pathway glioma came from Hoyt and Baghdassarian (1969), who reported the natural history of 36 patients with optic pathway gliomas, 21 of whom had NF1, over a 30-year period. They concluded that: (1) visual impairment at the time of diagnosis generally does not deteriorate, (2) excision of an intraorbital tumor is generally of no value and should be performed only to control proptosis, and (3) irradiation is of little or no benefit in these tumors. All of these conclusions, as will be subsequently reviewed, have stood the test of time.

In 1984, Lewis et al. reviewed the patients who had been evaluated by the Neurofibromatosis Program at the Baylor College of Medicine. They systematically studied the brain and orbits of 217 individuals with NF1 using CT. Although this was a heavily biased population of patients referred from around the country, they found optic pathway gliomas in 15% of the patients. These and other observations ultimately led to the inclusion of optic pathway glioma as one of the seven criteria approved by the NIH for the diagnosis of NF1 (National Institutes of Health 1987).

ANATOMY OF THE VISUAL PATHWAY

An accurate grasp of the anatomy of the visual pathway is necessary if one is to understand the pathogenesis of optic pathway gliomas and the various visual disturbances they cause. Figure 9-1 is a representation of the visual pathway. The optic nerve contains nerve fibers arising from the inner layer of the retina. The largest part of the optic nerve is extracranial, lying within the orbit (i.e., the intraorbital optic nerve). The nerve then enters the skull through the optic canal to become the intracranial optic nerve. The two optic nerves join to form the optic chiasm. Nerve fibers from the nasal half of the retina cross to the contralateral side of the brain, whereas fibers from the temporal half of the retina remain on the ipsilateral side. Together, these two groups of fibers join to form bilateral

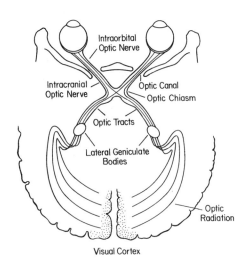

Figure 9-1. Visual pathway.

Table 9-1. Abnormalities on ophthalmologic examination in children with optic pathway gliomas

Decreased visual acuity
Decreased color vision
Afferent pupillary defect
Optic disk pallor
Papilledema
Visual field defect

optic tracts, each terminating in a lateral geniculate body. Finally, nerve fibers travel within the optic radiations and travel around the lateral ventricles into the visual cortex.

Most optic pathway gliomas in NF1 occur in the anterior visual pathway involving the intraorbital and intracranial portions of the optic nerve or the optic chiasm. Table 9-1 lists the various ophthalmologic signs encountered in patients with optic pathway gliomas. Although preservation of visual acuity is the ultimate goal in the management of these tumors, accurate reproducible measurements of visual acuity may be difficult to obtain in young children. Both decreased color vision and an afferent pupillary defect (Marcus Gunn pupil) are sensitive indicators of optic nerve pathology. An afferent pupillary defect can be detected using the swinging light test. When light is shone into the normal eye, both pupils constrict briskly. However, if the light is quickly shone into the abnormal eye, both pupils dilate because of the optic nerve pathology. An afferent pupillary defect will be detected only in children with unilateral optic nerve lesions. Visual-field defects will be bilateral if the tumor affects the optic chiasm or more posterior parts of the pathway. However, visual-field testing is unreliable in children under 7 and is best reserved for following older children with known chiasmal lesions. Finally, optic nerve atrophy is a late sign; thus, its absence does not preclude the presence of a glioma anywhere in the visual pathway.

PATHOLOGY

Optic pathway gliomas in NF1 are universally WHO grade I pilocytic astrocytomas. Grossly, these tumors are typically white to tan and rubbery, often with a great deal of mucus. There may be occasional cystic degeneration (Kleihues et al. 1995). The abundant mucus within these lesions may account for the rare reports of spontaneous tumor regression in some of these patients (Brzowski et al. 1992).

Histologically, these tumors are identical to pilocytic astrocytomas that occur elsewhere in the CNS. The majority of the tumor cells are elongated (fusiform or "pilocytic") with coarse fibrillary cytoplasmic processes that contain glial fibrillary acidic protein. The tumor cells form both densely fibrillary, cellular regions as well as less cellular more loosely textured areas. Fusiform eosinophilic club-shaped structures (Rosenthal fibers) and eosinophilic intracytoplasmic protein granular bodies are regularly found, as they are in other pilocytic tumors of the CNS (Kleihues et al. 1992).

Attempts have been made in the past to distinguish histologically between optic pathway tumors seen in children with NF1 and the sporadic tumors not associated with NF1. Two distinct architectural growth patterns have previously been described. Some tumors exhibit perineural circumferential growth in which the tumor consists of proliferating foci of astrocytes with mucin and microcystic degeneration. The subarachnoid space is widened without extension into the dura. In transection, architecturally normal nerve can be demonstrated surrounded by tumor. In contrast, an intraneural pattern of growth has been described in which the fibrovascular trabeculae of the nerve were stretched by astrocytes proliferating among the axons. The pia mater is fused to the arachnoid and dura with obliteration of the subarachnoid space. On cross section, no normal optic nerve can be identified. Stern et al. (1979, 1980) found the circumferential pattern of growth in 17 of 18 tumors taken from patients with NF1 and the intraneural pattern in 14 of 16 non-NF1 optic pathway gliomas. It is unclear at present whether this distinction is real and, if it is real, what its importance is.

It has been suggested that optic pathway gliomas are benign hamartomas rather than true neoplasms. In reviewing their experience over a 30-year period in 1969, Hoyt and Baghdassarian noted these tumors' apparent self-limited growth pattern and suggested that they were congenital, nonneoplastic lesions. However, as the above histologic features show, these tumors are true neoplasms. In addition, an actuarial analysis of 623 cases of optic pathway gliomas has shown that these tumors have a continuous spectrum of growth rates ranging from very slow to extremely rapid (Alvord and Lofton 1988). The extent to which the presence of NF1 may modify these growth rates will be discussed below.

MOLECULAR BIOLOGY

The majority of information regarding the molecular biology of the *NF1* gene in astrocytes derives not from studies on the optic nerve, but from studies of brain astrocytes and sporadic astrocytomas. In this regard, the role of the *NF1* gene as a negative growth regulator for astrocytes has only recently been investigated. In resting astrocytes from adult human and rodent brains, the expression of the *NF1* gene is nearly undetectable on both the RNA and protein levels (Daston et al. 1992; Gutmann et al. 1996; Nordlund et al. 1993). Neurofibromin, in contrast, is abundant in neurons and oligodendrocytes (Daston et al. 1992). However, in response to several physiologic and pathophysiologic stimuli, *NF1* gene expression can be dramatically upregulated in astrocytes (Hewett et al. 1995). Treatment of astrocytic cultures in vitro with proinflammatory cytokines or with agents that stimulate the protein kinase A pathway result in increased *NF1* gene expression. In addition, increased *NF1* gene expression is also observed in vivo in response to cerebral ischemia (Giordano et al. 1996). These results collectively suggest that neurofibromin expression is tightly regulated in astrocytes and may function as a negative growth regulator during critical times of astrocytic growth and differentiation.

Analysis of a small number of brains from individuals with NF1 has demonstrated increased numbers of glial fibrillary acidic protein (GFAP)–immunoreactive astrocytes in the brain (Nordlund et al. 1995). This postmortem study suggested that reduced *NF1* gene expression results in increased numbers of astrocytes. Recent observations have confirmed these findings in mice in which one copy of the *NF1* gene has been genetically altered and demonstrate increased astrocyte proliferation (Gutmann et al. in press; Rizvi et al. 1999). Support for the notion that reduced *NF1* gene expression in astrocytes leads to increased astrocyte proliferation and increased numbers of astrocytes in the brains of individuals with NF1 derives from morphometric studies on white matter regions in brains from children with NF1 (Greenwood et al. 1997; Said et al. 1996). In these studies, a statistically significant increase in the white matter as compared with gray matter regions was demonstrated in children affected with NF1.

Future studies on the role of neurofibromin in regulating astrocyte growth will be required to determine whether reduced but not absent neurofibromin expression results in the formation of astrocytomas. Given that most optic pathway gliomas in children with NF1 are not progressive, symptomatic optic pathway gliomas may result from additional genetic alterations that cooperate with the loss of *NF1* gene expression. The identification of these cooperating genetic events may provide insights into the molecular pathogenesis of these progressive symptomatic optic pathway gliomas.

The role of neurofibromin as a regulator of p21 *ras* in astrocytes relevant to the control of cell proliferation has only recently been addressed. In studies on sporadic astrocytomas from individuals without NF1, increased activity of p21 *ras* has been observed (Gutmann et al. 1996). Previous studies demonstrated that one of the functions of neurofibromin is to reduce p21-*ras* activity. The increase in p21-*ras* activity in the sporadic tumors results from increased epidermal growth factor receptor signaling. These results suggest two mechanisms for increased p21-*ras* activity relevant to astrocyte growth: (1) increased epidermal growth factor signaling, and (2) loss of neurofibromin expression. Future studies on astrocytomas from individuals with NF1 will be required to address the relationship between p21-*ras* activity and astrocyte proliferation.

CLINICAL CHARACTERISTICS

INCIDENCE

Estimates of the incidence of optic pathway gliomas in children with NF1 vary widely, depending on the mechanism of case ascertainment. The only population-based study was performed by Huson et al. (1988) in southeast Wales. After a thorough search for patients with NF1 was done by contacting general practitioners and reviewing inpatient and outpatient hospital records, 135 patients with

NF1 were identified, 2 of whom were found to have optic pathway glioma, for a prevalence of 1.5%. However, patients in this study were not systematically evaluated for the presence of asymptomatic tumors.

As previously mentioned, Lewis et al. (1984) identified 33 optic pathway gliomas in 217 patients with NF1, for an overall incidence of 15%. This was the first series that attempted to overcome past obstacles in deriving any meaningful data about these tumors in NF1. Its strengths included (1) a strict case definition of NF1, (2) the availability and use of CT in all patients, and (3) strict radiographic criteria for the identification of tumors. Its main weakness was in the source of its patients; as the Baylor program was one of the first multidisciplinary NF clinics in the country, it naturally may have attracted patients with more severe disease, creating a referral bias.

In two studies, Listernick et al. (1989, 1994) also performed screening neuroimaging on all children with confirmed NF1. Although a certain amount of referral bias is impossible to eliminate, these patients may have better represented the pediatric NF1 population at large. The most common manifestation of NF1 was café-au-lait spots, and only a few patients with tumors had overt complications of NF1 that might precipitate early referral, such as plexiform neurofibromas (18%) or orthopedic abnormalities (9%). As in Lewis's patients, Listernick and associates also found a 15% incidence of optic pathway gliomas, excluding children who presented with ophthalmologic symptoms. However, only 52% of the children who had radiographically identifiable optic pathway gliomas ultimately showed any signs or symptoms of their tumors. Therefore, the true incidence of symptomatic optic pathway glioma in NF1 is probably somewhere between 1.5% (Huson's prevalence figure) and 7.5%.

Two intriguing epidemiologic observations deserve comment. First, the female:male ratio of children with tumors in both series by Listernick et al. (1989, 1994) was 2:1. Second, there appears to be a lower incidence of optic pathway gliomas among African-American children with NF1, suggesting the presence of genes that influence the expression of NF1 clinical features. The existence of hormonal factors or modifying genes responsible for these observations remains to be elucidated.

AGE AT PRESENTATION

Optic pathway gliomas, whether or not they are associated with NF1, occur mainly in young children. Rush et al. (1982) reviewed the medical records of 85 patients with histologically confirmed tumors over a 55-year period; the mean age was 10.9 years. Similarly, Wright et al. (1989) identified 31 patients over a 16-year period with a mean age of 10.2 years. The incidences of NF1 in these series were 20% and 48%, respectively. All these tumors had been identified as the result of symptoms. On the other hand, Lewis et al. (1984) found a mean age of 20.8 years for patients with both NF1 and optic pathway tumors. Sixty-six percent of these tumors were unsuspected and were found on screening neuroimaging, probably having been present without causing symptoms for a long time.

Listernick et al. (1989, 1994) showed that the period of greatest risk for the development of symptomatic optic pathway glioma in NF1 is during the first 6 years of life. They found that the median age for the detection of these tumors was 4.2 years. Specifically, all patients with symptoms related to their tumors at the time of diagnosis were identified before 6 years of age. They described four children in whom optic pathway gliomas developed, after they had had previously normal neuroimaging findings, at a mean age of 3.6 years (Listernick et al. 1992). This argues that the development of a symptomatic tumor after the age of 6 years is extremely unusual.

SIGNS AND SYMPTOMS AT PRESENTATION

Optic pathway gliomas may be discovered because of (1) symptoms that prompt a patient to seek medical attention, (2) signs found on either physical or ophthalmologic examination, or (3) screening neuroimaging examinations of individuals with NF1. If all patients with NF1 were to undergo routine screening neuroimaging, anywhere from one half (Listernick et al. 1994) to two thirds (Lewis et al. 1984) of all the discovered optic pathway tumors would never cause any symptoms or signs. Said another way, will develop visual problems in one third of these patients with NF1 found to have optic pathway tumors.

Perhaps the most dramatic presentation of an optic pathway glioma is that of progressive proptosis. These children generally have poor or no vision in the affected eye. Most studies document proptosis in approximately 30% of the children with symptomatic tumors (Kuenzle et al. 1994; Listernick et al. 1994; Lund and Skovby 1991). Such tumors may grow rapidly over a relatively short period of time. Figure 9-2 is the initial CT scan of a 3-month-old girl with NF1; the optic nerves are thin and normal, perhaps with slight dural ectasia. Figure 9-3 is an MRI scan performed in the same child 17 months later; note the massive enlargement of the optic nerve causing a proptotic globe. Clearly, these tumors are biologically distinct from the quiescent optic nerve tumors seen in many other patients.

The majority of children with symptomatic optic pathway glioma will have visual abnormalities at the time of diagnosis. Estimates of abnormal visual examinations range from 33% (Lewis et al. 1984) to 89% (Lund and Skovby 1991). Signs may include an afferent pupillary defect, optic nerve atrophy, papilledema, strabismus, or defects in color vision. Most important, young children may have marked decrements in visual acuity without any symptoms. Listernick et al. (1989) reported on six children with visual acuity ranging from 20/40 to 20/300 who had no ophthalmologic complaints. This underscores the need for thorough annual eye examinations in all young children with NF1 (see below).

Children with optic pathway gliomas involving the optic chiasm are at risk for the development of precocious puberty. This was the presenting symptom in 30% of the patients with tumors in one series (Listernick et al. 1994). The first sign of precocious puberty will be accelerated linear growth (Fig. 9-4). As will be discussed below, these data make it clear that all young children with NF1

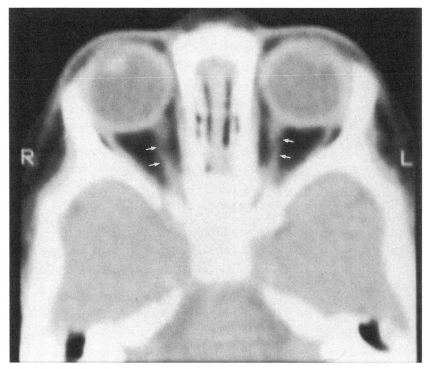

Figure 9-2. CT (axial without contrast) scan of the optic pathways in a 3-year-old girl. Thin, normal-appearing optic nerves are evident, perhaps with slight dural ectasia (arrows).

should have annual assessments of growth using standard growth charts and should be monitored for signs of premature sexual development.

LOCATION OF TUMOR

Optic pathway gliomas in NF1 almost always involve the anterior visual pathway (i.e., the intraorbital optic nerve, the intracranial optic nerve, and the optic chiasm). Conversely, these tumors rarely extend into the optic tracts (Table 9-2). The 48% incidence of postchiasmal extension reported by Kuenzle et al. (1994) is unusual. Bilateral optic nerve tumors (Fig. 9-5) are a hallmark of NF1.

NATURAL HISTORY

As mentioned previously, elucidation of the natural history of optic pathway gliomas in NF1 has been hindered by the inclusion of children who did not have NF1 (before the advent of strict diagnostic criteria in 1988) and by the rendering of overly aggressive treatment. Thus, studies performed before the past 10 years offer limited useful information.

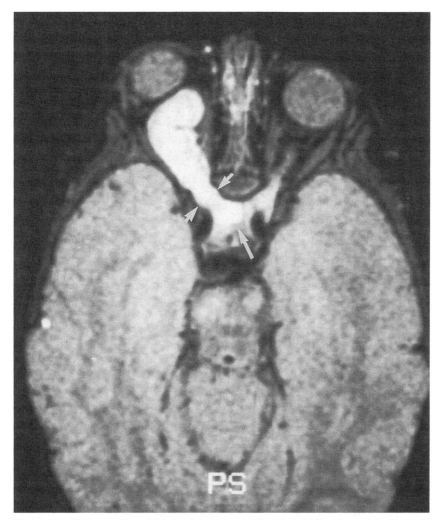

Figure 9-3. MRI scan (T_2-weighted axial with contrast) of the child in Figure 9-2, 17 months later. A large, lobulated enhancing right optic nerve glioma is evident, producing proptosis of the globe with extension into the optic chiasm (large arrow) and enlargement of the right optic nerve canal (small arrows).

Wright et al. (1989) were the first to point out that the natural history of optic pathway gliomas in children with NF1 might be more benign than that of sporadic tumors. Of 16 children whose tumors exhibited no growth over a 16-year period, 11 had NF1, whereas only 4 of 15 children who had actively growing tumors had NF1. These were specifically optic nerve tumors, as opposed to chiasmal tumors, primarily presenting with proptosis. Importantly, Wright pointed out that after a seemingly short period of rapid growth leading to proptosis, most NF1 tumors remained quiescent for long periods of time.

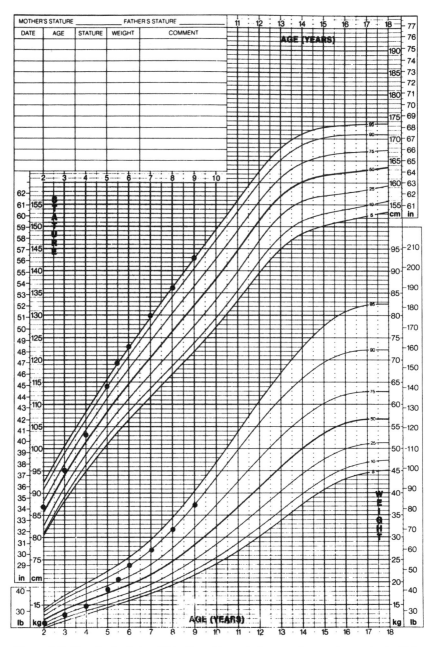

Figure 9-4. Growth chart of a child with a chiasmal glioma and precocious puberty. Note accelerated linear growth beginning between 4 and 5 years of age.

Table 9-2. Location of optic pathway gliomas in NF1

Study	Unilateral Optic Nerve	Bilateral Optic Nerve Only	Optic Chiasm Only	Optic Nerve +Chiasm	Optic Chiasm +Optic Tracts
Lewis et al. 1984	17/33 (52%)	5/33 (15%)	6/33 (18%)	5/33 (5%)	0 (0%)
Lund and Skovby 1991	3/16 (19%)	1/16 (6%)	1/16 (6%)	4/16 (25%)	7/16 (44%)
Pascual-Castroviejo et al. 1994	9/31 (29%)	0 (0%)	0 (0%)	16/31 (52%)	6/31 (19%)
Kuenzle et al.1994	7/21 (33%)	0 (0%)	0 (0%)	4/21 (19%)	10/21 (48%)
Listernick et al. 1995	11/33 (33%)	4/33 (12%)	4/33 (12%)	12/33 (37%)	2/33 (6%)

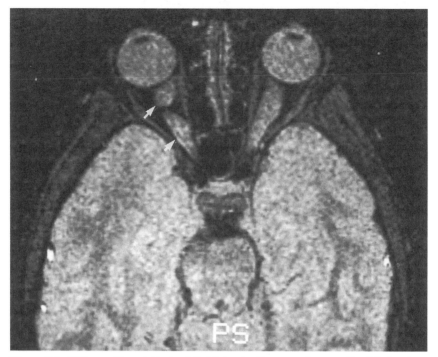

Figure 9-5. MRI scan (T$_2$-weighted axial). Bilateral optic nerve gliomas with a lobulated fusiform glioma with kinking involving right nerve (arrows) and a diffuse glioma of the left nerve.

Listernick et al. (1994) showed that optic pathway gliomas in children with NF1 infrequently progress once the tumors have come to medical attention. They observed 33 children with NF1 and optic pathway gliomas; the mean length of the follow-up period has now extended for over 8 years. Sixteen (48%) of the tumors never caused any symptoms or signs; these were all discovered by screening neuroimaging of asymptomatic children. Most important, of the 17 children who had symptomatic tumors, there was demonstrable growth of the tumor on neuroimaging or progression of visual disturbances in only 3 children. Even some tumors that had experienced rapid growth with proptosis before diagnosis failed to progress during the follow-up period. The 3 children who had progressive disease all had chiasmal involvement; 2 of these children had only minimal progression. One child with an intraorbital glioma was seen at age 1.8 years with proptosis and essentially no vision in the affected eye; after surgical removal of the optic nerve, she had evidence of a contralateral tumor on MRI with normal vision that has not changed for over 10 years. In a second child with a chiasmal tumor that was discovered on examination for precocious puberty bilateral optic disk pallor developed during the 7-year follow-up period with no change in tumor size or visual acuity. Tumor growth and decreasing visual acuity and visual fields significant enough to require intervention developed in only one child who had an intraorbital and chiasmal tumor. Similar results have been found by Kuenzle et al. (1994).

The accumulated data suggest that optic pathway gliomas in NF1 behave in a fairly predictable manner and fall into one of two groups. About half the tumors never cause any symptoms or signs; they would be discovered only by screening neuroimaging. The second group of tumors experience a period of growth culminating in a patient's reporting symptoms or in a physical sign (e.g., proptosis, decreased visual acuity, precocious puberty) leading to discovery; once found, these tumors rarely progress or cause any subsequent problems. In addition, the period of greatest risk for the development of symptomatic tumors is during the first 6 years of life, and significant tumor growth after this age is unusual. These data have profound implications as to how we approach both asymptomatic and symptomatic children with NF1 and optic pathway tumors, as will be discussed below.

PRECOCIOUS PUBERTY

Children with optic pathway gliomas are at risk for the development of precocious puberty. The onset of puberty is considered precocious if it occurs before the age of 7 in girls or before the age of 9 in boys. The currently accepted theory is that lesions located near the hypothalamus interfere with tonic CNS inhibition of the hypothalamic–pituitary–gonadal axis, resulting in premature onset of puberty. In a comprehensive study of children with NF1 cared for in a large multidisciplinary clinic, precocious puberty was diagnosed in 7 of 219 children (3%). All of these children had optic pathway gliomas that involved the optic chiasm; precocious puberty occurred in 39% of such children (Habiby et al. 1995). Precocious puberty may be the presenting sign of a chiasmal glioma in as many as 30% of all the children with NF1 gliomas (Listernick et al. 1994). This may underrepresent the incidence, as many of the children in the report were still very young and were at risk for the development of precocious puberty. Each child's clinical presentation was that of accelerated linear growth (see Fig. 9-4), underscoring the need for all children with NF1 to have annual assessments of growth using standard growth charts, particularly children with optic pathway gliomas.

It has been debated whether precocious puberty is a complication of NF1 per se or whether it occurs only within the context of a patient who has a chiasmal glioma, a common scenario in NF1. Previous reports of NF1 and precocious puberty in the absence of a glioma may have erroneously included children with McCune–Albright syndrome (the triad of polyostotic fibrous dysplasia, endocrine hyperfunction, and hyperpigmented skin lesions), in whom café-au-lait spots and precocious puberty may occur. In addition, older reports have lacked both CT and MRI technology, leaving open the possibility of undetected tumors. Habiby et al. (1995) found precocious puberty occurring exclusively in children with NF1 who had chiasmal gliomas. More recently, Cnossen et al. (1997) reported three children with NF1 and precocious puberty, only one of whom had an optic pathway glioma. The other two children had normal MRIs. While this may represent a real association, it may also be the chance simultaneous occurrence of these two relatively common conditions.

If precocious puberty is suspected in a child with NF1, bone age should be determined radiologically. An advanced bone age when compared to chronologic age is the hallmark of precocious puberty. Serial measurements of luteinizing hormone following intravenous administration of luteinizing hormone–releasing hormone (LHRH) is the standard by which precocious puberty is diagnosed. However, Habiby et al. (1995) showed that, as a screening tool, one can rely on a single elevated measurement of a highly sensitive luteinizing hormone immuno-chemiluminometric assay. A positive result would still need to be confirmed using provocative testing. Early detection is important, as both the accelerated linear growth and the development of secondary sexual characteristics can be curtailed. Such children usually respond well to treatment with a long-acting luteinizing hormone–releasing hormone agonist. Following an initial stimulation of gonadotropin release, prolonged use of such an agent leads to down-regulation of gonadotropin levels and eventual suppression of sex hormone production by the gonads. This returns the body to its prepubertal state and prevents premature epiphyseal closure, maximizing ultimate adult height. Finally, all children with NF1 and precocious puberty should undergo MRI testing to search for the presence of an optic pathway glioma.

IMAGING METHODS

COMPUTERIZED TOMOGRAPHY

The advent of CT heralded the beginning of an era of noninvasive neuroimaging, greatly facilitating the care of patients with NF1. Typical features of an optic nerve glioma on CT scan include tubular thickening of the optic nerve, often associated with a sinuous intraorbital course and one or more "kinks" (Fig. 9-6). The kinking is probably due to the large amount of mucin in the glioma, making it very pliant. These tumors have well-circumscribed margins due to lack of invasion of the dura (Jakobiec et al. 1984); contrast enhancement is almost uniformly present. Chiasmal tumors associated with NF1 have similar characteristic findings when they extend forward into the optic nerves. However, discrete globular tumors within or adjacent to the optic chiasm are generally not associated with NF1 (Fletcher et al. 1986). Despite their clear value, CT scans are limited in their ability to detect both intracanalicular and optic tract extension of tumor.

MAGNETIC RESONANCE IMAGING

MRI with contrast enhancement is presently the method of choice for diagnostic imaging of the CNS in individuals with NF1. MRI permits the use of serial examinations without exposing the patient to repeated doses of ionizing radiation. Equally important, MRI provides superior contrast resolution around the edges of a tumor, enabling sharper evaluation of tumor borders. As seen in Figure 9-7,

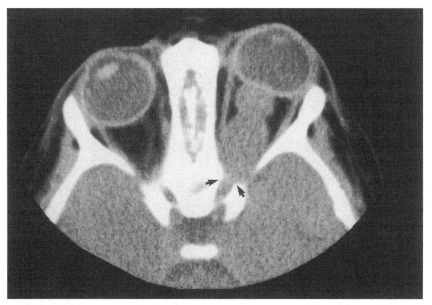

Figure 9-6. CT scan (axial with contrast). Large, mildly enhancing, lobulated left optic nerve glioma with kinking and extension into the anterior opening of the left optic nerve canal (arrows).

the characteristic MRI finding of an optic nerve glioma is a fusiform tumor of high signal intensity surrounding a core of lower signal intensity on T_2-weighted images (Haik et al. 1987; Imes and Hoyt 1991). As with CT scans, the intraorbital tumors will appear tortuous and "kinked." MRI will generally demonstrate a diffusely thickened optic chiasm when imaging chiasmal tumors in children with NF1 (Fig. 9-8); globular tumors or exophytic masses are less common in NF1 than in sporadic tumors. MRI is superior to CT in delineating the extent of tumor spread within the chiasm and posteriorly along the optic tracts and optic radiation (Fig. 9-9).

Previous experience with CT scans had demonstrated optic nerves that were described as "thickened" or "tortuous"; these were interpreted as optic nerve gliomas. MRI elegantly demonstrates a thickened optic nerve sheath or dural ectasia that is separate from a normal optic nerve (Van Es et al. 1996). This correlates well with the previously described histology of perineural arachnoidal proliferation (Stern et al. 1980) or optic nerve dural ectasia (Lövblad et al. 1994).

Magnetic resonance spectroscopy enables assessment of the biochemical composition of focal areas within the brain. In preliminary studies, spectroscopic patterns of NF1 gliomas differed from those found in normal areas of the brain, potentially offering the physician a sensitive tool that would delineate tumor spread and distinguish tumor from "unidentified bright objects," the areas of increased signal intensity seen on the T_2-weighted images of many individuals

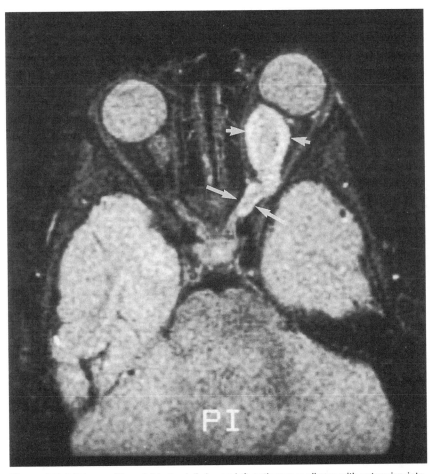

Figure 9-7. MRI scan (T_2-weighted axial). Large left optic nerve glioma with extension into anterior aspect of the intracanalicular portion of the nerve, producing enlargement of the anterior aspect of the optic nerve (large arrows) with kinking, and effacement of the left globe. The enhancement with increased signal is along the periphery of the optic nerve glioma (small arrows). There is no extension into the optic chiasm.

with NF1 (Castillo et al. 1995). Further study is necessary before the use of spectroscopy can be clinically applicable.

VISUAL EVOKED POTENTIALS

Visual evoked potentials (VEPs) have been proposed as a useful screening tool for the management of asymptomatic children with NF1. North et al. (1994) evaluated 30 children with NF1, 10 who had optic pathway gliomas (7 of 10 had abnormal visual acuity), and 20 who had normal visual pathways, using pattern-shift VEPs. They found a sensitivity of 90% and a specificity of 60% for the

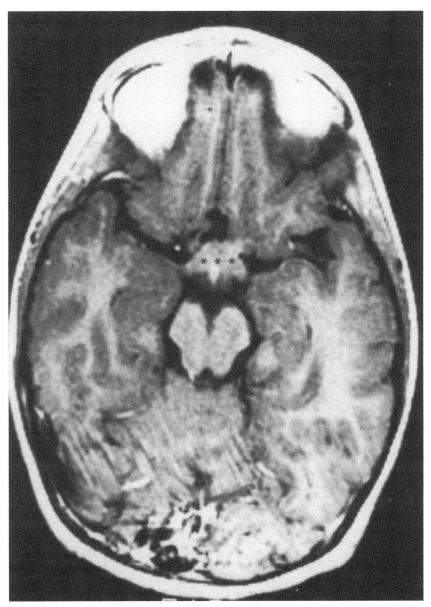

Figure 9-8. MRI scan (T_1-weighted axial with contrast). Small, mildly enhancing chiasmal glioma (asterisks).

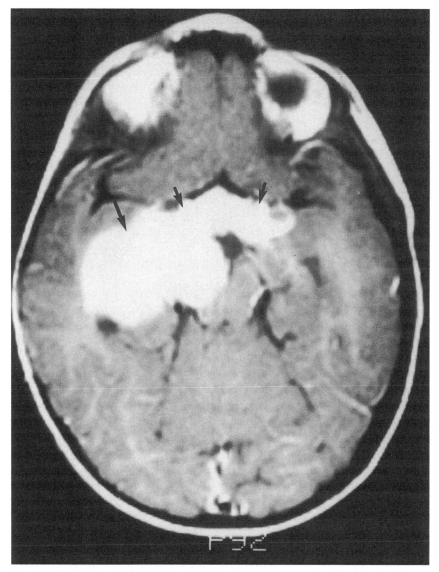

Figure 9-9. MRI scan (T_1-weighted axial with contrast). Large, markedly enhancing glioma involving optic chiasm (small arrows) with extension into right optic tract (large arrow).

detection of tumors. The only child under 5 years of age who had a glioma was evaluated using light-emitting diode goggles, a device for which normative data were not available. North and associates acknowledged that reliable results may not be obtained in children younger than 5 years, the peak age for optic pathway glioma. Even if one were willing to accept a high false positive rate of 40%, other studies have reported much lower sensitivities using VEP to detect tumors

(Rossi et al. 1994). Regardless, there is little, if any, utility in using VEPs to screen all asymptomatic children with NF1, and data regarding VEPs' usefulness in following children with known tumors are lacking.

NF1-ASSOCIATED VERSUS SPORADIC OPTIC PATHWAY GLIOMA

It has never been clear whether the clinical manifestations and natural history of optic pathway glioma associated with NF1 differ from those of sporadic tumors. Although some reports demonstrated longer survival in children with NF1 (Rush et al. 1982; Wright et al. 1989), conflicting results have also been reported (Imes and Hoyt 1986). Improper identification of patients with NF1 and the lack of availability of noninvasive neuroimaging techniques may have hampered the accurate classification of patients in the past. Indeed, authors often failed to distinguish between these two groups in their analyses. As such, previous recommendations regarding follow-up or treatment of these tumors are difficult to apply, as generally these two groups of patients have been lumped together.

Both Listernick et al. (1995) and Deliganis et al. (1996) looked at a combined total of 80 patients with optic pathway gliomas to delineate the effect that NF1 might have on the natural history of these tumors. Strict attention was paid to the NIH diagnostic criteria for NF1 in both studies. Remarkably similar results were seen in the two studies (Table 9-3). Decreased visual acuity was commonly found in both groups at presentation. While NF1-associated optic pathway gliomas often presented with proptosis or precocious puberty, symptoms of increased intracranial pressure with associated hydrocephalus were found almost exclusively in patients with sporadic tumors. Nystagmus and strabismus were generally seen only in the sporadic group.

Tumor location was distinctly different in the two groups. Optic tract involvement was far more common in non-NF1 tumors, and hydrocephalus was found exclusively in this group. Figure 9-10 shows a typical sporadic optic nerve glioma; note the large, globular suprasellar mass with marked hydrocephalus. As

Table 9-3. Distinguishing characteristics of NF1 optic pathway tumors (OPTs) and non-NF1 OPTs

	NF1 OPTs	Non-NF1 OPTs
Initial signs	Proptosis Precocious puberty Decreased visual acuity	Increased intracranial pressure/hydrocephalus Nystagmus Strabismus Decreased visual acuity
Tumor location	Intraorbital optic nerve common Multicentric Optic nerve ±chiasm	Intraorbital optic nerve rare Unicentric Optic tract ±chiasm
Tumor growth during follow-up period	Uncommon	Common

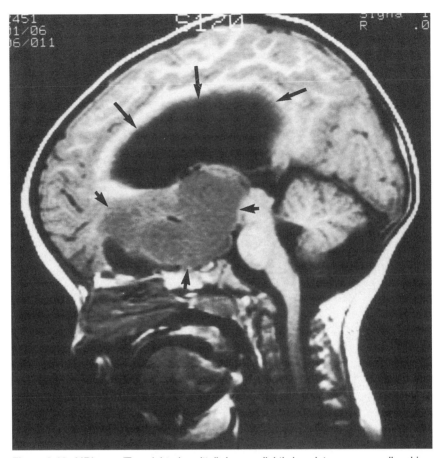

Figure 9-10. MRI scan (T_1-weighted sagittal). Large, slightly hypointense suprasellar chiasmal glioma (small arrows) producing hydrocephalus with enlargement of lateral ventricles (large arrows) in a patient who does not have NF1.

in previous studies, bilateral optic nerve tumors were a hallmark of NF1. Listernick et al. (1995) noted that all tumors confined to the intraorbital optic nerve in childhood were associated with NF1. Although isolated optic nerve glioma may be found in patients who do not have NF1, most such cases have involved older patients; this entity may be biologically distinct from tumors found in young children regardless of the presence of NF1.

Probably the most important distinction is found in these tumors' natural history. Following presentation, tumor progression, as defined by tumor growth or deteriorating visual function, was uncommon in NF1-associated tumors but common with sporadic tumors. Deliganis et al. (1996), who reported longer follow-up intervals than Listernick, found a much longer mean time before tumor progression in the patients with NF1. However, Deliganis and colleagues were unable to document any differences in overall survival between the two groups. Regardless of the results, these findings underscore the need for treatment protocols and research on these tumors in children to take into account the presence of NF1 in the planning stages and again when reporting results.

SCREENING NEUROIMAGING FOR ASYMPTOMATIC CHILDREN WITH NF1

There has been considerable debate regarding the role of screening tests (neuroimaging and visual evoked potentials) in the care of asymptomatic children with NF1. Routine "screening" would be important if it led to early detection of optic pathway gliomas and if early initiation of therapy prevented complications. Although many asymptomatic tumors might be identified through such an approach, the vast majority would not progress to the point of requiring treatment. A longitudinal study of children with NF1 in whom screening neuroimaging was performed failed to identify any tumors in which early detection altered the patient's clinical course (Listernick et al. 1994). Over half of the detected tumors never grew or caused any symptoms, while the vast majority of symptomatic optic pathway gliomas never required treatment. Overall, only 3 of 26 children showed any evidence of tumor progression following diagnosis and only 2 required treatment. Both of these children had abnormal eye examinations and would have been identified even if screening neuroimaging had not been performed.

One might advocate an approach of screening neuroimaging only for very young children, the group at high-risk for the development of optic pathway gliomas. However, even in three children in whom gliomas subsequently developed after having had normal neuroimaging studies, a screening strategy was unable to prevent complications of these tumors (Listernick et al. 1992). A strategy of repeated MRI examinations at frequent intervals would be extremely costly and still might not allow intervention before symptoms occurred. As discussed above, the data on the sensitivity of visual evoked potentials is conflicting, and their current reliability under the age of 5 is questionable. Thus, the preponderance of evidence suggests that screening of asymptomatic children with NF1 to detect optic pathway gliomas fails to improve clinical outcome and should not be performed. Emphasis should be placed on the clinical examination. This recommendation was endorsed by the NF1 Optic Pathway Glioma Task Force of the National Neurofibromatosis Foundation (Listernick et al. 1997).

TREATMENT OF THE ASYMPTOMATIC CHILD WITH NF1

Although screening neuroimaging is not recommended, the Task Force highlighted the need for serial ophthalmologic examinations, particularly in young children with NF1. These examinations should be performed by either a pediatric ophthalmologist or an ophthalmologist familiar with NF1. All children who are found to have unexplained ophthalmologic abnormalities should then un-

Table 9-4. Suggested ophthalmologic screening protocol for children with NF1 who do not have ocular symptoms

---

1. All children 6 years of age and under should have yearly full exams.
2. All newly diagnosed patients with NF1 should have full exams.
3. The following schedule may be used for all children older than 6 years
    who are being seen regularly in a NF referral center:
    Age 8 years: Abbreviated exam*
    Age 10 years: Full exam†
    Age 13 years: Abbreviated exam
    Age 16 years: Full exam
    Age 20 years: Abbreviated exam
    Age 25 years: Full exam
4. Full ophthalmologic examinations should be performed whenever
    signs or symptoms suggest an ophthalmologic abnormality.

---

*An abbreviated examination includes assessment of visual acuity, color vision, and slit-lamp examination.

†A full ophthalmologic examination for a child with NF1 includes assessment of visual acuity, color vision, slit-lamp examination, and ophthalmoscopy.

dergo MRI examination of the head and orbits with contrast enhancement. A suggested ophthalmologic screening protocol is proposed in Table 9-4. This protocol takes into account the observation that essentially all symptomatic optic pathway gliomas arise during the first 6 years of life. These recommendations are primarily based on longitudinal data generated by studies performed by Listernick et al. (1989, 1992, 1994).

A complete ophthalmologic examination of a child with NF1 should include assessment of visual acuity, color vision, visual fields, ophthalmoscopy, and slit-lamp examination. Visual acuity assessments include fixation patterns (infants and toddlers), Allen picture cards or Lippman "HOTV" matching game (cooperative preschool children), and linear Snellen test-equivalent (school-age children) with optical correction where appropriate. Ocular alignment and rotations, pupillary light responses, and refractive status with cycloplegia are also recommended. Ophthalmoscopy should include indirect and, when possible, direct examinations.

Finally, all children with NF1 should undergo longitudinal assessment of growth using standardized growth charts. As precocious puberty may be the first manifestation of a chiasmal glioma, even in the presence of a normal ophthalmologic examination, the physician should be alert to the finding of accelerated linear growth.

MANAGEMENT OF SYMPTOMATIC OPTIC PATHWAY GLIOMA

The prime dictum of medicine is to do no harm. In the past, many children with NF1 and optic pathway gliomas have been treated with unnecessary, overly aggressive therapy in large part due to a lack of understanding of the natural history of these tumors. As we now know that the large majority of these tumors in children with NF1 will not progress following discovery, many children can be followed closely without any specific intervention. Table 9-5 outlines a suggested schedule for following such children once a decision has been made to defer treatment. MRI with contrast enhancement is the preferred method for following these tumors. There is insufficient information available to endorse the routine use of either magnetic resonance spectroscopy or visual evoked potentials. Finally, all children with chiasmal gliomas should be followed closely for the development of accelerated linear growth or secondary sexual characteristics that would indicate the presence of precocious puberty. As the treatment of children with optic pathway gliomas and NF1 is highly dependent on the location of the tumor, the specifics of these differences will be discussed below.

INTRAORBITAL GLIOMAS

The vast majority of intraorbital optic nerve gliomas in patients with NF1 never progress once they have come to medical attention. This is especially true of those isolated intraorbital tumors that happened to be found by "screening" neuroimaging; these tumors rarely have associated visual deficits. As such, these children can be followed without any intervention using a protocol such as the one in Table 9-5. Although the required duration of follow-up studies is unclear, accumulating data suggest that they are unlikely to experience significant progression after 6 years of age.

Another group of patients will present with rapidly progressive proptosis and an eye with little or no vision. They will have a large intraorbital tumor causing proptosis, perhaps with involvement of the intracranial optic nerve, but without any evidence of chiasmal involvement (see Fig. 9-7). The main concern in these patients is retrograde spread of the tumor to the optic chiasm with associated de-

Table 9-5. Follow-up of children with NF1 and optic pathway glioma

Time Interval following Diagnosis	MRI Scan	Ophthalmologic Exam*
Diagnosis	X	X
3 months	X	X
6 months		X
9 months	X	X
12 months		X
15 months	X	
18 months		X
24 months	X	X
36 months	X	X
Yearly, thereafter	†	X

*A full ophthalmologic exam consists of assessment of visual acuity, color vision, slit-lamp examination, and ophthalmoscopy. Interval visual field evaluations should be performed when the child is old enough that reliable examinations can be obtained.

†The data are insufficient to make a clear recommendation regarding the intervals for MRI examinations after the first 2 years following diagnosis. However, assuming there has been no evidence of progression, the intervals between neuroimaging can be gradually lengthened.

creased vision in the contralateral eye. However, there are neither well-documented cases of this happening nor any evidence that surgical removal of tumor is necessarily effective in preventing spread. Thus, the surgery can be reserved for cosmetic purposes in a child with severe proptosis. Painful proptosis is also an indication for surgery in a nonseeing eye.

Treatment should be reserved for the few patients who have intraorbital gliomas with either residual useful vision and/or evidence of radiologic or ophthalmologic progression. There is evidence that radiotherapy will, at least transiently, stop further tumor progression (Flickinger et al. 1988). However, it is difficult to extract from the literature how many of these patients had NF1 tumors that would never have progressed. In general, radiation therapy should not be used in such young patients due to the well-described cognitive and endocrinologic side effects. Rather, a trial of chemotherapy, as discussed below, would be a prudent first step. It should be recognized that while there has been a great deal of accumulated data on the utility of chemotherapy in the treatment of chiasmal gliomas, there is as yet little published data of its utility in the treatment of isolated optic nerve tumors.

CHIASMAL GLIOMAS

Although symptomatic chiasmal gliomas in children with NF1 are more likely to progress following identification than are intraorbital tumors, a substantial majority of such tumors remain quiescent. In one study, only 3 of 18 tumors that involved the optic chiasm progressed and, in general, the degree of progression was minimal (Listernick et al. 1994). Thus, the initial management of most chiasmal gliomas should involve an observation period such as one outlined in Table 9-5.

Once the decision to treat has been made, several options are available. Surgery has a limited role in treating chiasmal tumors as it may increase both visual and neurologic morbidity. Occasionally, surgical debulking of an exophytic tumor mass or cystic component may benefit the patient. However, this is more common in sporadic non-NF1 associated tumors. Biopsy is rarely necessary in patients with NF1; tumors limited to the optic pathway are almost universally low-grade juvenile pilocytic astrocytomas.

Radiation therapy has long been the mainstay in the treatment of chiasmal gliomas. Many of these studies fail to adequately distinguish between NF1 associated and sporadic tumors (Horwich and Bloom 1985; Kovalic et al. 1990). Tumors destined to remain quiescent were irradiated; lack of progression was incorrectly interpreted as a response to therapy rather than as a result of the tumor's innately benign nature. In addition, a variety of studies have demonstrated that 5- and 10-year disease-free control in patients with progressive optic pathway gliomas, with or without NF1, will be better in patients who receive radiation therapy. However, at 20 years, the overall disease-free survival rates are essentially equivalent between the patients who received radiation therapy and those who did not.

Several concerns arise with the use of radiation therapy in children with NF1. As many of the children requiring treatment are young (less than 6 years), there is a significant risk of both endocrinologic (growth hormone deficiency, panhypopituitarism) and neurocognitive sequelae. There are theoretical concerns that radiation of children with NF1 may either cause mutation of a low-grade tumor to a higher-grade glioma or result in secondary malignancies in normal brain within the radiation portal. Finally, the rare NF1 tumors that extend posteriorly into the optic tracts and optic radiation may be too diffuse for inclusion within a radiation portal. For all these reasons there has been growing interest in the use of chemotherapy for these tumors.

Although a number of single-agent and multiple-agent chemotherapeutic regimens have been used, most recent attention has focused on the use of carboplatin alone or in combination with vincristine. Carboplatin-induced tumor shrinkage was accompanied by striking improvement in visual fields and visual acuity with return of color discrimination in a girl with NF1 and a progressive chiasmal tumor (Charrow et al. 1993). Packer et al. (1997) reported 78 children with a mean age of 3 years who had newly diagnosed, progressive low-grade gliomas, 58 of which involved the optic chiasm. They were treated with a combination of carboplatin and vincristine. Progression-free survival rates were 75% at 2 years and 68% at 3 years; 44% of the patients clearly responded to treatment. There was no difference in progression-free survival rates between the children who had NF1 and those who had sporadic tumors. Although these data are highly encouraging, chemotherapy should still be considered an investigational means of therapy. Chemotherapy should not be regarded as curative, but rather as a means by which tumor growth may be delayed until children are older, when radiation therapy can be employed with fewer potential side effects. Alternatively, it is possible that in children with NF1 the use of chemotherapy during these tumors' period of rapid growth (below the age of 6 years) may be sufficient treatment and obviate the need for any further treatment later. Only with further study and long-term follow-up will these questions be answered.

REFERENCES

Alvord E and Lofton S. 1988. Gliomas of the optic nerve or chiasm: outcome by patients' age, tumor site, and treatment. *J Neurosurg* 68:85–98.

Brzowski AE, Bazan C, Mumma JV, and Ryan SG. 1992. Spontaneous regression of optic glioma in a patient with neurofibromatosis. *Neurology* 42:679–81.

Castillo M, Green C, Kwock L, Smith K, Wilson D, Schiro S, and Greenwood R. 1995. Proton MR spectroscopy in patients with neurofibromatosis type 1: evaluation of hamartomas and clinical correlation. *AJNR Am J Neuroradiol* 16:141–7.

Charrow J, Listernick R, Greenwald MJ, Das L, and Radkowski MA. 1993. Carboplatin-induced regression of an optic pathway tumor in a child with neurofibromatosis. *Med Pediatr Oncol* 21:680–4.

Cnossen MH, Stam EN, Cooiman LCMG, Simonsz HJ, Stroink H, Oranje AP, Halley DJJ, de Goede-Bolder A, Niermeijer MF, and de Muinck Keizer-Schrama SMPF. 1997. Endocrinologic disorders and optic pathway gliomas in children with neurofibromatosis type 1. *Pediatrics* 100:667–70.

Daston MM, Scrable H, Norlund M, Sturbaum AK, Nissen LM, and Ratner N. 1992. The protein product of the neurofibromatosis type 1 gene is expressed at highest abundance in neurons, Schwann cells and oligodendrocyte. *Neuron* 8:415–28.

Davis FAD. 1940. Primary tumors of the optic nerve (a phenomenon of Recklinghausen's disease). *Arch Ophthalmol* 23:957–1022.

Deliganis AV, Geyer JR, and Berger MS. 1996. Prognostic significance of type 1 neurofibromatosis (von Recklinghausen disease) in childhood optic glioma. *Neurosurgery* 38:1114–9.

Emmanuel C. 1902. Ueber die bezeihungen der Sehnervengeschwülste zur elephantiasis neuromatodes und über Sehnervengliome. *Arch Ophthalmol* 53:129.

Fletcher WA, Imes RK, and Hoyt WF. 1986. Chiasmatic gliomas: appearance and long term changes demonstrated by computed tomography. *J Neurosurg* 65:154–9.

Flickinger JC, Torres C, and Deutsch M. 1988. Management of low-grade gliomas of the optic nerve and chiasm. *Cancer* 61:635–42.

Giordano MJ, Mahadeo DK, He YY, Geist RT, Hsu C, and Gutmann DH. 1996. Increased expression of the neurofibromatosis 1 (NF1) gene product, neurofibromin, in astrocytes in response to cerebral ischemia. *J Neurosci Res* 43:246–53.

Greenwood RS, Said SM, Yeh T-L, El-Fatatry MA, Tupler LA, and Krishnan. 1997. Changes in the brain volume in children with neurofibromatosis 1. *Ann Neurol* 42:500–1.

Gutmann DH, Geist RT, Wright DE, and Snider WD. 1995. Expression of the neurofibromatosis 1 (NF1) isoforms in developing and adult rat tissues. *Cell Growth Differ* 6:315–22.

Gutmann DH, Giordano MJ, Mahadeo DK, Lau N, Silbergold D, and Guha A. 1996. Increased neurofibromatosis 1 gene expression in astrocytic tumors: positive regulation by p21-ras. *Oncogene* 12:2121–7.

Gutmann DH, Loehr A, Zhang Y, Kim J, Henkemeyer M, and Cashen A. Haploinsufficiency for the neurofibromatosis 1 (NF1) tumor suppressor results in increased astrocyte proliferation. *Oncogene* (in press).

Habiby R, Silverman B, Listernick R, and Charrow J. 1995. Precocious puberty in children with neurofibromatosis type 1. *J Pediatr* 126:364–7.

Haik BG, Saint Louis L, Bierly J, Smith ME, Abramson DA, Ellsworth RM, and Wall M. 1987. Magnetic resonance imaging in the evaluation of optic nerve gliomas. *Ophthalmology* 94:709–17.

Hewett SJ, Choi DW, and Gutmann DH. 1995. Increased expression of the neurofibromatosis 1 (NF1) tumor expression gene protein, neurofibromin, in reactive astrocytes in vitro. *Neuroreport* 6:1505–8.

Horwich A and Bloom HJG. 1985. Optic gliomas: radiation therapy and prognosis. *Int J Radiat Oncol Biol Phys* 6:1067–79.

Hoyt WF and Baghdassarian SA. 1969. Optic glioma of childhood: natural history and rationale for conservative management. *Br J Ophthalmol* 53:793–8.

Huson SM, Harper PS, and Compston DAS. 1988. Von Recklinghausen neurofibromatosis: a clinical and population study in southeast Wales. *Brain* 111:1355–81.

Imes RK and Hoyt WF. 1986. Childhood chiasmal gliomas: update on the fate of patients in the 1969 San Francisco study. *Br J Ophthalmol* 70:179–82.

———. 1991. Magnetic resonance imaging signs of optic nerve gliomas in neurofibromatosis 1. *Am J Ophthalmol* 111:729–34.

Jakobiec FA, Depot MJ, Kennerdell JS, Shults WT, Anderson RL, Alper ME, Citrin CM, Housepian EM, and Trokel SL. 1984. Combined clinical and computed tomographic diagnosis of orbital glioma and meningioma. *Ophthalmology* 91:137–55.

Kleihues P, Soylemezoglu F, Schäuble B, Scheithauer BW, and Burger PC. 1995. Histopathology, classification, and grading of gliomas. *Glia* 15:211–21.

Kovalic JJ, Grigsby PW, Shepard MJ, Fineberg BB, and Thomas PR. 1990. Radiation therapy for gliomas of the optic nerve and chiasm. *Int J Radiat Oncol Biol Phys* 18:927–32.

Kuenzle C, Weissert M, Roulet E, Bode H, Schefer S, Huisman T, Landau K, and Boltshauser E. 1994. Follow-up of optic pathway gliomas in children with neurofibromatosis type 1. *Neuropediatrics* 25:295–300.

Lewis RA, Gerson LP, Axelson KA, Riccardi VM, and Whitford RP. 1984. von Recklinghausen neurofibromatosis: incidence of optic gliomata. *Ophthalmology* 91: 929–35.

Listernick R, Charrow J, and Greenwald M. 1992. Emergence of optic pathway gliomas in children with neurofibromatosis type 1 after normal neuroimaging results. *J Pediatr* 121:584–7.

Listernick R, Charrow J, Greenwald MJ, and Esterly NB. 1989. Optic gliomas in children with neurofibromatosis type 1. *J Pediatr* 114:788–92.

Listernick R, Charrow J, Greenwald MJ, and Mets M. 1994. Natural history of optic pathway tumors in children with neurofibromatosis type 1: a longitudinal study. *J Pediatr* 125:63–6.

Listernick R, Darling C, Greenwald M, Strauss L, and Charrow J. 1995. Optic pathway tumors in children: the effect of neurofibromatosis type 1 on clinical manifestations and natural history. *J Pediatr* 127:718–22.

Listernick R, Louis DN, Packer RJ, and Gutmann DH. 1997. Optic pathway gliomas in children with neurofibromatosis 1: consensus statement from the NF1 Optic Pathway Glioma Task Force. *Ann Neurol* 41:143–9.

Lövblad KO, Remonda L, Ozdoba C, Huber P, and Schroth G. 1994. Dural ectasia of the optic nerve sheath in neurofibromatosis type 1: CT and MR features. *J Comput Assist Tomogr* 18:728–30.

Lund AM and Skovby F. 1991. Optic gliomas in children with neurofibromatosis type 1. *Eur J Pediatr* 150:835–8.

Michael V. 1873. Ueber eine hyperplasie des chiasma und des rechten nervus opticus bei elephantiasis. *Arch Ophthalmol* 19:145.

National Institutes of Health. 1988. *Neurofibromatosis.* National Institutes of Health Consensus Development Conference Statement.

Nordlund M, Gu X, Shipley MT, and Ratner N. 1993. Neurofibromin is enriched in endoplasmic reticulum of CNS neurons. *J Neuroscience* 13:1588–1600.

Nordlund ML, Rizvi TA, Brannan CI, and Ratner N. 1995. Neurofibromin expression and astrogliosis in neurofibromatosis (type 1) brains. *J Neuropathol Exp Neurol* 54:588–600.

North K, Cochineas C, Tang E, and Fagan E. 1994. Optic gliomas in neurofibromatosis type 1: role of evoked potentials. *Pediatr Neurol* 10:117–23.

Packer RJ, Ater J, Allen J, Phillips P, Geyer R, Nicholson HS, Jakacki R, Kurczynski E, Needle M, Finlay J, Reaman G, and Boyett JM. 1997. Carboplatin and vincristine chemotherapy for children with newly diagnosed progressive low-grade gliomas. *J Neurosurg* 86:747–54.

Pascual-Castroviejo I, Bermejo AM, Martín VL, Pascual CR, and Pascual SI. 1994. Optic gliomas in neurofibromatosis type 1: presentation of 31 cases. *Neurologia* 9:173–7.

Rizvi TA, Akunuru S, de Courten-Myers G, Switzer RC, Nordlund ML, and Ratner N. 1999. Region-specific astrogliosis in brains of mice heterozygous for mutations in the neurofibromatosis type 1 (Nf1) tumor suppressor. *Brain Research* 816:111–23.

Rossi LN, Pastorino G, Scotti G, Gazocchi M, Maninetti MM, Zanolini C, and Chiodi A. 1994. Early diagnosis of optic glioma in children with neurofibromatosis type 1. *Child Nerv Syst* 10:426–9.

Rush JA, Younge BR, Campbell RJ, and MacCarty CS. 1982. Optic glioma: long-term follow-up of 85 histopathologically verified cases. *Ophthalmology* 89:1213–9.

Said SMA, Yeh T-L, Greenwood RS, Whitt JK, Tupler LA, and Krishnan KRR. 1996. MRI morphometric analysis and neuropsychological function in patients with neurofibromatosis. *Neuroreport* 7:1941–4.

Stern J, DiGiacinto GV, and Housepian EM. 1979. Neurofibromatosis and optic glioma: clinical and morphological correlations. *Neurosurgery* 4:524–8.

Stern J, Jakobiec FA, and Housepian EM. 1980. The architecture of optic nerve gliomas with and without neurofibromatosis. *Arch Ophthalmol* 98:505–11.

Van Es, North KN, McHugh K, and DeSilva M. 1996. MRI findings in children with neurofibromatosis type 1: a prospective study. *Pediatr Radiol* 26:478–87.

Wright JE, NcNab AA, and McDonald WI. 1989. Optic nerve glioma and the management of optic nerve tumours in the young. *Br J Ophthalmol* 73:967–74.

10

Other Malignancies

David H. Gutmann, M.D.,-Ph.D.,
and James G. Gurney, Ph.D.

NEUROFIBROMATOSIS 1 (NF1) AS A SYNDROME WITH INHERITED PREDISPOSITION TO CANCER

Neurofibromatosis type 1 (NF1) has long been recognized as a syndrome with an inherited predisposition to cancer, because both benign and malignant tumors develop at an increased frequency in individuals with NF1. Because of this increased incidence of tumor development, the *NF1* gene has been hypothesized to function as a tumor-suppressor gene (negative growth regulator). *NF1*, like other tumor-suppressor genes, functions to negatively regulate cell growth such that abnormalities in *NF1* gene function lead to increased cell proliferation and the development of tumors. As with other tumor-suppressor gene disorders, individuals with NF1 harbor one normal and one mutated copy of the *NF1* gene in all cells in their body (Fig. 10-1). The development of tumors is the result of somatic mutations in the one remaining wild-type (normal) *NF1* gene, rendering both copies of the *NF1* gene nonfunctional (Knudson 1971, 1993). This loss of *NF1* gene (neurofibromin) expression leads to dysregulated cell growth and may represent one of the initial events in tumor formation in affected individuals.

The most common malignancies seen in individuals affected with NF1 are astrogliomas (astrocytomas and gliomas) and malignant peripheral nerve sheath tumors (MPNSTs) (Poyhonen et al. 1997; Shearer et al. 1994). These tumor types are discussed elsewhere in the book. This chapter will focus on several of the less common malignancies seen in individuals with NF1 as well as discuss the risk of secondary malignancy in NF1 and the genetic epidemiology of cancer in NF1.

NF1 CANCER EPIDEMIOLOGY

The majority of tumors in individuals with NF1 are benign growths, such as neurofibromas (Riccardi 1992). However, a small percentage of tumors are classified as cancers and behave in a malignant fashion (Tables 10-1 and 10-2). There

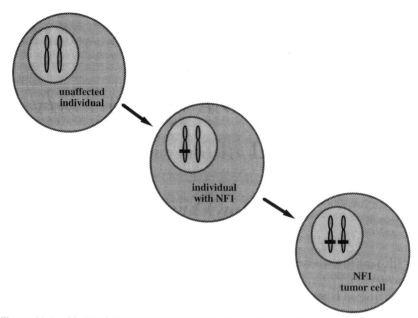

Figure 10-1. Model of the progression to malignancy. The Knudson hypothesis envisions that two genetic events are required for the development of a tumor in an individual with NF1. In individuals without NF1, two copies of the *NF1* gene located on chromosome 17 are functional. In individuals with NF1, one copy of the *NF1* gene is mutated (either inherited from an affected parent or arising de novo as a new mutation). The mutated *NF1* gene is denoted by the black box. In all cells in the body of an individual with NF1, one functional copy of the *NF1* gene exists. For tumors to develop, a second somatic mutation must occur in the remaining wild-type *NF1* gene to render both copies of the *NF1* gene nonfunctional. It is presumed that the loss of both copies of the *NF1* gene leads to dysregulated cell growth and the formation of a tumor.

is a general consensus that patients with NF1 have disproportionately high rates of not only benign neurologic tumors, but also malignancies of the nervous system. Because of the relative rarity of both NF1 and cancer (especially in younger populations for the latter), and because there are no large, comprehensive, population-based NF1 registries from which to initiate analytic epidemiologic studies, there are substantial methodologic difficulties in conducting informative research on this potential relationship (Bader 1986; Hope and Mulvihill 1981; Matsui et al. 1993; Schneider et al. 1986; Shearer et al. 1994). As such, the vast majority of evidence related to the elevated cancer risk in patients with NF1 is based on case reports and case series, with their inherent specialized selection, rather than on population-based studies, which ideally are not as vulnerable to problems related to clinical referral patterns or other selection biases.

Despite these limitations, a body of evidence supports the contention that individuals with NF1 are at increased risk for the occurrence of CNS malignancies (Friedman and Birch 1997; Ilgren et al. 1985). For example, Maris et al. (1997)

Table 10-1. Cancers associated with NF1 in four large series

Study	Astrocytoma, Including Optic Pathway Glioma (%)	MPNST (%)	Pheochromocytoma (%)	Rhabdomyosarcoma (%)	Leukemia (%)
Huson et al. 1998	2.2	1.4	0.7	1.4	0
North 1993	9	1	0	0	0
Riccardi 1992	15	4.3	0.2	0	0
Sorenson et al. 1986	7.5	1.9	1.4	0	0.5

Table 10-2. NF1 associated with malignancy

Malignancy	Individuals with NF1 (%)
Astrocytoma	
Optic pathway glioma	12.5
Other CNS sites	1.0–1.6
Sarcoma	
MPNST	31.4
Other sarcomas	1.76–4.2
Leukemia	
Juvenile chronic myeloid leukemia	1.7
Myelodysplastic syndromes	7.14
Rhabdomyosarcoma	1.36

reviewed the tumor registry of the Children's Hospital of Philadelphia and identified 5782 primary malignancies from 1960 to 1994, including 64 (1.1%) cancers that were diagnosed in children known to have NF1. CNS malignancies accounted for 35 (55%) of the malignant tumors and MPNSTs for an additional 16 (25%) among those with NF1.

Limited insight can be drawn from evaluating population-based case–control studies of brain cancer (intracranial tumors) in which the frequency of NF1 is estimated. For instance, Wrensch et al. (1997) compared 492 adults with incident primary astroglial tumors (ICD-O morphology codes 9380 to 9481) with 443 control adults. From reports by patients (n = 2) or their proxies (n = 1), neurofibromatosis (type not specified) was concurrently present in 3 patients with malignant brain tumor, but no control subjects. Based on reports from mothers in the West Coast Childhood Brain Tumor Study (Preston-Martin et al. 1996), there were 5 children with NF1 among 540 cases of brain tumor, as compared with no children with NF1 among 801 controls (unpublished data). Of the 5 case children with NF1, 2 had anaplastic astrocytomas, 1 had a glioblastoma, 1 had a malignant glioma, and 1 had a MPNST. Gold et al. (1994), using reports from fathers, found 4 children with NF1 among 361 childhood cases of brain tumor, as compared with no NF1 among 1086 matched control children. These and other (Matsui 1993) case-control studies suggest that NF1 is more common in populations of patients with brain cancer than in similar populations with no brain cancer, and that NF1 may be associated with approximately 1% of malignant brain tumors. However, such studies give no estimate of the increased risk of CNS malignancies among individuals with NF1.

An indication of the increased risk for CNS malignancies may be apparent from a retrospective cohort study of 212 individuals with NF1 who were hospitalized in Denmark between 1924 and 1944 and followed through a variety of record sources until 1983 (Sorensen et al. 1986). Compared with expected population estimates, the standardized incidence ratio (relative risk) for all malignancies combined was 4.0 (95% CI, 2.8–5.6). Of the 57 malignancies identified in the NF1 cohort, 21 (37%) were of the central nervous system and 6 (11%) were of the peripheral nervous system. It is obvious that the proportion of nervous system tumors was greatly overrepresented as compared with the common epithelial cancers that predominate in adult populations. Because this study was limited to patients with NF1 who were identified as a result of hospitalization for that disorder, it is unclear to what extent the observed pattern represents nonhospitalized individuals with NF1 in Denmark during the same period.

Blatt et al. (1986) retrospectively evaluated the frequency and distribution of tumors in 121 children with NF1 between 1953 and 1984 at Children's Hospital of Pittsburgh. Of the 22 (20%) "clinically significant" tumors among the cohort, 18 were of the central nervous system. This included 9 optic gliomas and 5 other astrocytomas. As is common in the literature, Blatt and associates distinguished optic gliomas from malignancies. Optic gliomas are usually low-grade pilocytic astrocytomas with fairly benign behavior (Heideman et al. 1997; Russell and Rubinstein 1989). There is inconsistency in the literature, however, regarding which CNS tumors should be classified as benign and which malignant. All astrocytomas, including pilocytic, are considered malignancies by the U.S. National Cancer Institute's Surveillance, Epidemiology, and End Results (SEER) Program. The classification of brain tumors, which has been evolving over the years, is controversial and has been the subject of considerable debate (Heideman et al. 1997). Thus, divergent estimates of the incidence of CNS cancer in populations of patients with NF1 may, to a degree, reflect differences in the manner in which optic gliomas and other low-grade astrocytomas are classified in a given series.

NEURAL CREST-DERIVED TUMORS

Early observations regarding the tissue origins of the diverse clinical manifestations of NF1 led several investigators to classify NF1 as a "neurocristopathy" (Bolande 1981). This label was applied to NF1 largely because several of the clinical manifestations of the disorder involve tissues and cell types that derive from the developing neural crest. However, it is now well appreciated that NF1 is not a neurocristopathy in that many of the manifestations of NF1 occur in tissues that do not derive from the neural crest.

The pigmentary abnormalities (café-au-lait spots, skinfold freckling, and Lisch nodules) and the most common tumor type (neurofibroma) are derived from melanocytes and Schwann cells, respectively. These two cell types take their origin from the developing neural crest. Support for this notion comes from studies that analyzed the expression of neurofibromin in the developing and adult chick (Stocker et al. 1995). *NF1* expression is abundant in early neural crest–derived progenitor cells and tissues. These observations raise the possibility that loss of *NF1* expression leads to dysregulated growth of neural crest–derived tissues and the development of specific malignancies, in particular, medullary thyroid cancer, malignant melanoma, and pheochromocytoma.

Scattered reports in the literature have suggested an association between neural crest–derived tumor syndromes and NF1 (Cantor et al. 1982; Chakrabarti et al. 1979; Daly et al. 1970; Griffiths et al. 1983; Ruppert et al. 1996; see also Chapter 12). One of these syndromes, multiple endocrine neoplasia 1 (MEN1) has been reported in rare individuals with NF1. Review of existing published case reports on such an association revealed five patients with NF1 and carcinoid; four with NF1 and hyperparathyroidism; three with NF1, pheochromocytoma, and duodenal carcinoids; one with NF1, pheochromocytoma, and thyroid cancer; and one with NF1, pheochromocytoma, and somatostatinoma. These rare reports underscore the improbability of a true association between NF1 and MEN1-like syndromes.

Studies on the molecular pathogenesis of multiple endocrine neoplasia syndromes demonstrated defects in the RET receptor tyrosine kinase. This receptor is a natural ligand for glial-derived neurotrophin factor (GDNF) and signals through the *ras* pathway. The possibility that neurofibromin might participate in this RET signaling pathway remains to be elucidated. Should neurofibromin function as a *ras* regulator in this signaling pathway, a role for the *NF1* gene might emerge relevant to the development of these neural crest tumors.

MEDULLARY THYROID CANCER

Medullary thyroid cancers (MTCs) are thyrocalcitonin-producing tumors with a neural crest derivation. These tumors arise from parafollicular C cells. There are case reports in the literature in which individuals with NF1 have associated thyroid cancer (Hasegawa et al. 1984). Despite these reports, there are no data to substantiate an association between MTC and NF1. Further work is required in this area.

MELANOMA

Melanin-producing cells derive from the embryonic neural crest. As several clinical manifestations of NF1 result from pigmentary abnormalities (café-au-lait spots, skinfold freckling, and Lisch nodules), it is possible that abnormalities in pigmentary cell development result from defects in *NF1* gene function. There are a small number of case reports of individuals with NF1 and melanoma (Mastrangelo et al. 1979; Specht and Smith 1988; To et al. 1989). In a large series of 900 individuals with melanoma, only one individual met diagnostic criteria for NF1 (Mastrangelo et al. 1979). In addition, several hospital-based studies on individuals affected with NF1 have failed to demonstrate any cases of melanoma.

Although no strong case can be made for an increased incidence of melanoma in individuals affected with NF1, there may be a role for the *NF1* gene in the molecular pathogenesis of sporadic malignant melanoma. Several studies have examined metastatic melanoma tumor cell lines from individuals without NF1 (Andersen et al. 1993; Johnson et al. 1993; The et al. 1993). In these studies, 25 to 30% of such tumors have reduced or absent *NF1* expression as detected on both the RNA and protein levels. In addition, DNA alterations affecting the *NF1* gene have been demonstrated in a select subset of these tumors. Further examination of several of these cell lines failed to demonstrate elevated levels of activated GTP-bound *ras* (Johnson et al. 1993; The et al. 1993). These results suggest that loss of *NF1* expression may be associated with the development of these cancers. Since these studies were performed on cell lines and not fresh tumor specimens, it is possible that these findings overestimate the contribution of the *NF1* gene to the development of these tumors. To this end, no mutations in the GAP domain of the *NF1* gene and no loss of heterozygosity were observed in 87 informative sporadic melanomas (Gomez et al. 1996).

One of the essential enzymes important for the production of melanin is regulated on the transcriptional level by neurofibromin. In one in vitro study, neurofibromin was shown to regulate the transcription of the tyrosinase gene (Suzuki et al. 1994). Moreover, this DNA regulatory function of neurofibromin is localized to the GTPase-activating protein (GAP) domain. These results collectively suggest that neurofibromin might play a role in the differentiation of melanocytes. It is possible that alterations in *NF1* gene expression might lead to loss of cellular differentiation and predispose to tumor formation, but no data exist to support this notion.

PHEOCHROMOCYTOMAS

Of all neural crest–derived tumors, the strongest case can be made for a true association between NF1 and pheochromocytomas. Among patients with pheochromocytomas, the proportion of individuals with NF1 has been estimated between 4 and 23% (Fernandez-Calvet and Garcia-Mayor 1994; Kalff et al. 1982; Meyer and Gifford 1978; Schlumberger et al. 1992). Several studies have demonstrated an increased incidence of pheochromocytomas in individuals with NF1, ranging from 0.2 to 1.4% (see Table 10-1). In one series of 18 patients with NF1 and hypertension, pheochromocytomas were identified in 10 individuals (Kalff et al. 1982). Although in this study pheochromocytomas were detected in patients with NF1 with an age range of 15 to 62 years, younger patients tended to have causes of hypertension other than pheochromocytomas.

Pheochromocytomas are derived from chromaffin cells of neural crest origin (reviewed in Werbel and Ober 1995). Approximately 85 to 95% of pheochromocytomas are located in the adrenal medulla, occurring with equal frequency in the right and left adrenal gland. Ten percent of tumors are bilateral and 10% are malignant. The diagnosis of a malignant pheochromocytoma cannot be reliably established by histologic appearance and is instead dependent on the presence or absence of metastases. Pheochromocytomas are typically well-encapsulated highly vascular tumors that range in size from 2 to 3000. Histologic analysis demonstrates pheochromocytes with marked cellular and nuclear pleiomorphism. A fine granular and basophilic cytoplasm is apparent after hematoxylin and eosin staining. Fixation in dichromate solution and staining with the Schmorl method produces the characteristic olive green coloration (chromaffin reaction). Although pheochromocytomas most commonly occur in the adrenal gland, they may also be found in the aortic bodies, mediastinum, and the organ of Zuckerkandl at the aortic bifurcation. The average age of detection in individuals with NF1 is 38 years, a figure not dissimilar from that observed in the general population.

Patients experiencing symptoms resulting from a pheochromocytoma may manifest with sustained or paroxysmal hypertension, unexplained agitation and anxiety, tachycardia, excessive perspiration and flushing, or headache. Markedly elevated levels of epinephrine are associated with paroxysmal hypertension, while elevated levels of norepinephrine are more commonly seen with sustained hypertension. In addition, abnormalities of glucose regulation, both hypoglycemia and hyperglycemia, are common.

Pheochromocytomas are a heterogeneous group of hormone-secreting tumors. Therefore, there is no one single test that achieves 100% sensitivity. Diagnostic evaluation should include a 24-hour urine collection to quantitate the excretion of vanillylmandelic acid and specific catecholamines (metanephrine, epinephrine, and norepinephrine). Other tests, including the clonidine suppression test or measurements of chromagranin A, can also be used. Localization of the tumor follows the finding of an abnormal biochemical test. Three procedures are routinely used. The most sensitive study was MRI (100%) followed by CT (94%) and radionuclide scans (88%), although CT detected 100% of abdominal pheochromocytomas (reviewed in McGrath et al. 1998). MRI and CT scans have been reported to have accuracies of 85 to 95% in detecting masses with a spatial resolution of 1 cm or smaller. Initial focus is on the adrenal glands, where 90% of these tumors are located. Extra-adrenal sites should be sought in the face of a normal adrenal MRI study and elevated catecholamines. Repeat determinations may be necessary if a high degree of suspicion exists. Radionuclide scans (^{131}I-metaiodobenzylguanidine) are sometimes employed to determine the precise location of the tumors, but have lower accuracy (86–94%) than CT or MRI scans. Once identified, prompt surgical removal is warranted to avoid the potentially life-threatening complications of untreated pheochromocytoma. Preoperative management should begin at least 7 days before surgery to control blood pressure and to expand plasma volume. The treatment of malignant pheochromocytomas includes chemotherapeutic regimens that have been successful in neuroblastoma, such as vincristine, cyclophosphamide, and dacarbazine.

Molecular analysis of pheochromocytomas from individuals with NF1 has demonstrated loss of heterozygosity for markers surrounding the *NF1* gene (Xu et al. 1992). Loss of neurofibromin expression has been observed in tumors with genetic evidence of *NF1* gene alterations (Gutmann et al. 1994). In addition, pheochromocytomas in individuals without NF1 also demonstrate loss of *NF1* gene expression (Gutmann et al. 1993b). Approximately one third (35%) of pheochromocytomas from individuals with no clinical evidence of NF1 demonstrated reduced *NF1* RNA or neurofibromin expression. As discussed in Chapter 5, multiple alternatively spliced exons exist with the *NF1* gene that may contribute to the generation of neurofibromin functional diversity (Gutmann et al. 1993c). Exon 23a encodes a highly basic sequence of 21 amino acids that is inserted into the GAP domain. Normal adrenal gland predominantly expresses *NF1* mRNA containing exon 23a in contrast to the majority of pheochromocytomas that express *NF1* mRNA lacking this exon (Gutmann et al. 1995a). The significance of this *NF1* RNA isoform switch is unknown, but raises the possibility that this change in isoform expression may relate to the pathogenesis of these tumors.

Several insights into the pathogenesis of pheochromocytomas have derived from studies on mice with targeted disruptions of the *NF1* gene. In mice heterozygous for an *Nf1* gene mutation (*Nf1+/–*), pheochromocytomas develop in 15% of mice after 15 months of age (Jacks et al. 1994). One fourth of these tumors are present bilaterally. Analysis of these pheochromocytomas has demonstrated loss of expression of the one remaining wild-type *Nf1* gene, proving that the development of these tumors requires complete loss of neurofibromin expression. These observations are consistent with Knudson's (1993) hypothesis and are in complete agreement with results obtained with human pheochromocytoma tumors.

EMBRYONAL TUMORS

Several embryonal tumors have been reported in association with NF1. These include neuroblastoma, Wilms tumor, and rhabdomyosarcoma.

NEUROBLASTOMA

Neuroblastomas represent another neural crest–derived adrenal medullary tumor. There are a few cases of neuroblastoma reported in association with NF1 (Bolande and Towler 1970; Hayflick et al. 1990; Knudson and Amromin 1966). Matsui reported three cases of neuroblastoma in children with NF1 and cancer while other studies have failed to find any such associations (Matsui et al. 1993). At present, the evidence strongly argues against an association between neuroblastoma and NF1.

Several studies have examined *NF1* expression in sporadic neuroblastoma tumor cell lines derived from patients without NF1 (Johnson et al. 1993; The et al. 1993). In two such studies, 20 to 25% of sporadic neuroblastoma cell lines demonstrated loss of *NF1* expression on the RNA and protein levels. As was reported for the melanoma tumor cell lines, no alterations in *ras*-GTP levels were observed in these neurofibromin-deficient tumors. These results suggest that neurofibromin loss may be associated with the development of neuroblastomas by altering growth unrelated to the *ras* pathway.

WILMS TUMOR

Several cases of Wilms tumor in association with NF1 have been reported in the literature (Walden et al. 1977). However, several hospital-based studies have failed to demonstrate cases of Wilms tumor in individuals affected with NF1. In 342 consecutive Wilms tumor cases, three individuals with NF1 were found (Stay and Vawter 1977). These tumors were all observed in children 3 years of age or younger. A secondary cancer (malignant peripheral nerve sheath tumor) developed in one of these children, who received both chemotherapy and radiation. Although the existing evidence does not support a true association between Wilms tumor and NF1 (Hope and Mulvihill 1981), such children with NF1 and embryonal tumors appear to be more susceptible to the development of secondary malignancies after chemotherapy and radiation treatments (Maris et al. 1997).

Wilms tumor derives from the metanephric tubule that requires interaction with the neural tube during embryonic development. The relationship between *NF1* expression in the developing kidney or neural tube and the specification of the metanephric tubule is unclear. Future studies examining the signaling pathways that are aberrant in Wilms tumors may suggest how defects in neurofibromin might result in the formation of these embryonal tumors.

RHABDOMYOSARCOMA

Many cases of rhabdomyosarcoma in association with NF1 have been reported in the literature (Gutjahr et al. 1986; Hope and Mulvihill 1981; Mata et al. 1981; Shearer et al. 1994). In a national case–control study of 249 children (< 21 years of age) in the United States with rhabdomyosarcomas, Yang et al. (1995) reported 5 children (2%) with concurrent NF1 as compared with no NF1 among 302 control children ($p = .02$). All of the 5 NF1 patients had embryonal rhabdomyosarcomas and were younger than 3 years of age (including 3 who were in their first year of life); 4 of the patients were male. These results are consistent with an earlier population-based series of 157 children with soft-tissue sarcomas (including 103 rhabdomyosarcomas) by Hartley and associates (1988) from England. In a retrospective review, they determined that 4 patients had NF1 and another 9 possibly had NF1. Of the 4 that were almost certainly NF1, all had rhabdomyosarcomas, all were male, and all were younger than 13 months of age.

The results of these population-based studies are entirely consistent with findings from several clinical series. In one such series, over 1% of individuals with NF1 were found to have a rhabdomyosarcoma. Of 84 children diagnosed with rhabdomyosarcoma, 5 were found to meet diagnostic criteria for NF1 (McKeen et al. 1978). This observed figure was much larger than the 0.03 individuals predicted using the 1:3000 to 1:4000 frequency figure for NF1 in the general population and suggests a true association between rhabdomyosarcoma and NF1. Rhabdomyosarcoma, in the context of NF1, largely affects young individuals. A review of 20 reported cases in the literature revealed that 14 individuals with NF1 and rhabdomyosarcoma were younger than 18 years of age. These tumors have been reported most commonly in the extremities, bladder, prostate, and orbit as well as in other sites (Table 10-3). Most of the rhabdomyosarcomas reported in children with NF1 were embryonal rhabdomyosarcomas. This distribution of tumor location does not differ from that reported for individuals without NF1.

Support for an association between NF1 and rhabdomyosarcoma derives from three lines of indirect evidence: (1) muscles of the head region are derived from the neural crest, (2) *NF1* gene expression is detected in the developing myotomes and muscle during embryogenesis (Daston and Ratner 1993; Gutmann et al. 1995b; Stocker et al. 1995), and (3) a rare form of malignant peripheral nerve sheath tumor termed a "Triton tumor," observed in the context of NF1, has evidence of muscle transdifferentiation. Other support for the notion that rhab-

Table 10-3. Sites of rhabdomyosarcoma tumors in individuals with NF1

Location	Number of Cases
Extremities	5
Bladder	4
Prostate	3
Orbit	3
Vagina	2
Chest	2
Neck	1
Paraspinal	1
Palate	1
Retroperitoneum	1
Myocardium	1
Peritesticular region	1
Perianal region	1

domyosarcomas might result from abnormalities in *NF1* expression emanate from studies examining *NF1* expression in muscle. One isoform of neurofibromin derives from alternative splicing of exon 48a (Gutmann et al. 1993a). Expression of exon 48a containing *NF1* messenger RNA and protein is restricted to skeletal and cardiac muscle (Gutmann et al. 1995b). The finding of a muscle-specific isoform of neurofibromin suggests that the *NF1* gene might have specific functions during muscle cell differentiation. To this end, examination of muscle-cell differentiation in vitro has demonstrated an increase in *NF1* expression concomitant with myoblast fusion and growth arrest (Gutmann et al. 1994). These results collectively argue that neurofibromin might have a specific role in muscle-cell differentiation such that loss of neurofibromin expression might favor muscle-cell proliferation. Analysis of mice homozygous for a targeted disruption of the *Nf1* gene (*Nf1−/−*) demonstrates hypoplastic abdominal muscles (Brannan et al. 1993). Formal proof for the notion that neurofibromin is a critical growth regulator for muscle cells will require further experiments.

LEUKEMIA

Childhood leukemias have been reported in individuals with NF1 (Bader and Miller 1978; Brodeur 1994; Clark and Hutter 1982; Mosso et al. 1987). Although childhood myeloid leukemias are uncommon malignancies, individuals with NF1 have a greatly increased risk for myeloid cancers such as juvenile chronic myeloid leukemias (JCML) and myelodysplastic syndromes (MDS). Typically, lymphocytic leukemias predominate 4:1 over nonlymphocytic (myeloid) leukemias in children without NF1. However, in individuals affected with NF1, there is a 20:9 ratio of nonlymphocytic to lymphocytic leukemias (Bader and Miller 1978). Moreover, the most common leukemias in children with NF1 are JCML and MDS. In the study by Matsui, eight individuals affected with NF1 had nonlymphocytic leukemias, including myelodysplastic syndrome (two individuals), chronic myeloid leukemia (3), nonlymphocytic leukemia (2), and monocytic leukemia (1), as compared with four children with lymphocytic leukemia (Matsui et al. 1993). Most of the children with NF1 and malignant myeloid disorders reported in the literature are boys under 10 years of age. The age and sex distribution of myeloid and lymphocytic leukemias observed in children with NF1 is illustrated in Figure 10-2. Interestingly, a high proportion of the children with NF1 and myeloid leukemias inherited the mutant *NF1* gene from their mother (Shannon et al. 1992).

Previous work on JCML in children who do not have NF1 has demonstrated activating ras mutations. In the study by Farr, 8 of 34 children had *ras* mutations, while 5 had chromosome 7 abnormalities (Farr et al. 1991). None of the children with chromosome 7 abnormalities had ras mutations. This high proportion of activating *ras* mutations observed in JCML suggested that increased *ras* activity might also result from inactivating mutations in the *NF1* gene during the development of myeloid leukemias. Mutations in the *NF1* gene have been demonstrated in 14 children with JCML or MDS by loss-of-heterozygosity studies as well as by direct demonstration of *NF1* gene mutations (Kalra et al. 1994; Maris et al. 1997; Shannon et al. 1994). These results argue that activation of a growth factor pathway important for myeloid-cell proliferation can result from augmented *ras* activity secondary to activating mutations in *ras* or loss of neurofibromin expression (Fig. 10-3). In support of this notion, no children with activating *ras* mutations have been shown to have defects in the *NF1* gene.

In an attempt to investigate the pathogenesis of myeloid leukemias in the context of NF1, myeloid precursors were examined from mice homozygous for an *Nf1* gene mutation (*Nf1−/−*) (Bollag et al. 1996; Largaespada et al. 1996). In these elegant studies, loss of *Nf1* gene expression leads to increased myeloid precursor proliferation and increased sensitivity to granulocyte macrophage colony stimulating factor (GM-CSF). GM-CSF functions as a potent growth factor for myeloid precursor cells and functions in part through activation of the *ras* signal-

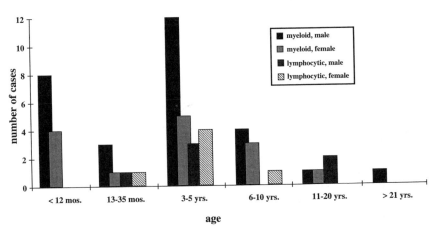

Figure 10-2. Distribution of leukemias in children with NF1. The number of cases of myeloid and lymphocytic leukemias in children with NF1 are graphically represented by age and divided into male and female. The majority of myeloid leukemias occur in boys under 10.

ing pathway. Loss of neurofibromin expression in these myeloid precursors re-sults in dramatic increases in *ras* activity in response to GM-CSF stimulation. In this fashion, defects in *NF1* function can lead to increased cell proliferation via alterations in the *ras* signaling pathway (see Fig. 10-3). These observations have

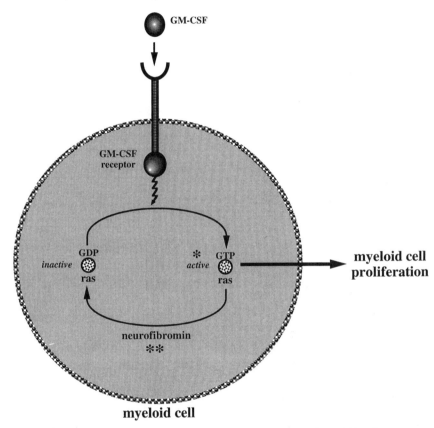

Figure 10-3. Activation of the *ras* pathway and the development of myeloid-cell tumors. Normally, the binding of granulocyte macrophage colony-stimulating factor (GM-CSF) to its receptor tyrosine kinase (GM-CSF receptor) results in the conversion of *ras* from its inac-tive GDP confirmation to its active GTP-bound confirmation. Activation of *ras* in this fashion promotes the proliferation of myeloid cells. Alternatively, activation of the platelet-derived growth factor (PDGF) receptor may also stimulate the proliferation of myeloid cells through the *ras* signaling pathway. Sustained or aberrant activation of *ras* leads to sustained prolif-eration of myeloid cells and the formation of myeloid malignancies. This can occur by two mechanisms. The first mechanism entails an activating mutation in *ras*, rendering it insensi-tive to GTP hydrolysis. These activating mutations lead to constitutive *ras* activity and prolif-eration of myeloid cells (*). Alternatively, inactivation of neurofibromin, whose normal role is to inactivate *ras*, would lead to an increase in the relative *ras* GTP levels within the cell (**). As before, constitutive activation of *ras*, as a result of defects in neurofibromin expression, would lead to an increase in the proliferation of myeloid cells and the development of myeloid cancers.

now been substantiated using bone marrow samples from children with NF1 and JCML or MDS (Bollag et al. 1996).

Several reports in the literature have suggested an association between NF1, juvenile xanthogranulomas (JXGs), and the development of JCML (Cooper et al. 1984; Morier et al. 1990). JXGs are soft, flat, yellow to pink-colored papules seen in individuals both with and without NF1 (Ackerman and Cohen 1991; Cohen and Hood 1989; Jensen et al. 1971). Although the pathogenesis of these skin lesions is unknown, they are thought to be composed of lipid-laden histiocytes and giant cells (Sonoda et al. 1985; Tahan et al. 1989). JXGs typically appear during the first year or two of life (70% are detected during first 12 months) and may be detected anywhere on the body, but are more commonly seen in the head region. Although typically restricted to the skin, they may appear in the eye, resulting in glaucoma. These lesions are not associated with hypercholesterolemia or accelerated cardiac disease. JXGs increase in both size and number for months or years and then regress and disappear completely by midadolescence. Analysis of the existing case reports has prompted clinicians to suggest that the finding of these skin lesions in individuals with NF1 is associated with a 20- to 30-fold increased risk of JCML developing (Zvulunov et al. 1995). However, further analysis of these cases does not substantiate a strong link between NF1, JXGs, and JCML. As JCML and MDS are exceedingly rare even in individuals affected with NF1, the finding of JXG does not warrant a search for an underlying myeloid malignancy (Gurney et al. 1996). To this end, Riccardi reported 14 cases of JXG among 614 individuals with NF1 (Riccardi 1992). No cases of JCML were reported in his series. In addition, analysis of the National Neurofibromatosis Foundation database, in conjunction with a worldwide survey of Neurofibromatosis Programs, uncovered 22 cases of NF1 and JXG (Friedman and Birch 1997). None of these children had signs or symptoms of a myeloid malignancy. These results strongly argue that JXG in the context of NF1 has little prognostic value in predicting the development of myeloid cancers.

SECONDARY MALIGNANCIES

One natural extension of the observation that NF1 is a tumor-suppressor gene disorder is that individuals with NF1 might be more likely to have secondary malignancies develop as a result of chemotherapy or radiation therapy treatments. These secondary malignancies are hypothesized to result from DNA damage to the wild-type *NF1* allele as a result of the therapy, rendering both copies of the *NF1* gene nonfunctional in that given cell. Loss of *NF1* gene expression as a result of these therapies might lead to the development of other malignancies. Review of the Children's Hospital of Philadelphia Tumor Registry over a 35-year period demonstrated several children with NF1 and a secondary malignancy (Maris et al. 1997). Secondary malignancy developed in all but one of these children as a result of cytotoxic chemotherapy. Interestingly, a related cohort of children with NF1 and cancer treated with radiation therapy had no secondary malignancies (Blatt et al. 1986). Further analysis of this database demonstrated that children with NF1 and embryonal tumors had a high incidence of secondary malignancies. To this end, secondary malignancies were observed in children with NF1 and Wilms tumor (two of two cases), neuroblastoma (two of three), and rhabdomyosarcoma (two of three). Similar observations have been made in children with NF1 and rhabdomyosarcoma (Heyn et al. 1993). This high risk of secondary malignancy may result from the use of combination therapy involving both multiagent chemotherapy and radiation treatments. Interestingly, myeloid leukemias and osteosarcomas comprised only 5% of the primary malignancies in children with NF1 but represented half of the secondary malignancies. These data lend credence to the notion that individuals with NF1 might be more prone to secondary malignancies that result from the treatment of the primary tumor.

Early studies on fibroblasts derived from individuals with NF1 demonstrated increased sensitivity to ionizing radiation as compared with fibroblasts taken from unaffected individuals (Kopelovich and Rich 1986; Woods et al. 1986). This increased sensitivity to radiotherapy might also contribute to the development of secondary malignancies. Compelling data from mice heterozygous for a targeted *Nf1* gene mutation (*Nf1+/−*) demonstrated a high rate of secondary malignancies after exposure to alkylating agents (cyclophosphamide). In these studies, secondary leukemias developed in eighteen of 38 *Nf1+/−* mice as compared with none of 32 *Nf1+/+* (normal) mice (Maghoub et al. 1997). No increased incidence of secondary leukemias was observed following etoposide (topoisomerase II inhibitor) treatment. These preliminary results may provide a model system for assessing the likelihood of developing a secondary malignancy in response to specific chemotherapy regimens.

When counseling families regarding possible chemotherapy protocols, clinicians should keep in mind that children with NF1 may be more prone to secondary malignancies. In this regard, aggressive chemotherapy for slower-growing tumors in patients with NF1 may predispose to the development of secondary malignancies in individuals who survive their primary malignancy. The decision to treat a patient with NF1 and a primary tumor is difficult and should be discussed with the family and a multidisciplinary team, including oncologists and radiation therapists. The prognosis of the primary cancer should be considered in the decision-making process, as aggressive chemotherapy of a slowly growing tumor or a widely metastatic cancer may not be warranted. Unfortunately, many of the malignancies associated with NF1 (MPNSTs and invasive pheochromocytomas) have generally poor prognoses and require chemotherapy. Survivors must be monitored closely for the development of secondary malignancy. Given the risk of secondary malignancy in NF1, it is reasonable to closely follow all patients for secondary tumors, regardless of treatment protocol, since it is not known whether any individual therapy (i.e., radiation or specific chemotherapy agents) has a higher associated risk of secondary malignancy. The design of future chemotherapy and radiation therapy protocols will need to take these concerns into consideration.

REFERENCES

Ackerman CD and Cohen BA. 1991. Juvenile xanthogranuloma and neurofibromatosis. *Pediatr Dermatol* 8:339–40.

Andersen LB, Fountain JW, Gutmann DH, Tarle SA, Glover TW, Dracopoli NC, et al. 1993. Mutations in the neurofibromatosis 1 gene in sporadic malignant melanomas. *Nat Genet* 3:118–21.

Bader JL. 1986. Neurofibromatosis and cancer. *Ann NY Acad Sci* 486:57–65.

Bader JL and Miller RW. 1978. Neurofibromatosis and childhood leukemia. *J Pediatr* 92:925–9.

Blatt J, Jaffe R, Deutsch M, and Adkins JC. 1986. Neurofibromatosis and childhood tumors. *Cancer* 57:1225–9.

Bolande RP. 1981. Neurofibromatosis—the quintessential neurocristopathy: pathogenetic concepts and relationships. *Adv Neurol* 29:67–75.

Bolande RP and Towler WF. 1970. A possible relationship of neuroblastoma to von Recklinghausen's disease. *Cancer* 26:162–75.

Bollag G, Clapp DW, Shih S, Adler F, Zhang YY, Thompson P, et al. 1996. Loss of NF1 results in activation of the Ras signaling pathway and leads to aberrant growth in haematopoietic cells. *Nat Genet* 12:144–8.

Brannan CI, Perkins AS, Vogel KS, Ratner N, Nordlund ML, Reid SW, Buchberg AM, Jenkins NA, Parada LF and Copeland NG. 1994. Targeted disruption of the neurofibromatosis type-1 gene leads to developmental abnormalities in heart and vanons neural-crest-derived tissues. *Genes and Development* 8:1019–29.

Brodeur GM. 1994. The NF1 gene in myelopoiesis and childhood myelodysplastic syndromes. *New England J Med* 330:637–8.

Cantor AM, Rigby CC, Beck PR, and Mangion D. 1982. Neurofibromatosis, phaeochromocytoma and somatostatinoma. *BMJ* 285:1618–9.

Chakrabarti S, Murugesan A, and Arida EJ. 1979. The association of neurofibromatosis and hyperparathyroidism. *Am J Surg* 137:417–20.

Clark RD and Hutter JJ. 1982. Familial neurofibromatosis and juvenile chronic myelogenous leukemia. *Human Genetics* 60:230–32.

Cohen BA and Hood A. 1989. Xanthogranuloma: report on clinical and histologic findings in 64 patients. *Pediatr Dermatol* 6:262–6.

Cooper PH, Frierson HF, Kayne AL, and Sabio H. 1984. Association of juvenile xanthogranuloma with juvenile myeloid leukemia. *Arch Dermatol* 120:371–5.

Daly D, Kaye M, and Estrada RL. 1970. Neurofibromatosis and hyperparathyroidism: a new syndrome? *Can Med J* 103:258–9.

Daston MM and Ratner N. 1993. Neurofibromin, a predominantly neuronal GTPase activating protein in the adult, is ubiquitously expressed during development. *Dev Dynam* 195:216–6.

Farr C, Gill R, Katz F, Gibbons B, and Marshall CJ. 1991. Analysis of ras gene mutations in childhood myeloid leukaemia. *Br J Haematol* 77:323–7.

Fernandez-Calvet L and Garcia-Mayor RVG. 1994. Incidence of pheochromocytoma in South Galicia, Spain. *J Intern Med* 236:675–7.

Friedman JM and Birch PH. 1997. Type 1 neurofibromatosis: a descriptive analysis of the disorder in 1728 patients. *J Med Genet* 70:138–43.

Gold EB, Leviton A, Lopez R, Austin DF, Gilles FH, Hedley-White ET, Kolonel LN, Lyon JL, Swanson GM, Weiss NS, West DW, and Aschenbrener C. 1994. The role of family history in risk of childhood brain tumors. *Cancer* 73:1302–11.

Gomez L, Rubio M-P, Martin MT, Vazquez J, Idoate M, Pastorfide G, et al. 1996. Chromosome 17 allelic loss and NF1-GRD mutations do not play a significant role as molecular mechanisms leading to melanoma tumorigenesis. *J Invest Dermatol* 106:432–6.

Griffiths DFR, Williams GT, and Williams ED. 1983. Multiple endocrine neoplasia associated with vin Recklinghausen's disease. *BMJ* 287:1341–3.

Gurney JG, Shannon KM, and Gutmann DH. 1996. Juvenile xanthogranuloma, neurofibromatosis 1 and juvenile chronic myeloid leukemia. *Arch Dermatol* 132:1390.

Gutjahr P, Dittrich M, Lauf R, and Riedmiller H. 1986. Embryonal rhabdomyosarcoma of 2 boys with von Recklinghausen's neurofibromatosis. *Aktuel Urol* 17:198–301.

Gutmann DH, Andersen LB, Cole JL, Swaroop M, and Collins FS. 1993a. An alternatively spliced mRNA in the carboxy terminus of the neurofibromatosis type 1 (NF1) gene is expressed in muscle. *Hum Mol Genet* 2:989–92.

Gutmann DH, Cole JL, Stone WJ, Ponder BAJ, and Collins FS. 1993b. Loss of neurofibromin in adrenal gland tumors from patients with neurofibromatosis type 1. *Genes Chromosomes Cancer* 10:55–8.

Gutmann DH, Cole JL, and Collins FS. 1994. Modulation of neurofibromatosis type 1 (NF1) gene expression during in vitro myoblast differentiation. *J Neurosci Res* 37:398–405.

Gutmann DH and Collins FS. 1993. The neurofibromatosis type 1 (NF1) gene: beyond positional cloning. *Arch of Neurol* 50:1185–93.

Gutmann DH, Geist RT, Rose K, Wallin G, and Moley JF. 1995a. Loss of neurofibromatosis type 1 (NF1) gene expression in pheochromocytomas from patients without NF1. *Genes Chromosomes Cancer* 13:104–9.

Gutmann DH, Geist RT, Rose K, and Wright DE. 1995b. Expression of two new protein isoforms of the neurofibromatosis type 1 gene product, neurofibromin, in muscle tissues. *Dev Dynam* 202:302–11.

Gutmann DH, Geist RT, Wright DE, and Snider WD. 1995c. Expression of the neurofibromatosis 1 (NF1) isoforms in developing and adult rat tissues. *Cell Growth Differ* 6:315–22.

Hartley AL, Birch JM, Marsden HB, Harris M, and Blair V. 1988. Neurofibromatosis in children with soft tissue sarcoma. *Pediatr Hematol Oncol* 5:7–16.

Hasegawa M, Tanaka H, Watanabe I, Uehara T, and Nasu M. 1984. Malignant schwannoma and follicular thyroid carcinoma associated with von Recklinghausen's disease. *J Laryngol Otol* 98:1057–61.

Hayflick SJ, Hofman KJ, Tunnessen WW, Leventhal BG, and Dudgeon DL. 1990. Neurofibromatosis 1: recognition and management of associated neuroblastoma. *Pediatric Dermatol* 7:293–5.

Heideman RL, Packer RJ, Albright LA, Freeman CR, and Rorke LB. 1997. Tumors of the central nervous system. In: Pizzo PA and Poplack DG, eds. *Principles and Practice of Pediatric Oncology,* 3rd ed. Philadelphia: Lippincott-Raven, pp. 633–97.

Heyn R, Haeberlen V, Newton WA, Ragab AH, Raney RB, Tefft M, et al. 1993. Second malignant neoplasms in children treated for rhabdomyosarcoma. *J Clin Oncol* 11:262–70.

Hope DG and Mulvihill JJ. 1981. Malignancy in neurofibromatosis. *Adv Neurol* 29:33–56.

Huson SM, Harper PS and Compston DAS. 1988. von Recklinghausen neurofibromatosis: a clinical and population study in South East Wales. *Brain* 111:1355–81.

Ilgren EB, Kinnier-Wilson LM, and Stiller CA. 1985. Gliomas in neurofibromatosis: a series of 89 cases with evidence for enhanced malignancy in associated cerebellar astrocytomas. *Pathol Ann* 20:331–58.

Jacks T, Shih TS, Schmitt EM, Bronson RT, Bernards A, and Weinberg RA. 1994. Tumor predisposition in mice heterozygous for a targeted mutation in NF1. *Nat Genet* 7:353–61.

Jensen NE, Sabharwal S, and Walker AE. 1971. Naevoxanthoendothelioma and neurofibromatosis. *Br J Dermatol* 85:326–30.

Johnson MR, Look AT, DeClue JE, Valentine MB, and Lowy DR. 1993. Inactivation of the *NF1* gene in human melanoma and neuroblastoma cell lines without impaired regulation of GTP-Ras. *Proc Natl Acad Sci USA* 90:5539–43.

Kalff V, Shapiro B, Lloyd R, Sisson JC, Holland K, Nakajo M, et al. 1982. The spectrum of pheochromocytoma in hypertensive patients with neurofibromatosis. *Arch Intern Med* 142:2092–8.

Kalra R, Paderanga DC, Olson K, and Shannon KM. 1994. Genetic analysis is consistent with the hypothesis that NF1 limits myeloid cell growth through p21-ras. *Blood* 84:3435–9.

Knudson AG. 1971. Mutation and cancer: statistical study of retinoblastoma. *Proc Natl Acad Sci USA* 68:820–3.

———. 1993. Antioncogenes and human cancer. *Proc Natl Acad Sci USA* 90:10914–21.

Knudson AG and Amromin GD. 1966. Neuroblastoma and ganglioneuroma in a child with multiple neurofibromatosis: Implications for the mutant origin of neuroblastoma. *Cancer* 19:1032–7.

Kopelovich L and Rich RF. 1986. Enhanced radiotolerance to ionizing radiation is correlated with increased cancer proneness of cultured fibroblasts from precursor states in neurofibromatosis patients. *Cancer Genet* 22:203–10.

Largaespada DA, Brannan CI, Jenkins NA, and Copeland NG. 1996. NF1 deficiency causes Ras-mediated granulocyte/macrophage colony stimulating factor hypersensitivity and chronic myeloid leukaemia. *Nat Genet* 12:137–43.

Mahgoub N, Taylor B, Le Beau M, Gratiot M, Carlson K, Jacks T, et al. A mouse model of alkylator-induced leukemia. *Blood* (in press).

Maris JM, Wiersma SR, Mahgoub N, Thompson P, Geyer RJ, Hurwitz CGH, et al. 1997. Monosomy 7 myelodysplastic syndrome and other second malignant neoplasms in children with neurofibromatosis type 1. *Cancer* 79:1438–46.

Mastrangelo MJ, Goepp CE, Patel YA, and Clark WH. 1979. Cutaneous melanoma in a patient with neurofibromatosis. *Arch Dermatol* 115:864–5.

Mata M, Wharton M, Geisinger K, and Pugh JE. 1981. Myocardial rhabdomyosarcoma in multiple neurofibromatosis. *Neurology* 31:1549–51.

Matsui I, Tanimura M, Kobayashi N, Sawada T, Nagahara N, and Akatsuka J-I. 1993. Neurofibromatosis type 1 and cancer. *Cancer* 72:746–54.

McGrath PC, Sloan DA, Schwartz RW, and Kenady DE. 1998. Advances in the diagnosis and treatment of adrenal tumors. *Curr Opin Oncol* 10:52–7.

McKeen EA, Bodurtha J, Meadows AT, Douglass EC, and Mulvihill JJ. 1978. Rhabdomyosarcoma complicated multiple neurofibromatosis. *J Pediatr* 93:992–3.

Morier P, Merot Y, Paccaud D, Beck D, and Frenk E. 1990. Juvenile chronic granulocytic leukemia, juvenile xanthogranulomas, and neurofibromatosis. *J Am Acad Dermatol* 22:962–5.

Mosso ML, Castello M, Bellani FF, DiTullio MT, Loiacono F, Paolucci G, Tamaro P, Terracini B and Pastore G. 1987. Neurofibromatosis and malignant childhood cancers: A survey in Italy, 1970–83. *Tumori* 73:209–12.

North K. 1993. Neurofibromatosis type 1: Review of the first 200 patients in an Australian clinic. *J Child Neurology* 8:395–402.

Okada E and Shozawa T. 1984. von Recklinghausen's disease (neurofibromatosis) associated with malignant pheochromocytoma. *Acta Pathol Jpn* 34:425–34.

Poyhonen M, Niemela S, and Herva R. 1997. Risk of malignancy and death in neurofibromatosis. *Arch Pathol Lab Med* 121:139–43.

Preston-Martin S, Gurney JG, Pogoda JM, Holly EA, and Mueller BA. 1996. Brain tumor risk in relation to electric blankets and heated water beds: results from the United States West Coast Childhood Brain Tumor Study. *Am J Epidemiol* 143:1116–22.

Riccardi VM. 1992. *Neurofibromatosis: Phenotype, Natural History and Pathogenesis.* 2nd ed. Baltimore: Johns Hopkins University Press.

Ruppert RD, Buerger LF, and Chang WWL. 1966. Pheochromocytoma, neurofibromatosis and thyroid carcinoma. *Metabolism* 15:537–41.

Russell DS and Rubinstein LJ. 1989. *Pathology of Tumours of the Nervous System.* Baltimore: Williams & Wilkins.

Schneider M, Obringer AC, Zackai E, and Meadows AT. 1986. Childhood neurofibromatosis: risk factors for malignant disease. *Cancer Genet Cytogenet* 21:347–54.

Schlumberger M, Gicquel C, Lumbroso J, Tenenbaun F, Comoy E, Bosq J, et al. 1992. Malignant pheochromocytoma: clinical, biological, histologic and therapeutic data in a series of 20 patients with distant metastases. *J Endocrinol Invest* 15:631–42.

Shannon KM, Watterson J, Johnson P, O'Connell P, Lange B, Shah N, et al. 1992. Monosomy 7 myeloproliferative disease in children with neurofibromatosis type 1: epidemiology and molecular analysis. *Blood* 79:1311–8.

Shannon KM, O'Connell P, Martin GA, Paderanga D, Olson K, Dinndorf P, et al. 1994. Loss of the normal NF1 allele from the bone marrow of children with type 1 neurofibromatosis and malignant myeloid disorders. *N Engl J Med* 330:597–601.

Shearer P, Parham D, Kovnar E, Kun L, Rao B, Lobe T, et al. 1994. Neurofibromatosis type 1 and malignancy: review of 32 pediatric cases treated at a single institution. *Med Ped Oncol* 22:78–83.

Sonoda T, Hashimoto H, and Enjoji M. 1985. Juvenile xanthogranuloma: clinicopathologic analysis and immunohistochemical study of 57 patients. *Cancer* 56:2280–6.

Sorensen SA, Mulvihill JJ, and Nielsen A. 1986. Long-term follow-up of von Recklinghausen neurofibromatosis: survival and malignant neoplasms. *New Engl J Med* 314:1010–5.

Specht CS and Smith TW. 1988. Uveal malignant melanoma and von Recklinghausen neurofibromatosis. *Cancer* 62:812–7.

Stay EJ and Vawter G. 1977. The relationship between nephroblastoma and neurofibromatosis (von Recklinghausen's disease). *Cancer* 39:2250–5.

Stocker KM, Baizer L, Coston T, Sherman L, and Ciment G. 1995. Expression of neurofibromin, a GTPase activating protein involved in p21-ras regulation, in migrating neural crest cells of avian embryos. *Dev Biol* 27:535–52.

Suzuki H, Takahashi K, Yasumoto H-i, and Shibahara S. 1994. Activation of the tyrosinase gene promoter by neurofibromin. *Biochem Biophys Res Commun* 205:1984–91.

Tahan SR, Pastel-Levy C, Bhan AK, and Mihm MC. 1989. Juvenile xanthogranuloma: clinical and pathologic characterization. *Arch Pathol Lab Med* 113:1057–61.

The I, Murthy AE, Hannigan GE, Jacoby LB, Menon AG, Gusella JF, et al. 1993. Neurofibromatosis type 1 gene mutations in neuroblastoma. *Nat Genet* 3:62–6.

To KW, Rabinowitz SM, Friedman AH, Merker C, and Cavanaugh CP. 1989. Neurofibromatosis and neural crest neoplasms: primary acquired melanosis and malignant melanoma of the conjunctiva. *Surv Ophthalmol* 33:373–9.

Walden PAM, Johnson AG, and Bagshawe KD. 1977. Wilms tumor and neurofibromatosis. *BMJ* 1:813.

Werbel SS and Ober KP. 1995. Pheochromocytoma: update on diagnosis, localization, and management. *Med Clin North Am* 79:131–53.

Woods WG, McKenzie B, Letourneau MA, and Byrne TD. 1986. Sensitivity of cultured skin fibroblasts from patients with neurofibromatosis to DNA-damaging agents. *Ann NY Acad Sci* 486:336–48.

Wrensch M, Lee M, Miike R, Newman B, Barger G, Davis R, Wiencke J, and Neuhaus J. 1997. Familial and personal medical history of cancer and nervous system conditions among adults with glioma and controls. *Am J Epidemiol* 145:581–93.

Xu W, Mulligan LM, Ponder MA, Liu L, Smith BA, Mathew CGP, et al. 1992. Loss of *NF1* alleles in phaeochromocytomas from patients with type 1 neurofibromatosis. *Genes Chromosomes Cancer* 4:337–42.

Yang P, Grufferman S, Khoury MJ, Schwartz AG, Kowalski Y, Ruymann FB, and Maurer HM. 1995. Association of childhood rhabdomyosarcoma with neurofibromatosis type 1 and birth defects. *Genet Epidemiol* 12:467–74.

Zvulunov A, Barak Y, and Metzker A. 1995. Juvenile xanthogranuloma, neurofibromatosis and juvenile chronic myelogenous leukemia. *Arch Dermatol* 131:904–8.

11

Skeletal System

Vincent M. Riccardi, M.D.

NF1 is a disease that involves both focal skeletal defects and the entire gamut of growth parameters characterizing the individual as a whole. The osseous skeleton is frequently involved in NF1, in terms of primary features, secondary features, and complications (Kraiem et al. 1988). Previous emphasis on skin and nervous system manifestations or on the presumed neural crest nature of NF1 has tended to minimize the attention paid to the skeletal involvement, especially in terms of what it may be telling us about pathogenesis.

Early twentieth-century literature pertaining to growth characteristics in the NF1 population is scant. In 1956, Crowe et al. addressed this point partially, characterizing 13 patients considered to have physical or sexual underdevelopment. Thirteen years later, Carey et al. (1979) noted that short stature was present in 3.8% of cases from 60 families. In 1981 (Riccardi 1981) and 1986 (Riccardi and Eichner 1986) short stature was definitively shown to be prevalent in the NF1 population: the mean sex- and age-corrected height percentile was noted to be 34, and at least 16% of patients with NF1 were noted to have heights at or below the third centile. In the 2nd edition of this book, Haeberlin and Riccardi characterized short stature among patients with NF1 (Haeberlin et al. 1990).

The skeletal system is affected by NF1 mutations in at least four different ways:

1. short stature,
2. macrocephaly,
3. dysplasia of vertebrae, flat bones, and long bones, and
4. erosion by adjacent plexiform neurofibromas.

SHORT STATURE

As early as 1981, we understood that the average height for a group of patients with patients with NF1 is much less than for a normal control group and that there is a significant excess of individuals with NF1 whose heights are below the third centile, corrected for sex and age. In addition, there is an excess of patients with a head circumference centile greater than 50 among those with height centiles less than 50. That is, there is a portion of patients with NF1 who have relative macrocephaly (vis-à-vis height) as well as a group who have absolute macrocephaly (i.e., head circumference above the 97th centile). These data suggest a difference, in at least some patients with NF1, between the factors that govern growth of the cranium and those that determine stature (Haeberlin et al. 1990).

The combined data demonstrate that a representative population of patients with NF1 manifests both short stature and macrocephaly. However, not every patient with NF1 is short, suggesting that the primary feature of short stature may occur on an all-or-nothing basis. Moreover, since only some patients with short stature also have macrocephaly, two independent mechanisms likely control the growth potential for height and head circumference.

Adjustments for the effects of sex and either socioeconomic status, race, severity grade, or family history showed significant differences in head circumference between males and females, but no such differences for height. Among patients with NF1, the respective proportions of short, average, and tall persons remain constant, indicating that NF1 short stature is not usually an age-related phenomenon. This in turn suggests that short stature is a primary feature of NF1, a constitutional aberration of skeletal growth, as opposed to an acquired defect that is more or less randomly superimposed on patients who otherwise would have normal growth patterns. The presence or degree of short stature does not correlate with any other feature of NF1, including head size. In Figure 11-1, de-

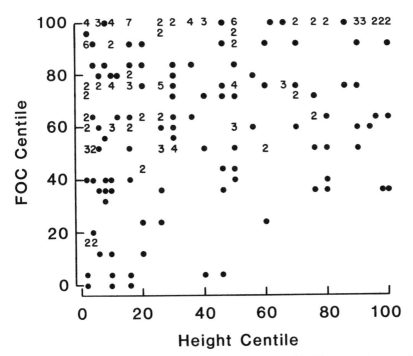

Figure 11-1. Scattergraph showing the number of patients with NF1 with various combinations of paired height and head circumference (fronto-occipital circumference; FOC) measurements, expressed as percentiles.

picting the relationship of head circumference centiles to height centiles for individual patients with NF1, we see that large heads are seen in all height categories. In Figure 11-2 we see that, for both males and females, there is an excess of individuals with a relatively large head and relatively short stature. This is consistent with the observation that, whereas NF1 height centile averages are more or less constant on a year-to-year basis, head circumference centile averages are not consistently elevated until after the fourth birthday.

SUMMARY OF HEIGHT STUDIES OF HAEBERLIN AND RICCARDI

The NF1 case population was selected from a pool of subjects with NF1 registered with the Baylor NF Program between April 1, 1978 and June 30, 1988.

Baseline Data

NF1 populations appear to be shorter than reference populations. Significant differences were found for both males and females. For both sexes, short stature is prevalent early in life and is present at all age levels. Race was not significantly different for either gender, although a trend is noticeable, with the Z-scores of Hispanic patients being farthest from the mean. Socioeconomic status, confounded by race, showed a significant difference only for the females ($p = .03$). Height for either sex was not influenced by family history or the severity of the disease. The disorder affects height in a similar manner for both sexes.

Serial Data

For individual patients with NF1, stature centile assignments seem to be consistent from one time period to the next.

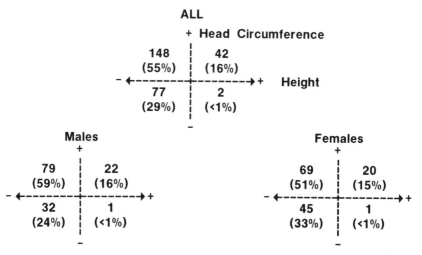

Figure 11-2. Quadrant plots of head circumference versus height standardized scores for 269 patients with NF1 (see Chapter 12).

Adult Data

With some exceptions, the population of adults with NF1 appeared to be shorter. This is consistent with the notion that the short stature characteristic of the NF1 population is present in all age ranges, even after the growth period of the first two decades.

Ethnicity

There is no question that there are racial and geographic influences on growth. For this reason, only patients born in the United States were included in the material reviewed here. These patients were a mixture of blacks, whites, and Hispanics, comprising, respectively, 15%, 74%, and 11% of the NF1 population. Comparisons were made to the NHANES II height data (Hamill et al. 1977; Najjar and Rowland 1987), which consisted of 17% blacks and an 83% mixture of Hispanics and whites. Race or ethnicity alone does not account for the short stature associated with NF1.

Socioeconomic Status

Individual growth pattern differences are unrelated to either economic or racial/ethnic status.

Parental Influence

The results showed no difference in height when comparing spontaneous mutations with inherited cases, for either sex. Short stature is a manifestation of NF1, independent of any other heritable factor. There was no indication of any maternal effect.

Severity Grade

The severity of disease did not significantly influence height.

SHORT STATURE AS A FEATURE OF NF1

From the foregoing, the following conclusions can be drawn (Figs. 11-3 and 11-4).

1. The distribution of NF1 height percentiles relative to the general population was significantly different. Both male and female patients with NF1 had yearly height averages consistently below the 25th percentile. Over one third of the NF1 population for both sexes fell below the 5th percentile.
2. Standardized test results were highly significant for identifying the NF1 population as being shorter than the reference population.
3. The cumulative frequencies on a year-by-year basis indicate that the patients with NF1 appear to be shorter.
4. All the data support the conclusion that the NF1 population is shorter than the reference group. Data from adults with NF1 and serial data from young patients are consistent with this conclusion and suggest that short stature is relatively constant for all age groups.

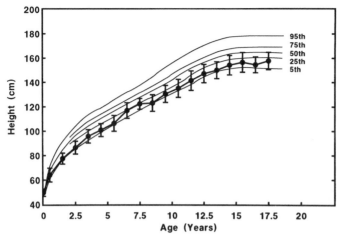

Figure 11-3. Average height measurements of 142 females with NF1 plotted on NHANES growth curves, from birth to 18 years of age.

This does not mean all patients with NF1 are short. Rather, the contrary would appear to be the case. Only a portion of patients with NF1 manifest short stature. By analogy with other primary features of NF1, it is likely that short stature is an all-or-nothing phenomenon, apparent in only a subpopulation of patients with NF1. For example, although optic pathway gliomas occur in 15% of patients with NF1 (Lewis et al. 1984; Listernick et al. 1989), for those in whom the tumor ultimately manifests, it is essentially an all-or-nothing matter. The same can be said about other NF1 features, including cognitive disabilities, plexiform neurofibromas, and neurofibrosarcomas.

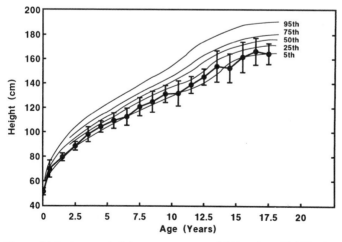

Figure 11-4. Average height measurements of 144 males with NF1 plotted on NHANES growth curves, from birth to 18 years of age.

SUMMARY

Short stature associated with NF1 appears to involve the axial skeleton and the limbs, and it is both proportionate and symmetric. Localized structural defects do not account for the short stature. Neither deficiencies of growth hormone nor anatomic lesions of the hypothalamus or pituitary gland have been shown to account for the short stature among patients with NF1. Thus, the mechanism or mechanisms to account for this feature of NF1 are unknown.

Additional research is certainly required, particularly longitudinal studies to determine growth rates, family studies to determine the influence of other genes and environmental factors, further studies of the growth hormone and other circulating and locally active growth factors, and finally, studies on the behavior and metabolism of bone-growth centers.

MACROCEPHALY

The head circumference measurement (i.e., the fronto-occipital circumference, or FOC), albeit only a substitute for actual brain size, is a practical and easy method for monitoring both skull and brain growth. In terms of FOC, macrocephaly is defined as an FOC ≥ 2 SD above the mean for sex and age. There are no apparent adverse consequences of the macrocephaly per se. The natural history and pathogenesis of macrocephaly in NF1 are discussed in Chapter 8.

The first study specifically designed to assess a growth parameter in an NF population was performed by Weichert et al. (1973). They determined that 3 of 20 boys (15%) and 5 of 7 girls (71%) had FOC measurements above the 98th percentile. Radiographic measurements of cranial volume for the same population increased the number of cases at or above the 98th percentile to 72% for males and 83% for females. The authors concluded that macrocranium may be a manifestation of NF1. Almost as an aside, four cases charting 2 SD below the mean height for age were mentioned; the authors suggested that, when considering macrocranium, one might also want to account for stature.

At about the same time, DeMeyer (1972) published a study focusing on the clinical features of unusual cases of macrocephaly. A summary chart grouped NF as a neurocutaneous disease under "anatomic macrocephaly." Norman (1972) reported a family with eight members diagnosed with NF1; six had "enlarged heads." Four years later, Holt and Kuhns (1976) determined radiographically that the cranial vault size of 23 of 50 selected hospital patients with NF1 measured above the 95th percentile. Carey et al. (1979) evaluated 59 families accounting for 130 individuals with NF1; the overall prevalence of macrocephaly was 35%.

In this context, and starting with data first cited in 1981 (Riccardi 1981) and in the second edition of this book, Haeberlin and Riccardi (Haeberlin et al. 1990) studied a series of patients with NF1 to document the head sizes of patients with NF1.

SUMMARY OF MACROCEPHALY STUDIES
OF HAEBERLIN AND RICCARDI

Baseline Data

Demographic data show that for both males and females, the distributions within the categories of age, race, socioeconomic status, family history, and severity grade are the same for head circumference data. In comparing the NF1 population to the reference population, there was no significant difference for either male or female head circumference at birth. Males attained significant differences at 4 years and continued to show the difference throughout most of the yearly age strata. Females showed extremely large heads at about 1 year but not thereafter.

Parental Influence

Parents' FOC measurements were available in only a few cases, not enough to assess formally at present. Therefore, comparison was made between cases of inherited disease and spontaneous mutations, assuming that the unaffected parents had average FOCs and that they would produce offspring with average FOC. There was no difference between the average standardized scores for spontaneous mutations compared to the inherited cases, for either sex. The data thus suggest that macrocephaly is a manifestation of NF1, independent of any other heritable factor. There was no indication of any maternal effect.

Severity Grade

The extent of disease, as represented by severity grade, did not significantly influence head circumference. If confounding growth factors were not originally excluded, grade would have been expected to influence the measurements, probably increasing the FOC measurements means.

Age

At almost every age level, the average NF1 head circumference plotted above the reference average. The chi-square statistic was significant for both males and females.

MACROCEPHALY AS A FEATURE OF NF1
(FIGS. 11-5, 11-6, 11-7, AND 11-8)

In a representative population of patients with NF1, macrocephaly is present. What has not been shown is that every patient with NF1 has macrocephaly. That not all NF1 cases have macrocephaly may indicate that an all-or-nothing mechanism is at play. Adjustments for the effects of sex and either socioeconomic status, race, severity grade, or family history, showed significant differences in head circumference between males and females, but not for height. Why should this occur for head circumference and not for height? Are more females excluded because of more severe confounding factors? Is there any greater mortality asso-

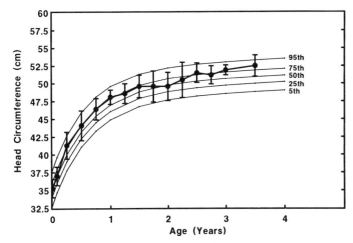

Figure 11-5. Average head circumference of 140 females with NF1 plotted on Fels Institute growth curves, from birth to 3.5 years.

ciated with enlarged head circumference for females over that for males? A longitudinal study could determine if and when growth changes occur in both the male and female NF1 populations.

DYSPLASIA OF FLAT BONES, VERTEBRAE, AND LONG BONES

CRANIOFACIAL DYSPLASIA

Dysplasia of the bones of the skull and face is common in NF1, ranging from simple skull asymmetry to localized defects (usually in the parietal and occipital

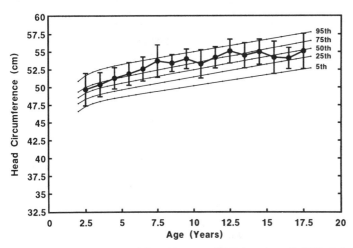

Figure 11-6. Average head circumference of 140 females with NF1 plotted on Fels Institute growth curves, from 2.5 to 17.5 years.

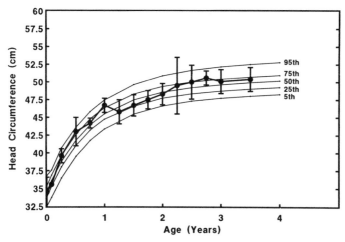

Figure 11-7. Average head circumference of 143 males with NF1 plotted on Fels Institute growth curves, from birth to 3.5 years.

regions) of various sizes (Fig. 11-9). Ordinarily, there are no adverse consequences. Distortions of the base of the skull, however, particularly those involving the foramen magnum, may ultimately lead to impingement on the brain stem or upper spinal cord, especially if there are associated anomalies of the atlas and axis (Ferner et al. 1989). Neurofibromas of the scalp may be associated with areas of cranial vault hypoplasia or aplasia (Duchateau and Lejour 1986).

The most consistent craniofacial bone dysplasia in NF1 involves the sphenoid wings (Fig. 11-10). Sphenoid wing dysplasia is almost always unilateral, and the

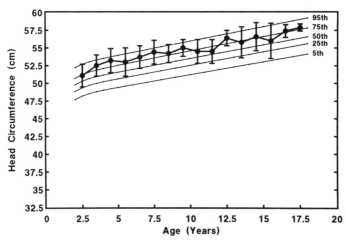

Figure 11-8. Average head circumference of 143 males with NF1 plotted on Fels Institute growth curves, from 2.5 to 17.5 years.

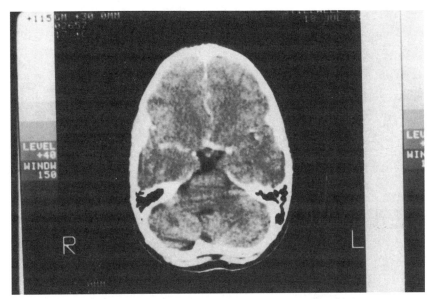

Figure 11-9. Cranial CT scan of a patient with NF1, showing right cerebellar hypoplasia subjacent to an area of skin hypoplasia hypotrichosis.

greater wing is distorted more often than the lesser wing. Identification of this defect by skull radiography may help establish the diagnosis of NF1 in patients who otherwise have only café-au-lait spots. There may or may not be associated neurofibromas. As a static local lesion it has no adverse consequences, but with progression (only sometimes associated with growth of local neurofibromas), the

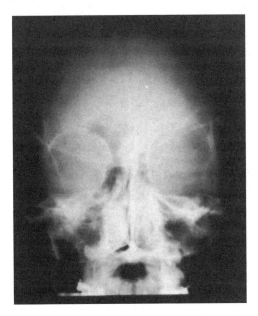

Figure 11-10. Skull radiograph of a patient with NF1, showing dysplasia of the sphenoid wing and other bones of the left orbit.

integrity of the posterior, inferior, and/or superior orbital walls may be seriously disrupted, leading to a pulsating enophthalmos and herniation of the brain into the orbital confines, requiring reconstructive surgery.

OTHER FLAT BONES

The sternum and ribs are frequently involved in NF1. The ribs are largely if not solely involved in a secondary manner, with aberrations reflecting erosions by adjacent neurofibromas and mechanical distortions from kyphoscoliosis, as is the sternum. Pectus excavatum involving the lower portion of the sternum is present in at least 50% of patients with NF1 of all ages; occasionally pectus carinatum is also seen.

Pectus excavatum varies in severity (Figs. 11-11 and Fig. 11-12), and its pathogenetic basis is uncertain. It may not even represent an intrinsic osseous defect, as opposed to a secondary consequence of deranged chest wall function. The presence of pectus excavatum in at least some alternative forms of NF (Fig. 11-13) suggests that the sternal abnormality is an important aspect of NF pathogenesis in general and as such adds credence to the importance of skeletal dysplasia as a primary element of NF1, specifically. The pelvic bones are not known to be abnormal in NF1 except by virtue of erosion and other secondary distortions from local neurofibromas, meningoceles, and/or scoliosis.

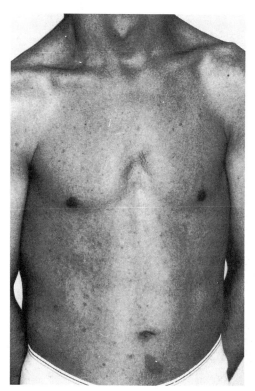

Figure 11-11. An adult male patient with NF1, showing lower sternal pectus excavatum.

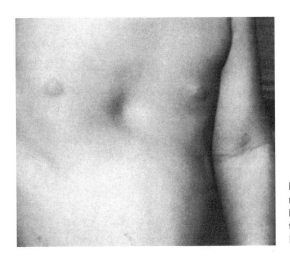

Figure 11-12. A preadolescent male patient with NF1, showing lower sternal pectus excavatum. *Source:* Riccardi 1987. Reprinted with permission.

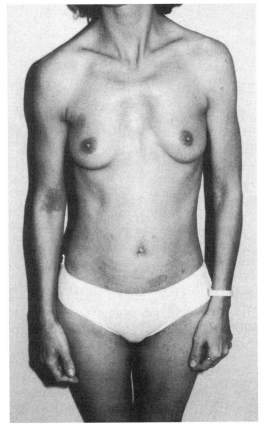

Figure 11-13. A patient with NF6, showing multiple café-au-lait spots, pectus excavatum, and the absence of neurofibromas.

VERTEBRAE

Vertebral involvement in NF1 involves scoliosis, often with kyphosis, the secondary destruction of vertebrae from paraspinal neurofibromas, vertebral scalloping, and congenital vertebral defects (Yaghmai, 1986). The mildest form of vertebral involvement in NF1 is scalloping, usually on the posterior (dorsal) surface of the vertebral body. This radiographically appreciated defect has no implications for ill health and does not necessarily imply the presence of paravertebral neurofibromas. It is sufficiently characteristic of NF1, however, that the presence of lumbar vertebrae scalloping may be used as additional evidence for the presence of the mutant NF1 gene (Casselman and Mandell 1979; Heard and Pasyne 1962; Holt 1978). Vertebral scalloping is not necessarily limited to NF1, but there are few data germane to this issue. Among the Clinical Research Program patients with NF1, lumbar vertebral scalloping was seen in approximately 10%.

Scoliosis in one form or another is probably present in at least 10% of patients with NF1, although age and factors such as changes due to a neurologic deficit or lower limb hypertrophy are not available. Scoliosis may merely be lateral ("S shaped") and involve any portion of the spinal column (lumbar, thoracic, cervical), but the type most characteristic of NF1 involves the lower cervical or upper thoracic spine, usually with a sharp anterior angulation (kyphoscoliosis; Fig. 11-14).

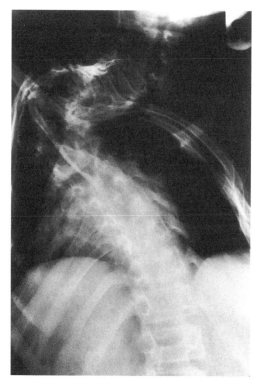

Figure 11-14. Lumbosacral spine radiograph of a patient with NF1, showing severe dystrophic kyphoscoliosis.

The early-onset, rapidly progressive scoliosis that is characteristic of NF1 is often referred to as a dystrophic scoliosis. Most patients in whom the dystrophic form of NF1-associated scoliosis ultimately develops have unremarkable spines clinically through early childhood; that is, this complication of NF1 usually does not develop before the age of 6 years or so. Conversely, if the dystrophic form of scoliosis is not apparent by the end of the first decade, it is unlikely to develop. An aberrant hair whorl over the spinal column of a patient with NF1, the "Riccardi" sign (Flannery and Howell 1987; Pivnick et al. 1997), is a reliable indicator of underlying dysplastic vertebrae and/or paraspinal plexiform neurofibromas (see Fig. 2-30).

Once scoliosis is apparent, however, it must be monitored closely for progression that may be rapid (over a period of months) and require bracing as a temporizing measure and, virtually always, surgery, including Harrington rod or other forms of internal fixation (Chaglassian et al. 1976; Dickson 1985; Shufflebarger 1989). The dystrophic (that is, the vigorously progressive) type of scoliosis/kyphoscoliosis of NF1 is not necessarily accounted for by paravertebral neurofibromas. Ordinarily, scoliosis is not merely a secondary complication of local neurofibromas; however, large or aggressively growing paravertebral neurofibromas may (but do not always) lead to scoliosis.

Of course, other types of scoliosis may be seen in NF1, including the type indistinguishable from the common multifactorial form, and which may merely be coincidental to the NF1.

Vertebral destruction due to paravertebral neurofibromas is not uncommon in NF1 and may be one of the most common causes of serious long-term morbidity and untimely death among patients with NF1. This problem can wreak havoc, particularly in the cervical region. Massive cervical neurofibromas, with and without overlying hyperpigmentation, can lead to neurologic compromise in four different ways, a consideration that must be respected when surgical therapy is anticipated. These four types of compromise are: (1) involvement of brachial plexus components and proximal peripheral nerves; (2) direct nerve-root involvement; (3) spinal-cord compression by the tumor mass itself; and (4) vertebral collapse and/or dislocation with resultant spinal-cord compression.

Deficits resulting from surgery must also be taken into account. Similar problems from paravertebral neurofibromas elsewhere along the spinal column also occur relatively frequently, especially in and around the lumbar and sacral plexuses. The cervical region lesions deserve special emphasis because they are usually outwardly obvious (by virtue of visible and palpable neck masses), and serious problems, ranging from local deficits through hemiparesis or quadriparesis to frank quadriplegia, frequently result (Isu et al. 1983).

These problems and the underlying neurofibroma develop and progress inexorably, often insidiously, up to a certain point, after which more rapid deterioration ensues, reflecting the summation of the multiple types of compromise itemized above. All patients with NF1 who have extensive paravertebral neurofibromas warrant close follow-up.

Vertebral dysplasia is often an element of the dystrophic form of NF1 scoliosis, and it frequently accompanies paraspinal neurofibromas. In addition, the vertebral dysplasia of NF1 may occur in the apparent absence of associated neurofibromas. In either case, the dysplasia may involve one vertebra or a group of them with varying degrees of severity, ranging from trivial radiographic findings to severe distortions that may lead to spinal-cord or nerve-root compression. Abnormalities involving the first and second cervical vertebrae may be particularly important for patients with NF1 who are undergoing general anesthesia for surgery, and in other settings as well. The suspicion or recognition of vertebral dysplasia on either routine or symptom-indicated spine radiography warrants close clinical and radiographic follow-up.

Meningeal defects, ranging from dural ectasia to meningoceles, may distort one or more vertebrae and lead to spinal-cord compromise (see Chapter 8). One important facet of such lesions is that they exemplify how vertebral and/or spinal-cord compromise may result from an NF1 mutation, even in the absence of neurofibromas or other such tumors.

LONG BONES

The tubular bones of the skeleton manifest the NF1 mutation in a variety of ways, including congenital pseudarthrosis, hypertrophic and or destructive changes associated with aggressively growing plexiform neurofibromas, and, perhaps, various types of metaphyseal and diaphyseal localized lytic defects.

Pseudarthrosis or "false-joint" abnormalities of the NF1 skeleton are usually limited to one site per person, and that site is most often a tibia (Fig. 11-15), although such lesions have also been reported in the femur, radius, ulna, and clavicle. Each presumably represents a congenital defect of bone formation even though it may not be appreciated clinically or radiographically for weeks, months, or years after birth. The clinical manifestations primarily involve bowing at the site, ranging in severity from trivial to overwhelming (Beneux et al. 1979). If the latter occurs, there may be a need to amputate the limb proximal to the lesion.

Treatment for all but the mildest lesions involves surgery, either to facilitate healing through local excisions and bone grafting or, not infrequently, amputation (Jacobsen et al. 1983). The use of internal fixation devices (Edge and Denham 1981), microvascular surgical techniques (DeBoer et al. 1988; Weiland and Daniel 1980), or the application of electric currents as an adjunct (Bassett et al. 1981) have not clearly influenced the overall outcome (Karski and Warda 1986); the final words have yet to be written. The Ilizarov procedure (Dal Monte and Donzelli 1987; Green 1988; Ilizarov and Frankel 1988; Louis et al. 1987; Prevot 1986) has held out great promise as a treatment approach, for both young patients and for older patients whose pseudarthrosis-associated deformities have been of long standing.

The nature of the primary lesion is unclear, though it is not a neurofibroma or other tumor of identifiable neural or Schwann-cell origin (Brown et al. 1977; Gregg et al. 1982; Holt and Wright 1948; Klatte et al. 1976). NF1 pseudarthrosis

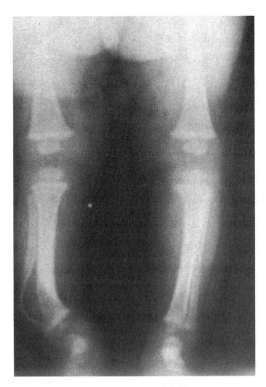

Figure 11-15. Plain radiograph of the lower extremities of a patient with NF1, showing moderately severe pseudarthrosis defects of the right tibia and fibula.

typically presents as a medial deviation of the distal third or quarter of the leg, with some degree of instability at the site. It may be apparent at birth but most often is recognized some weeks or months later. This feature of NF1 often is not appreciated by many otherwise astute clinicians when they examine infants with or at risk for NF1. Thus, I encourage all such clinicians to examine carefully each segment of the four limbs of an infant for deviations toward or away from the midline of the body. The radiographic appearances of both tibial pseudarthrosis and the milder bowing have been well characterized (Holt and Wright 1948; Hunt and Pugh 1961; Klatte et al. 1976). In other sites, particularly in non-weight-bearing bones, the presentation almost totally depends on the degree of bowing and therefore may be much later than for the tibial lesion.

Bowing without apparent pseudarthrosis must also be considered as part of the NF1 pseudarthrosis spectrum (Fig. 11-16). There is no logical or pathogenetic reason that this type of tibial bowing is anything other than the mildest end of the spectrum of the pseudarthroses. Moreover, what may appear to be merely trivial bowing in the first few months of life may be associated later with either a delay in ambulation or the development of a true pseudarthrosis consequent to weight-bearing or an otherwise minor injury. A practical consequence is the need to examine carefully each infant at risk for such bowing.

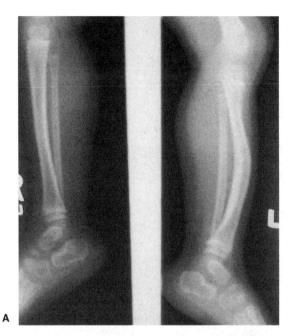

A

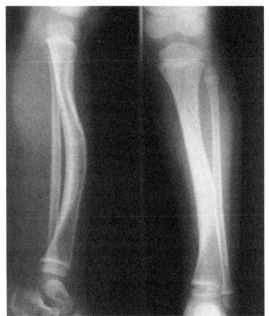

B

Figure 11-16. Plain radiographs of the left leg of a patient with NF1. (A) Mild tibial bowing at 6 months of age. (B) Minimal or no progression of the leg deformity at 12 months of age.

One set of observations is sobering in terms of fitting pseudarthrosis into the larger picture of NF1. In the second edition of this book, we reported on three infants with tibial pseudarthrosis and a maximum of two or three very pale, indistinct café-au-lait spots. It would not have been possible to diagnose NF1 based solely on the café-au-lait spots. However, in each instance a parent had unequivocal typical NF1. When last seen, each child was well beyond the 1-year-old age limit when the full complement of café-au-lait spots is ordinarily apparent, yet all three children still had a paucity of café-au-lait spots (two to four).

On the one hand, this observation suggests a reciprocal relationship between the number of café-au-lait spots and the presence of tibial pseudarthrosis, the first suggestion of a functional interrelation between NF1 lesions in different tissues. On the other hand, since there is no reason to consider that sporadic NF1 is different from inherited NF1, one must be very cautious about discounting NF1 in an infant with pseudarthrosis, one to three café-au-lait spots and no parent with NF1.

Among patients with NF1, the frequency of pseudarthrosis is probably about 1%, but major ascertainment and reporting biases are probably at play, and an accurate frequency remains to be established. Among 238 Clinical Research Program patients, there were 6 pseudarthroses (2.5%), including 5 tibial lesions (2.1%) and 1 radial lesion (0.4%). There is no apparent increased risk for recurrence of this defect once it has been identified in a given family. It is of interest that males are more likely to manifest pseudarthrosis than are females.

Benign isolated lytic defects, primarily of the cortex of the metaphysis or diaphysis of long bones of patients with NF1, may be more common than in the general population (Hunt and Pugh 1961; Klatte et al. 1976; Mandell et al. 1979), but this has not been definitely established (Holt 1978). Among the first 173 Clinical Research Program patients with NF1, 10% showed such defects, but so did 4 of 24 of their unaffected first-degree relatives. Based on these figures, and because these lesions had no clinical consequences, long-bone radiographs are no longer part of the routine NF evaluation. In addition, bony lytic lesions may be due to an overlying or adjacent diffuse plexiform neurofibroma (Fig. 11-17).

Occasionally, lytic lesions associated with local bone-growth disturbance may be seen in NF1. This type of lesion is shown in Figure 11-18. This young girl's left upper limb was significantly shortened by the humeral lesion, but there was no associated neurofibroma. Such lesions are of interest not only because they represent one of the features of NF1, but also because they point to primary skeletal involvement (i.e., dysplasia) as part of this disease. They also indicate an overlap of NF1 with the disorder known as Albright syndrome (Andersen and Sorensen 1988; Benedict et al. 1986; Riccardi 1987).

Albright syndrome is characterized by one or more café-au-lait spots, precocious puberty, and bony lytic lesions (Benedict et al. 1986; Riccardi 1987) (Fig. 11-19). Although the distinction between NF1 and Albright syndrome is ordinarily clear, there may be enough clinical overlap for confusion to arise (Andersen and Sorensen 1988). The oft-touted difference in the appearance of the border of

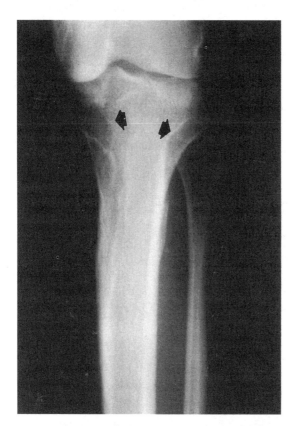

Figure 11-17. Radiograph of the knee region of a patient with NF1, showing bony changes (arrows) secondary to a diffuse plexiform neurofibroma.

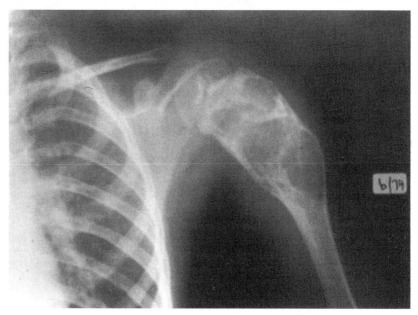

Figure 11-18. Radiograph of the left shoulder of a patient with NF1, showing cystic dysplasia of the proximal humerus.

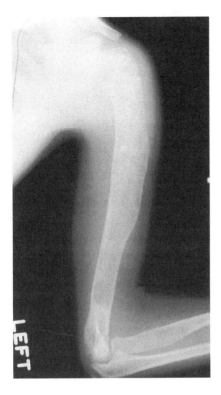

Figure 11-19. Radiograph of the left arm, showing polyostotic fibrous dysplasia of the humerus of a young girl with Albright syndrome.

café-au-lait spots in the two syndromes is not at all reliable (Riccardi 1982). Additional confusion may reflect the fact that von Recklinghausen's name is used to designate not only NF1, but also a separate bony disorder (Thannhauser 1944).

Both genu varum and genu valgum are frequently seen in NF1. At least 5% and probably as many as 10 to 15% of patients with NF1 manifest this type of problem (Figs. 11-20 and 11-21). In some instances, treatment with braces or even surgery may be warranted.

DYSPLASIA VERSUS SECONDARY EFFECTS, PARTICULARLY EROSION

Because of the extensive secondary abnormalities of the skeleton brought about by various types of neurofibromas, especially those of the diffuse plexiform variety, and the effects of scoliosis and neurologic deficits, the importance of a primary skeletal dysplasia in NF1 has been largely overlooked.

However, the data provided throughout this book and summarized in this chapter indicate that such a primary dysplasia accounts for the majority of the skeletal features of NF1. The primary craniofacial and vertebral aberrations are among the most common and straightforward. The sternal deformities, genu varum/valgum, pseudarthrosis of the tibia and other tubular bones, and the occasional lytic lesions also point to, or are at least consistent with, intrinsic defects

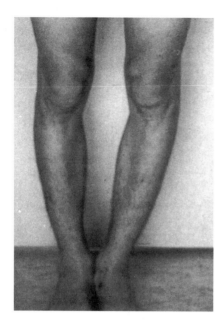

Figure 11-20. The lower limbs of a patient with NF1, showing moderately severe genu varum.

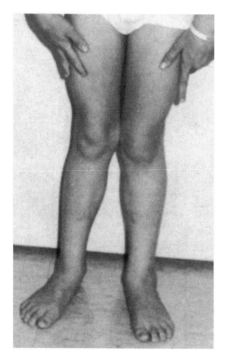

Figure 11-21. The lower extremities of a patient with NF1, showing moderately severe genu valgum.

of the NF1 skeleton. A great deal more clinical, pathologic, and basic science research is obviously warranted in this area.

Secondary bony changes due to overgrowth or destruction associated with a locally aggressive hypertrophic plexiform neurofibroma are well known. The involved bones may become enlarged, assume new shapes, or be resorbed. The exact reasons for these changes are not entirely clear, but they presumably reflect altered vascularity, direct invasion by neurofibroma cells, the mechanical pressure and weight of the tumor, and altered muscle insertions, origins, and actions. Such destructive changes, if severe enough, may determine the strategy for surgical treatment, including the need for amputation of a severely hypertrophied limb.

REFERENCES

Andersen LB and Sorensen SA. 1988. Diagnosis of von Recklinghausen's neurofibromatosis and the Albright syndrome. *Neurofibromatosis* 1:120–3.

Bassett CA, Caulo N, and Kort J. 1981. Congenital "pseudarthroses" of the tibia: treatment with pulsing electromagnetic fields. *Clin Orthop* 154:136–48.

Benedict PH, Szabo G, Fitzpatrick TB, and Sinesi SJ. 1986. Melanotic macules in Albright's syndrome and in neurofibromatosis. *JAMA* 205:618–26.

Beneux J, Rigault P, Poluliquen JC, et al. 1979. [Congenital curvatures and pseudarthroses of the leg in the child]. *Chir Pediatr* 20:99–113.

Brown GA, Osebold WR, and Ponseti IV. 1977. Congenital pseudarthrosis of long bones: a clinical, radiographic, histologic and ultrastructural study. *Clin Orthop* 128:228–42.

Carey JC, Laub JM, and Hall BD. 1979. Penetrance and variability in neurofibromatosis: a genetic study of 60 families. *Birth Defects Original Article Series,* vol. 15, no. 5B. New York: Liss, pp. 271–81.

Casselman ES and Mandell GA. 1979. Vertebral scalloping in neurofibromatosis. *Radiology* 131:89–94.

Chaglassian JH, Riseborough EJ, and Hall JE. 1976. Neurofibromatous scoliosis: natural history and results of treatment in 37 cases. *J Bone Joint Surg [Br]* 58:695–702.

Crowe FW, Schull WJ, and Neel JV. 1956. *A Clinical, Pathological, and Genetic Study of Multiple Neurofibromatosis.* Springfield, Ill.: Charles C Thomas, pp. 1–181.

Dal Monte A and Donzelli O. 1987. Tibial lengthening according to Ilizarov in congenital hypoplasia of the leg. *J Pediatr Orthop* 7:135–8.

DeBoer HH, Verbout AJ, Nielsen HK, and Van Der Eijken JW. 1988. Free vascularized fibular graft for tibial pseudarthrosis in neurofibromatosis. *Acta Orthop Scand* 59:425–9.

DeMeyer W. 1972. Megalencephaly in children. *Neurology* 22:634–43.

Dickson RA. 1985. Thoracic lordoscoliosis in neurofibromatosis: treatment by Harrington rod with sublaminar wiring: report of two cases. *J Bone Joint Surg [Am]* 67:822–3.

Duchateau J and Lejour M. 1986. Neurofibromatosis of the scalp associated with occipital bone aplasia. *Pediatr Radiol* 16:262–3.

Edge AJ and Denham RA. 1981. External fixation for complicated tibial fractures. *J Bone Joint Surg [Br]* 63:92–7.

Ferner RE, Honavar M, and Gullan RW. 1989. Spinal neurofibroma presenting as atlanto-axial subluxation in von Recklinghausen neurofibromatosis. *Neurofibromatosis* 2:43–6.

Flannery DB and Howell CG. 1987. Confirmation of the Riccardi sign. *Proc Greenwood Genet Ctr* 6:161.

Green SA. 1988. Ilizarov external fixation. *Bull Hosp Joint Dis Orthop Inst* 28:28–35.

Gregg PJ, Price BA, Ellis HA, and Stevens J. 1982. Pseudarthrosis of the radius associated with neurofibromatosis. *Clin Orthop* 171:175–9.

Haeberlin R, Riccardi SL, and Riccardi VM. 1990. Disjoining of height and head circumference measurements in pediatric patients with NF-1: implications for central nervous system pathogenesis. *Proc Greenwood Genet Ctr* 9:93–103.

Hamill PV, Drizd TA, and Johnson CL. 1977. *Growth Curves for Children, Birth to 18 Years, U.S., 1967–1973.* Vital and Health Statistics Series 11, no. 165. Washington, D.C.: U.S. Government Printing Office (DHHS Publish no. (PHS) 78-1650.).

Heard GE and Pasyne EE. 1962. Scalloping of vertebral bodies in von Recklinghausen's disease of the nervous system (neurofibromatosis). *J Neurol Neurosurg Psychiatry* 25:345–51.

Holt JF. 1978. Neurofibromatosis in children. *AJR Am J Roentgenol* 130:615–39.

Holt JF and Kuhns LR. 1976. Macrocranium and macroencephaly in neurofibromatosis. *Skeletal Radiol* 1:25–8.

Holt JF and Wright EM. 1948. The radiologic features of neurofibromatosis. *Radiology* 51:647–63.

Hunt JC and Pugh DG. 1961. Skeletal lesions in neurofibromatosis. *Radiology* 76:1–19.

Ilizarov GA and Frankel VH. 1988. The Ilizarov external fixator, a physiologic method of orthopedic reconstruction and skeletal correction: a conversation with Prof. G.A. Ilizarov and Victor H. Frankel. *Orthop Rev* 17:1142–54.

Isu T, Miyasaka K, Abe H, et al. 1983. Atlantoaxial dislocation associated with neurofibromatosis. *J Neurosurg* 58:451–3.

Jacobsen ST, Crawford AH, Millar EA, and Steel HH. 1983. The Syme amputation in patients with congenital pseudarthrosis of the tibia. *J Bone Joint Surg [Am]* 65:533–7.

Karski T and Warda E. 1986. [Diagnostic and therapeutic problems of congenital pseudarthrosis of the lower leg in children]. *Z Orthop* 124:13–8.

Klatte EC, Franken EA, and Smith JA. 1976. The radiographic spectrum in neurofibromatosis. *Semin Roentgenol* 11:17–33.

Kraiem C, Ihmid J, Allegue M, Bakir A, Tlili K, and Bakir D. 1988. Bone anomalies in von Recklinghausen disease. *J Radiol* 69:291–5.

Lewis RA, Riccardi VM, Gerson LP, Whitford R, and Axelson KA. 1984. von Recklinghausen neurofibromatosis: II. Incidence of optic nerve gliomata. *Ophthalmology* 91:929–35.

Listernick R, Charrow J, Greenwald MJ, and Esterly NB. 1989. Optic glioma in children with neurofibromatosis type I. *J Pediatr* 114:788–92.

Louis R, Jouve JL, and Borrione F. 1987. Anatomic factors in the femoral implantation of the Ilizarov external fixator. *Surg Radiol Anat* 9:5–11.

Mandell GA, Dalinka MK, and Goleman BG. 1979. Fibrous lesions in the lower extremities in neurofibromatosis. *Am J Radiol* 133:1135–8.

Najjar MF and Rowland M. 1987. *Anthropometric Reference Data and Prevalence of Overweight, US, 1976 to 1980.* Vital and Health Statistics Series 11, no. 238. Washington, D.C.: U.S. Government Printing Office (DHHS Publish no. (PHS) 87-1688).

Norman ME. 1972. Neurofibromatosis in a family. *Am J Dis Child* 123:159–60.

Pivnick EK, Lobe TE, Fitch SJ, and Riccardi VM. 1997. Hair whorl as an indicator of a mediastinal plexiform neurofibroma. *Pediatr Dermatol* 14:129–31.

Prevot J. 1986. [Axial correction of the limbs in children by the Ilizarov method (2 cases)]. *Rev Chir Orthop* 72(Suppl 2):19–21.

Riccardi VM. 1981. von Recklinghausen neurofibromatosis. *N Engl J Med* 305:1617–27.

———. 1982. The multiple forms of neurofibromatosis. *Pediatr Rev* 3:292–8.

———. 1987. Neurofibromatosis and the Albright syndrome. *Dermatol Clin* 5:193–203.

Riccardi VM and Eichner JE. 1986. *Neurofibromatosis: Phenotype, Natural History, and Pathogenesis.* Baltimore: Johns Hopkins University Press, pp. 1–305.

Shufflebarger HL. 1989. Cotrel-Dubousset instrumentation in neurofibromatosis spinal problems. *Clin Orthop* 245:24–8.

Thannhauser SJ. 1944. Neurofibromatosis (von Recklinghausen) and osteitis fibrosa cystica localisata and disseminata (von Recklinghausen). *Medicine (Baltimore)* 23:105–48.

Weichert K, Dine M, Corning H, and Silverman F. 1973. Macrocranium and neurofibromatosis. *Radiology* 107:163–6.

Weiland AJ and Daniel RK. 1980. Congenital pseudarthrosis of the tibia: treatment with vascularized autogenous fibular grafts. A preliminary report. *Johns Hopkins Med J* 147:89–95.

Yaghmai I. 1986. Spine changes in neurofibromatosis. *Radiographics* 6:261–85.

12

Vascular and Endocrine Abnormalities

J. M. Friedman, M.D., Ph.D.

CARDIOVASCULAR SYSTEM

Hypertension occurs in association with NF1 and may have several different causes, including pheochromocytoma and renal artery stenosis. Renal artery stenosis is one manifestation of a vasculopathy that may be localized or generalized in patients with NF1. Other important manifestations include aortic coarctation and cerebral vascular disease. The pathogenesis of NF1 vasculopathy is poorly understood.

Congenital heart disease has been reported among patients with NF1 but is uncommon. The most frequent congenital cardiac lesion among patients with NF1 is valvular pulmonic stenosis, which appears to be an uncommon manifestation of the *NF1* mutation. It is unclear whether other forms of congenital heart disease or hypertrophic cardiomyopathy are pathogenically associated with NF1. The cardiovascular system can also be affected secondarily by adjacent neurofibromas or other manifestations of NF1.

HYPERTENSION

Hypertension can develop in patients with NF1 at any age but is more common in older adults than in children. The prevalence by age among 2163 NF1 probands in the National Neurofibromatosis Foundation International Database and 594 in the Neurofibromatosis Institute Database is shown in Figure 12-1. Among these patients, the frequency of hypertension was only about 1% in children under 10 years of age and increased to more than 18% after age 60. High blood pressure was seen with similar frequencies in patients with NF1 in other studies. Hypertension was documented in 4.5% of 200 patients in an Australian series (North 1993). Familial occurrence of hypertension and its complications in association with NF1 has been reported (Bertrand et al. 1992).

Hypertension is also common in the general population, in which the frequency varies greatly by age and race. No studies are available that directly compare the prevalence of hypertension among patients with NF1 and other people of similar age from the same population. Treatment of hypertension is important

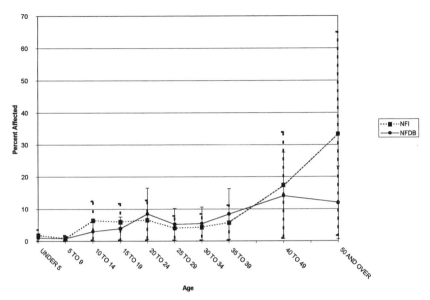

Figure 12-1. Frequency of hypertension among 2163 patients with NF1 from the National Neurofibromatosis Foundation International Database and among 594 patients with NF1 from the Neurofibromatosis Institute Database. The vertical bars indicate the 95% confidence interval of the point estimates.

in patients with NF1, just as it is in other patients, because hypertension is associated with increased mortality in adults with NF1 (Zöller et al. 1995).

Hypertension is especially common during pregnancy in women with NF1. High blood pressure was recorded at the first prenatal assessment in 5 of 10 women with NF1 studied during their first pregnancies by Swapp and Main (1973) and in 16 of 19 pregnancies in 10 affected women reported by Sharma et al. (1991).

Renovascular Hypertension
Abnormalities of the renal arteries are a frequent cause of hypertension in children with NF1 (Castanon Garcia-Alix et al. 1992; Devaney et al. 1991; Ferner 1994; Halpern and Currarino 1965; Hirayama et al. 1996; Huffman et al. 1996; Huson et al. 1989; Schürch et al. 1975; Westenend et al. 1994; Zochodne 1984). Renovascular hypertension may also present during pregnancy (Swapp and Main 1973; Horyn et al. 1988; Pilmore et al. 1997; Hagymásy et al. 1998) or at other times in adulthood (Faggioli et al. 1992; Huson et al. 1989; Pollard et al. 1989; Tenschert et al. 1985). This form of high blood pressure should be considered in any patient with NF1 who has hypertension.

Definite diagnosis of renal arterial abnormalities often requires arteriography and renal vein renin determinations (Daniels et al. 1987; Deal et al. 1992). However, less invasive imaging procedures can provide valuable indications of the presence of such lesions. Tests that are used for this purpose include renal duplex ultrasound examination (using both B-mode and Doppler imaging), captopril-induced radionuclide renogram, rapid-sequence intravenous pyelogram, digital subtractive angiography, and magnetic resonance angiography. Measurement of plasma renin in a peripheral vein is generally not useful in identification of renal artery anomalies, although performing such measurements before and after a test dose of captopril may provide a worthwhile screen (Wilcox 1993).

A variety of renal arterial lesions has been reported in patients with NF1 and hypertension. Renal artery stenosis is most common (Devaney et al. 1991; Guthrie et al. 1982; Halpern and Currarino 1965; Pollard et al. 1989; Watson and Osofsky 1981), but saccular aneurysm formation (Daniels et al. 1987; Faggioli et al. 1992; Huffman et al. 1996) and intrarenal parenchymal vessel abnormalities (Finley and Dabbs 1988; Pollard et al. 1989; Westenend et al. 1994) may also be seen. It seems likely that renal artery anomalies in NF1 are a manifestation of the vasculopathy that characterizes this disease (see below). A less frequent manifestation of this process is coarctation of aorta, which can also cause hypertension (Halpern and Currarino 1965; Donaldson et al. 1985).

Renovascular hypertension can usually be treated by surgical repair of the abnormal renal arteries, revascularization of the kidney, or unilateral nephrectomy (Hirayama et al. 1996; Ing et al. 1995; Pilmore et al. 1997; Schürch et al. 1975; Westenend et al. 1994). Aortorenal bypass, renal autotransplantation, and percutaneous angioplasty have also been used successfully (Casalini et al. 1995; Fossali et al. 1995; Pollard et al. 1989; Watano et al. 1996).

Pheochromocytoma

Pheochromocytoma is a well-recognized but uncommon cause of hypertension in patients with NF1 (Brasfield and Das Gupta 1972; Crowe et al. 1956; Ferner 1994; Manger and Gifford 1977; Riccardi 1992). It is important to rule out pheochromocytoma in adults with NF1 and hypertension, especially if the high blood pressure is episodic and associated with intermittent palpitations, tachycardia, headache, excessive perspiration, unexplained anxiety, or orthostatic hypotension. If untreated, pheochromocytoma can produce severe high blood pressure and even death. Diagnosis and management of pheochromocytomas are discussed in Chapter 10.

Other Causes of Hypertension

Hypertension in most patients with NF1 is "essential" (i.e., has no apparent cause). Neither pheochromocytoma nor renal artery anomalies are usually found (Gutmann et al. 1995; North 1993; Virdis et al. 1994). Brain tumor or coarctation of the aorta may cause hypertension in patients with NF1, but such lesions are uncommon. Of nine patients with NF1 and hypertension who were between 1 and 23 years of age studied by Virdis et al. (1994), two had renal artery stenosis, and none had a pheochromocytoma. Of the seven patients who did not have renal artery stenosis, one had a hypothalamic glioma, a second had a glioma of the thalamus, and a third had an optic chiasm glioma. It is not clear that the brain tumors caused the hypertension in these patients, but brain tumors appear to have exacerbated hypertension in other patients with NF1 (Guthrie et al. 1982). Excessive norepinephrine secretion and consequent hypertension sometimes develop in patients with NF1 who have massive cervical neurofibromas (Riccardi 1992).

VASCULOPATHY

Mutations of the *NF1* gene can cause a severe vasculopathy (Feyrter 1949; Halpern and Currarino 1965; Reubi 1944, 1945; Salyer and Salyer 1974). The process most often affects arterial vessels, with involvement of vessels ranging in size from the aorta to arteries as small as 50 μm in diameter. The systemic circulation is affected much more often than the pulmonary arteries, although the latter may be involved (Latour et al. 1981). The outflow tract of the heart itself may also be affected (Rosenquist et al. 1970). Involvement of the veins is much less common but has been reported (Finley and Dabbs 1988; Lehrnbecher et al. 1994).

Most patients with NF1 and vasculopathy have involvement of multiple vessels (Casalini et al. 1995; Dubure et al. 1984; Devaney et al. 1991; Glenn et al. 1952; Halper and Factor 1984; Halpern and Currarino 1965; Kurien et al. 1997; Latour et al. 1981; Lehrnbecher et al. 1994; Muhonen et al. 1991; Pellock et al. 1980; Pentecost et al. 1981; Planché et al. 1983; Rowen et al. 1975; Schürch et al. 1975; Sobata et al. 1988; Syme 1980; Taboada et al. 1979; Tenschert et al. 1985; Tomsick et al. 1976; Wertelecki et al. 1982; Westenend et al. 1994; Zachos et al. 1997). The lesions vary from stenosis to aneurysmal dilation. The condition is sometimes progressive, with lesions becoming more severe with time or recurring after effective treatment (Kurien et al. 1997; Pentecost et al. 1981; Planché et al. 1983).

The overall frequency of vasculopathy among patients with NF1 is not known. Symptomatic involvement is uncommon (Brasfield and Das Gupta 1972), but many occurrences may remain asymptomatic throughout life (Salyer and Salyer 1974). Vasculopathy is most often recognized in patients with NF1 in childhood or early adulthood, but some patients are older when they became symptomatic (Huffman et al. 1996; Leier et al. 1972; Sasaki et al. 1995; Tenschert et al. 1985). Complications of NF1 vasculopathy often become clinically apparent during or just after pregnancy (Horyn et al. 1988; Pilmore et al. 1997; Sobata et al. 1988; Tapp and Hickling 1969).

Vessels involved by NF1 vasculopathy may rupture, producing serious or fatal hemorrhage, but this is uncommon. Bleeding into muscles, the neck, the mediastinum, the retroperitoneal space, the gastrointestinal tract, or other viscera may occur (Brady and Bolan 1984; Larrieu et al. 1982; Lehrnbecher et al. 1994; Leier et al. 1972; Serleth et al. 1998; Tapp and Hickling 1969; Waxman et al. 1986). Another important clinical manifestation of vasculopathy in patients with NF1 is hypertension, as discussed above.

NF1 vaculopathy may involve the cerebral arteries (Barrall and Summers 1996; Horikawa et al. 1997; Levisohn et al. 1978; Sasaki et al. 1995; Sobata et al. 1988; Toboada et al. 1979; Tomsick et al. 1976; Wertelecki et al. 1982). Symptoms result from cerebral ischemia, hemorrhage, or infarction. Patients often present with acute hemiplegia or other neurologic manifestations. The diagnosis, pathogenesis, and management of cerebral vascular disease associated with NF1 are discussed in Chapter 8.

Salyer and Salyer (1974) described four classes of histopathologic changes in NF1 vasculopathy:

1. a pure intimal type, characterized by focal nodules of spindle and polygonal cells in the intima and thinning of the media of small arteries (Reubi 1944, 1945);
2. an advanced intimal type, with eccentric fibrous thickening and small aggregates of spindle cells in the intima, often with accompanying fibrosis of the media (Feyrter 1949);
3. an intimal-aneurysmal type, with marked fibrous thickening of the intima and loss of smooth muscle and elastica fragmentation in the media (Reubi 1944, 1945); and
4. a nodular or epithelial type, with small clusters of spindle and epithelial cells in the media or throughout all three layers of the arterial wall (Reubi 1944, 1945; Feyrter 1949).

Mixed, intermediate, and variant forms occur in many cases, suggesting that these lesions are pathologically related (Salyer and Salyer 1974). They may all result from proliferation of cells in the arterial walls, with the apparent histologic differences resulting from variations in severity, maturation, and the extent of subsequent healing.

Although it was originally suggested that the foci of spindle and epithelial cells seen in NF1 vasculopathy arise from Schwann cells (Feyrter 1949; Salyer and Salyer 1974), most pathologists now interpret these lesions as being composed largely of cells that arise from the walls of the arteries themselves (Greene et al. 1974; Holt and Wright 1948; Meszaros et al. 1966; Westenend et al. 1994). Origin of the vascular lesions from the arterial wall would imply an effect of the *NF1* mutation on tissue of mesodermal origin. The demonstration of neurofibromin expression in blood vessel endothelial and smooth muscle cells of rats, cattle, and early chick and quail embryos (Ahlgren-Beckendorf et al. 1993; Norton et al. 1995; Stocker et al. 1995) is consistent with this interpretation.

The lesions of NF1 vasculopathy are distinct from secondary involvement of the vessels by compression or invasion by neurofibromas and from the abnormal vasculature that may be seen within neurofibromas themselves (Brady and Bolan 1984; Francis and Mackie 1987; Glenn et al. 1952; Greene et al. 1974; Halpern and Currarino 1965; Keenan et al. 1982; Larrieu et al. 1982; Leier et al. 1972; Noubani et al. 1997; Shelton 1983; Wan 1988). Such tumor-associated vessels may also rupture and produce serious or even fatal bleeding. This is especially true of neurofibromas involving the gastrointestinal tract.

CONGENITAL HEART DISEASE

Various kinds of congenital heart disease have been reported in patients with NF1, but the overall frequency is low. It has, therefore, been controversial whether the concurrence of congenital heart disease with NF1 reflects an occasional manifestation of the *NF1* mutation or merely the coincidence of two different disorders. It now seems clear that *NF1* mutations can cause valvular pulmonic stenosis, at least in some families. Whether other kinds of congenital heart disease occur more frequently than expected among patients with NF1 remains uncertain.

Pulmonic Stenosis

Watson Syndrome. Pulmonic stenosis, multiple café-au-lait spots, and dull intellect are the cardinal features of Watson syndrome (Allanson et al. 1991; Watson 1967; see Chapter 2). Affected patients may also have other manifestations of NF1. Watson syndrome is transmitted as an autosomal dominant trait. It appears to be an allelic variant of NF1, but one in which the phenotype is less variable than typically occurs in NF1.

Pulmonic stenosis has been described in more than one affected relative in three families with Watson syndrome (Allanson et al. 1991; Leão and Ribeiro da Silva 1995; Watson 1967). Features of NF1 occur in other members of these families who do not have pulmonic stenosis, so heart disease is a variable manifestation in these kindreds. The pulmonic stenosis occurs at the level of the valve in all cases of Watson syndrome in which the lesion has been delineated (Allanson et al. 1991; Leão and Robeiro da Silva 1995; Watson 1967). Pathologic description of the pulmonic abnormality has been reported in only two cases (Watson 1967). In one instance, the lesion was described as severe valvular stenosis with no unusual features. In the other case, gross hypertrophy of the infundibulum was seen in association with severe valular stenosis.

The recognition that Watson syndrome results from mutations of the *NF1* gene raises the possibility that pulmonic stenosis may also occur with increased frequency among other patients with NF1. Observations in another phenotypic variant, the NF1–Noonan syndrome, support this notion.

NF1–Noonan Syndrome. Noonan syndrome is characterized by short stature, typical facies, and congenital heart disease (Allanson 1987; Noonan 1994; Sharland et al. 1992; see Chapter 2). Pulmonic stenosis occurs in about half of all patients with Noonan syndrome. Noonan syndrome can be transmitted as an autosomal dominant trait, and in some affected families, it appears to result from mutations of the *NF1* locus (Colley et al. 1996; Kayes et al. 1994; Stern et al. 1992; Tassabehji et al. 1993). However, most patients with Noonan syndrome do not have NF1, and Noonan syndrome is not linked to the *NF1* locus in most affected families (see Chapter 2).

Pulmonic stenosis occurs in some patients with the NF1–Noonan syndrome (Colley et al. 1996; Neiman et al. 1974; Tassabehji et al. 1993). The family reported by Neiman and associates (1974) included a boy with pulmonic valvular stenosis and features of NF1 but not Noonan syndrome, a girl with coarctation of the aorta and NF1–Noonan syndrome, and their mother, who had NF1–Noonan syndrome with pulmonic stenosis. Most patients with NF1–Noonan syndrome do not have any cardiovascular malformation (Allanson et al. 1985; Colley et al. 1996; Mendez 1985; Meschede et al. 1993; Opitz and Weaver 1985; Stern et al. 1992).

Pulmonic Stenosis in Patients with NF1 Who Do Not Have Watson Syndrome or the NF1–Noonan Syndrome. Pulmonic stenosis is the kind of congenital heart disease seen most often in patients with NF1 and is clearly more frequent than in the general population. Kaufman et al. (1972) first pointed out the association between NF1 and pulmonic stenosis. They observed congenital heart disease in six patients with NF1. The lesion was pulmonic stenosis in five of these six individuals, and the obstruction was shown to be at the level of the valve in four of them. None of these patients was noted to have features of Noonan syndrome or Watson syndrome. The association of café-au-lait spots and pulmonic stenosis had previously been noted by Pernot et al. (1971), and it is likely that at least some of the patients described by Pernot had NF1. Colley and associates (1996) found pulmonic stenosis in 9 (2.0%) of 453 patients with NF1 from 235 families. Four of the patients with pulmonic stenosis had NF1–Noonan syndrome and two had Watson syndrome. Three patients with NF1 had neither Watson syndrome nor the NF1–Noonan syndrome phenotype.

Pulmonic stenosis was observed in at least 15 of 2550 patients with NF1 from the National Neurofibromatosis Foundation International Database (Friedman et al. 1997). Individuals diagnosed as having Watson syndrome were excluded from this analysis. The frequency of pulmonic stenosis among these patients was 11 times greater than that expected in the general population (Ferencz et al. 1985).

An interesting additional observation in this study is that 12 of the 15 patients with NF1 with pulmonic stenosis were male (Friedman et al. 1997). All four of the patients with NF1 and proven valvular pulmonic stenosis reported by Kaufman et al. (1972) were male, and most patients reported with Watson syndrome or NF1–Noonan syndrome and pulmonic stenosis are also male (Neiman et al. 1974; Allanson et al. 1991; Tassabehji et al. 1993; Leão and Ribeiro da Silva 1995).

Hypertrophic Cardiomyopathy

Hypertrophic cardiomyopathy is characterized by left ventricular hypertrophy without obvious cause (Coonar and McKenna 1997; Maron 1997). The ventricular chamber itself is usually not dilated, but there is often associated asymmetrical septal hypertrophy and dynamic narrowing of the subaortic region during systole. Hypertrophic cardiomyopathy often has a genetic etiology. Mutations of the β-cardiac myosin heavy-chain gene, the cardiac troponin T gene, the cardiac myosin-binding protein C gene, or the α-tropomyosin gene all can cause dominantly inherited hypertrophic cardiomyopathy (Coonar and McKenna 1997; Maron 1997).

Hypertrophic cardiomyopathy is usually asymptomatic, but echocardiography is useful in detecting subclinical manifestations (Coonar and McKenna 1997; Maron 1997). Characteristic echocardographic changes can reliably be demonstrated in asymptomatic adults who carry inherited forms of hypertrophic cardiomyopathy, but incomplete penetrance has been documented for some mutations. Most children under 12 years of age who have a dominantly inherited hypertrophic cardiomyopathy mutation have normal echocardiograms. The prevalence of symptomatic hypertrophic cardiomyopathy in the general population is estimated to be about 20 in 100,000 (Codd et al. 1989). Echocardiographic evidence of hypertrophic cardiomyopathy is about 10 times more frequent (Maron et al. 1995).

Hypertrophic cardiomyopathy has been reported in several patients with NF1 (Elliott et al. 1976; Fitzpatrick and Emanuel 1988; Hosokawa et al. 1986; Sachs et al. 1984; Salvadori et al. 1986; Schräder et al. 1986; Waxman et al. 1986). Two sibs with hypertrophic cardiomyopathy and NF1 were described by Fitzpatrick and Emanuel (1988). Other members of this family had NF1 but no apparent heart disease.

No systematic survey of patients with NF1 for subclinical echocardiographic manifestations of hypertrophic cardiomyopathy has been reported, and the prevalence of hypertrophic cardiomyopathy among patients with NF1 is unknown. Available data are inadequate to determine whether hypertophic cardiomyopathy is an occasional feature of NF1 or if the reported concurrences are merely coincidental. The observation that muscle-specific isoforms of neurofibromin are expressed in the heart (Gutmann et al. 1995; Huynh et al. 1994; Suzuki et al. 1996) is consistent with the possibility that *NF1* mutations may sometimes cause cardiomyopathy.

Other Kinds of Congenital Heart Disease

Coarctation of the aorta has been reported repeatedly in patients with NF1 (Beggs et al. 1981; Debure et al. 1984; Donaldson et al. 1985; Friedman et al. 1997; Guthrie et al. 1982; Kurien et al. 1997; Latour et al. 1981; Planché et al. 1983; Rowen et al. 1975; Schürch et al. 1975; Senning and Johansson 1960; Tenschert et al. 1985; Welch and McKusick 1993). Often the aortic narrowing is seen in association with stenosis of other major arterial vessels or with abnormalities of the cerebral vasculature (Debure et al. 1984; Guthrie et al. 1982; Kurien et al. 1997; Latour et al. 1981; Planché et al. 1983; Rowen et al. 1975; Schürch et al. 1975; Tenschert et al. 1985; Welch and McKusick 1993). This observation suggests that aortic coarctation may be a manifestation of NF1 vasculopathy (see above).

Other congenital cardiovascular anomalies have also been observed in patients with NF1. The lesions described include atrial septal defects, ventricular septal defects, aortic stenosis, tetralogy of Fallot, complex congenital heart disease and vascular ring (Fischberg et al. 1996; Friedman et al. 1997; Kaufman et al. 1972; Lin and Garver 1988; Neiman et al. 1974; Stoll et al. 1995). It seems likely that many of these occurrences are just coincidental. However, it is interesting to note that mice homozygous for a targeted disruption of *Nf1,* the murine homolog of the human *NF1* gene, die as embryos with severe cardiovascular malformations (Brannan et al. 1994).

OTHER CARDIAC ABNORMALITIES

Neurofibromas may develop within the heart in patients with NF1, although this is quite rare (McAllister and Fenoglio 1978). Neurofibromas may also obstruct blood flow in the heart or a major vessel by external compression or invasion (Fischberg et al. 1996; Glenn et al. 1952; Halpern and Currarino 1965; Noubani et al. 1997). In other instances, erosion of a major vessel by a neurofibroma and consequent severe hemorrhage have been observed (Larrieu et al. 1982; Brady and Bolan 1984).

Mitral-valve prolapse has been reported a few times in patients with NF1 (Bensaid et al. 1986; Etches and Pickering 1978; Scotto di Uccio et al. 1988). Mitral-valve prolapse is common, however, and it seems most likely that these occurrences are just coincidental. The same explanation probably accounts for the observation of restrictive cardiomyopathy in one patient with NF1 (Benotti et al. 1980). The interpretation of apical cardiac sympathetic denervation in two patients with NF1 with coronary artery spasm and myocarditis is uncertain (Nogami et al. 1991).

ENDOCRINE SYSTEM

Children with NF1 are often shorter and have somewhat larger heads than expected for age. No endocrine cause for these effects on growth has been found. Growth in patients with NF1 is discussed in detail in Chapter 11.

The onset of puberty may be earlier or later than expected in children with NF1. In many but not all such cases, an alteration in the onset of puberty can be related to the presence of an optic chiasm glioma or other brain tumor. Both men and women with NF1 usually are normally fertile, but pregnancy in women with NF1 may be complicated by various manifestations of the disease. Neurofibromas may increase in size and number in pregnant women, but regression of some of these lesions occurs after delivery. The effect of pregnancy on most other features of NF1 has not been clearly delineated.

Pheochromocytoma and somatostatinoma are two hormone-secreting tumors that occur with increased frequency among patients with NF1. Other endocrine problems appear to be uncommon among patients with NF1.

GROWTH

The average height of individuals with NF1 is less than expected for age, but the reduction in height is usually mild. More than 80% of patients with NF1 have heights less than the population mean, but only 5 to 7% have severe short stature (height more than 3 SD below the mean). Chapter 11 provides a full discussion of growth in children with NF1.

The cause of the decreased height in NF1 is not known. Linear growth is proportionate and symmetrical, and the effect is seen at all ages. Growth hormone deficiency was found in 3 (2.5%) of 122 children with NF1 in one study (Cnossen et al. 1997), but such hormonal abnormalities do not appear to be the cause of the relatively small stature in most patients with NF1.

The average head size, which is conventionally measured as the fronto-occipital circumference, is greater in patients with NF1 than expected for age. (See Chapters 8 and 11 for a full discussion.) The cause of macrocephaly in patients with NF1 is unknown. A few cases are associated with hydrocephalus, but usually no cause is apparent.

The weight of patients with NF1 is usually normal, but this has not been systematically studied. Severe obesity is distinctly uncommon among patients with NF1 (Riccardi 1992). The explanation for this is not known but could reflect the same process that affects growth in height during childhood.

ONSET OF PUBERTY

Most patients with NF1 undergo normal pubertal development. Puberty may, however, occur prematurely or be delayed. The frequency of true precocious or delayed puberty ranges from 1 to 4% in patients with NF1 (Riccardi 1992; Friedman and Birch 1997). Premature puberty is particularly likely to occur in patients with NF1 who have optic chiasm gliomas or other brain tumors in the region of the hypothalamus (Cnossen et al. 1997; Habiby et al. 1995; Holt 1978; Iraci et al. 1980; Kelly et al. 1998; Laue et al. 1985; Listernick et al. 1995; Saxena 1970; Tertsch et al. 1979). Pubertal disturbances are much less common among patients with NF1 who do not have optic gliomas or other predisposing CNS lesions, but several such cases have been reported (Cnossen et al. 1997; Laue et al. 1985; Zacharin 1997). No cause has been recognized for the abnormal onset of puberty in these children.

True gynecomastia has been observed in association with underlying neurofibromas of the chest wall in a boy with NF1 who did not have premature genital maturation (Solomon et al. 1976). This must be differentiated from true gynecomastia without neurofibromas of the chest wall and from pseudogynecomastia in which neurofibroma of a breast causes it to enlarge without proliferation of the mammary epithelium (Lipper et al. 1981).

PREGNANCY

Although patients with NF1 as a group have decreased genetic fitness (i.e., reduced reproductive success) in comparison with the general population (see Chapter 4), both men and women with NF1 usually have normal fertility. This apparent paradox probably reflects the fact that some patients with NF1 die early in life, do not marry, or do not reproduce despite their potentially normal fertility. An adult with NF1 who lacks obvious anatomic or physiologic compromise can be expected to have a normal ability to have children. Conversely, infertility cannot be attributed to NF1 unless a mediating lesion is identified.

Although most pregnancies for healthy women with NF1 are normal (Dugoff and Sujansky 1996; Jarvis and Crompton 1978; Weissman et al. 1993), serious complications can occur. Pelvic or genital neurofibromas, especially if they are large, can complicate or preclude vaginal delivery in a pregnant woman with NF1 (Dugoff and Sujansky 1996; Griffiths and Theron 1978). Unexplained fetal growth retardation has been observed in a few pregnancies in women with NF1 (Blickstein and Lancet 1987; Weissman et al. 1993), but it is not clear that this complication occurs more often than expected in the general population (Dugoff and Sujansky 1996). Cesarean delivery may be necessary more often for pregnant patients with NF1 than for other women (Dugoff and Sujansky 1996; Weissman et al. 1993).

Women who have NF1 and high blood pressure may have serious exacerbation of their symptoms when they become pregnant (Edwards et al. 1983; Geisler and Lloyd 1963; Horyn et al. 1988). Eclamptic seizures have been reported in pregnant women with NF1 (Sharma et al. 1991; Sherman and Schwartz 1992). Women with NF1, hypertension, and poor fetal outcomes such as growth retardation, placental abruption, or stillbirth in one pregnancy may be more likely to have similar complications in future pregnancies as well (Bertrand et al. 1992; Horyn et al. 1988; Sharma et al. 1991). One family has been reported in which three women with NF1 all had hypertension during pregnancy and poor fetal outcomes (Bertrand et al. 1992).

Pregnancy is often associated with exacerbation of NF1. The number and size of dermal neurofibromas increases throughout pregnancy in many women (Douvier et al. 1987; Dugoff and Sujansky 1996; Horyn et al. 1988; Swapp and Main 1973). Enlargement of plexiform neurofibromas during pregnancy has also been reported (Ansari and Nagamani 1976). Regression of at least some of these tumors occurs after delivery. Café-au-lait spots and freckling do not seem to be influenced by pregnancy. Preexisting brain tumors have enlarged and become symptomatic during pregnancy in patients with NF1 (Boiten et al. 1987; Douvier et al. 1987). The appearance and rapid growth of malignant peripheral nerve sheath tumors have also been reported during pregnancy in NF1 patients (Ginsburg et al. 1981; Puls and Chandler 1991). Fortunately, such complications are rare.

HORMONE-PRODUCING TUMORS

Pheochromocytoma

Pheochromocytomas are neoplasms that arise in the adrenal medulla or various other organs associated with the sympathetic nervous system. The tumors are called pheochromocytomas if they secrete norepinephrine or other catecholamines. Paragangliomas are histologically identical tumors that are nonsecretory and arise outside of the adrenal medulla.

Pheochromocytomas are rare tumors, but they occur more often in patients with NF1 than in others. The incidence in the general population is estimated to be about 0.4 per 100,000 per year (Wu et al. 1997). The frequency among patients with NF1 in most series is 0.1 to 1.5%, with higher frequencies in older patients (Brasfield and Das Gupta 1972; Crowe et al. 1956; Huson et al. 1989; Manger and Gifford 1977; Mulvihill 1994; Okada and Shozawa 1984; Riccardi 1992; Wolkenstein et al. 1996; Zöller et al. 1997). In most published series (Jansson et al. 1988; Linnoila et al. 1990; Loh et al. 1997; Manger and Gifford 1977) between 1% and 10% of patients with pheochromocytomas have been found to have NF1. The diagnosis, management, and pathogenesis of pheochromocytomas are discussed in Chapter 10.

It is probably not useful to screen asymptomatic patients with NF1 for pheochromocytoma on a routine basis. Riccardi et al. (1985) did not find any cases of pheochromocytoma among 194 patients with NF1 screened for pheochromocytoma with 24-hour urine measurements of epinephrine and norepinephrine. Similarly, in another series (Wolkenstein et al. 1996) no abnormalities were found on 24-hour urine catecholamine screening in 83 patients with NF1 without hypertension.

Carcinoid Tumors

Carcinoid tumors are neoplasms that contain a variety of peptide hormones. Most carcinoids arise in the wall of the gastrointestinal tract, but they may also be found in the pancreas, lung, ovary, or elsewhere. Some carcinoids, especially those of the small intestine and proximal colon, exhibit chromaffin staining and were thought to be of neural crest origin. However, this theory is no longer generally accepted (Baylin 1990; Le Douarin 1982; Vinik and Perry 1997).

Most carcinoids grow slowly and remain asymptomatic for years. When symptoms do occur, they may result from local obstruction, metastasis, or secretion of serotonin and related vasoactive peptides by the tumors. Cutaneous flushing and diarrhea are the most common features of excessive hormone release by a carcinoid tumor.

Carcinoid tumors occur in the general population with an incidence of about 1.5 cases per 100,000 per year (Vinik and Perry 1997) but are more common among patients with NF1 (Burke et al. 1989; Cantor et al. 1982; Dawson et al. 1984; Dayal et al. 1986; Griffiths et al. 1983, 1987; Hough et al. 1983; Huson et al. 1989; Kapur et al. 1983; Mulvihill 1994; Ohtsuki et al. 1989; Scully et al. 1989; Simmons et al. 1987; Wheeler et al. 1986; Wolkenstein et al. 1996; Yoshida et al. 1991). Black patients with NF1 may be more likely than white patients to develop carcinoid tumors (Burke et al. 1990). Most carcinoid tumors diagnosed in patients with NF1 are recognized between the fourth and sixth decades of life (Griffiths et al. 1987; Yoshida et al. 1991).

Carcinoid tumors diagnosed in patients with NF1 usually arise in or near the ampulla of Vater (Griffiths et al. 1987; Yoshida et al. 1991; Ferner 1994), but tumors in this location may be more likely to produce jaundice and come to medical attention. Almost all carcinoid tumors that have been studied from patients with NF1 contain somatostatin (Burke et al. 1990; Dayal et al. 1986; Griffiths et al. 1987; Yoshida et al. 1991). These carcinoid tumors have a glandular or tubular histopathologic appearance and often contain psammoma bodies, features that are otherwise uncommon in carcinoid tumors (Burke et al. 1989, 1990; Dayal et al. 1986; Griffiths et al. 1987). Carcinoid tumors in patients with NF1 may metastasize (Burke et al. 1990; Dayal et al. 1986; Griffiths et al. 1987; Hough et al. 1983). Patients with NF1 may also have multiple primary carcinoid tumors (Burke et al. 1990; Dawson et al. 1984; Hough et al. 1983).

Patients with NF1 who have a pheochromocytoma are especially likely to have a carcinoid tumor as well, and vice versa (Cantor et al. 1982; Griffiths et al. 1983, 1987; Stephens et al. 1987; Wheeler et al. 1986). In one series of 27 patients with NF1 with duodenal carcinoid tumors, 6 (22%) also had pheochromocytoma (Griffiths et al. 1987). This is much higher than the 0.1 to 1% frequency of pheochromocytoma estimated for patients with NF1 in general (Brasfield and Das Gupta 1972; Crowe et al. 1956; Manger and Gifford 1977; Riccardi 1992; Salyer and Salyer 1974). It is unclear whether this association reflects a propensity of certain NF1 mutations to produce both neoplasms, an unrecognized hormonal interconnection between the two tumors, or simply the increased likelihood of detecting one of these tumors in a patient who is undergoing extensive evaluation for the other. In any case, the association suggests that a pheochromocytoma should be sought in any patient with NF1 who is found to have a carcinoid tumor, and that a carcinoid tumor should be sought in any patient with NF1 who is found to have a pheochromocytoma.

Other Hormone-Secreting Tumors

Parathyroid adenomas have been reported among patients with NF1 (Chakrabarti et al. 1979; Daly et al. 1970; Freimanis et al. 1984; Zöller et al. 1997), but it is not clear that such reports represent a pathogenic association rather than just coincidence.

Medullary carcinoma of the thyroid gland is a neoplasm of the calcitonin-secreting C-cells, which are neural crest derivatives (Le Douarin 1982). Medullary thyroid carcinoma has been observed in patients with NF1 (Pagès et al. 1970; Yoshida et al. 1991; Zöller et al. 1997), but this cancer does not appear to occur much more often than would be expected by chance (Hope and Mulvihill 1981). Papillary and follicular thyroid cancers have also been reported in patients with NF1 but do not appear to be unusually common (Brasfield and Das Gupta 1971; Corkill and Ross, 1969; Hasegawa et al. 1984; Nakamura et al. 1986; Ruppert et al. 1966; Zöller et al. 1997).

About 2 to 5% of patients with NF1 develop massive nodular plexiform neurofibromas of the neck (Riccardi 1992). The tumors are found in and about the cervical spinal cord and adjacent soft tissues and are usually accompanied by large numbers of subcutaneous neurofibromas elsewhere in the body (Fig. 12-2). Riccardi (1992) described three such patients who had otherwise unexplained excessive norepinephrine secretion. He proposed that the source of the excessive norepinephrine in these patients was the large neurofibromas. This proposal is consistent with the observation that norepinephrine can be demonstrated in neurofibroma tissues (Rubenstein et al. 1981).

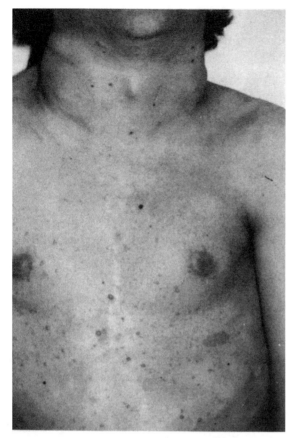

Figure 12-2. Massive cervical nodular plexiform neurofibromas in an 18-year-old man with NF1 and otherwise unexplained excessive secretion of norepinephrine.

OTHER ENDOCRINE ABNORMALITIES

Other endocrine abnormalities are uncommon among patients with NF1. Although patients with NF1 may have thyroid dysfunction (Brasfield and Das Gupta 1971), this does not seem to be a feature of the disease. No other endocrine problem has been recognized as occurring with a frequency greater than that expected in the general population. Diabetes mellitus is infrequently observed among patients with NF1 (Riccardi 1992). This might be related to the infrequent occurrence of obesity among patients with NF1.

REFERENCES

Ahlgren-Beckendorf JA, Maggio WW, Chen F, and Kent TA. 1993. Neurofibromatosis 1 mRNA expression in blood vessels. *Biochem Biophys Res Commun* 197:1019–24.
Allanson JE. 1987. Noonan syndrome. *J Med Genet* 24:9–13.

Allanson JE, Hall JG, and Van Allen MI. 1985. Noonan phenotype associated with neurofibromatosis. *Am J Med Genet* 21:457–62.

Allanson JE, Upadhyaya M, Watson GH, Partington M, MacKenzie A, Lahey D, MacLeod H, Sarfarazi M, Broadhead W, Harper PS, and Huson SM. 1991. Watson syndrome: is it a subtype of type 1 neurofibromatosis? *J Med Genet* 28:752–6.

Ansari AH and Nagamani M. 1976. Pregnancy and neurofibromatosis (von Recklinghausen's disease). *Obstet Gynecol* 47(suppl):25S–29S.

Barrall JL and Summers CG. 1996. Ocular ischemic syndrome in a child with moyamoya disease and neurofibromatosis. *Surv Ophthalmol* 40:500–4.

Baylin SB. 1990. "APUD" cells: Fact and fiction. *Trends Endocrinol Metab* 1:198–204.

Beggs I, Shaw DG, Brenton DP, and Fisher C. 1981. An unusual case of neurofibromatosis: cystic bone lesions and coarctation of the aorta. *Br J Radiol* 54:416–8.

Benotti JR, Grossman W, and Cohn PF. 1980. Clinical profile of restrictive cardiomyopathy. *Circulation* 61:1206–12.

Bensaid J, Gueret P, Virot P, Vergnoux H, Lacroix P, and Thiry M. 1986. Maladie de Recklinghausen et prolapsus valvulaire mitral. *Presse Med* 15:1424.

Bertrand C, Ville Y, and Fernandez H. 1992. Hérédité hypertensive gravidique dans la maladie de Recklinghausen: une famille. *Presse Med* 21:2142–4.

Blickstein I and Lancet M. 1987. Fetal growth retardation as a complication of pregnancy in patients with neurofibromatosis. *Am J Obstet Gynecol* 157:343.

Boiten J, Jansen ENH, and de Graaff R. 1987. von Recklinghausen neurofibromatosis (VRNF) and pregnancy: a single case study. *Clin Neurol Neurosurg* 89:181–4.

Brady DB and Bolan JC. 1984. Neurofibromatosis and spontaneous hemothorax in pregnancy: two case reports. *Obstet Gynecol* 63:35S–37S.

Brannan CI, Perkins AS, Vogel KS, Ratner N, Nordlund ML, Reid SW, Buchberg AM, Jenkins NA, Parada LF, and Copeland NG. 1994. Targeted disruption of the neurofibromatosis type-1 gene leads to developmental abnormalities in heart and various neural crest-derived tissues. *Genes Dev* 8:1019–29.

Brasfield RD and Das Gupta TK. 1972. von Recklinghausen's disease: a clinicopathological study. *Ann Surg* 175:86–104.

Burke AP, Federspiel BH, Sobin LH, Shekitka KM, and Helwig EB. 1989. Carcinoids of the duodenum: a histologic and immunochemical study of 65 tumors. *Am J Surg Pathol* 13:828–37.

Burke AP, Sobin LH, Shekitka KM, Federspiel BH, and Helwig EB. 1990. Somatostatin-producing duodenal carcinoid in patients with von Recklinghausen's neurofibromatosis: a predilection for black patients. *Cancer* 65:1591–5.

Cantor AM, Rigby CC, Beck PR, and Mangion D. 1982. Neurofibromatosis, phaeochromocytoma, and somatostatinoma. *BMJ* 285:1618–9.

Casalini E, Sfondrini MS, and Fossali E. 1995. Two-year clinical follow-up of children and adolescents after percutaneous transluminal angioplasty for renovascular hypertension. *Invest Radiol* 30:40–3.

Castanon Garcia-Alix M, Berga Fauria C, Ninot Sugranes S, Mortera Perez C, and Mulet Melia J. 1992. [Neurofibromatosis as a cause of arterial hypertension in children]. *An Esp Pediatr* 37:228–32.

Chakrabarti S, Murugesan A, and Arida EJ. 1979. The association of neurofibromatosis and hyperthyroidism. *Am J Surg* 137:417–20.

Cnossen MH, Stam EN, Cooiman LCMG, Simonsz HJ, Stroink H, Oranje AP, Halley DJ, de Goede-Bolder A, Niermeijer MF, and de Muinck Keizer-Schrama SMPF. 1997. Endocrinologic disorders and optic pathway gliomas in children with neurofibromatosis type 1. *Pediatrics* 100:667–70.

Codd MB, Sugrue DD, Gersh BJ, and Melton LJ. 1989. Epidemiology of idiopathic dilated and hypertrophic cardiomyopathy: a population-based study in Olmsted County, Minnesota, 1975–1984. *Circulation* 80:564–772.

Colley A, Donnai D, and Evans DGR. 1996. Neurofibromatosis/Noonan phenotype: a variable feature of type 1 neurofibromatosis. *Clin Genet* 49:59–64.

Coonar AS and McKenna WJ. 1997. Molecular genetics of familial cardiomyopathies. *Adv Genet* 35:285–324.

Corkill AGL and Ross CF. 1969. A case of neurofibromatosis complicated by medulloblastoma, neurogenic sarcoma, and radiation-induced carcinoma of the thyroid. *J Neurol Neurosurg Psychiatry* 32:43–7.

Crowe FW, Schull WJ, and Neel JV. 1956. *A Clinical, Pathological, and Genetic Study of Multiple Neurofibromatosis.* Springfield, Ill.: Charles C Thomas.

Daly D, Kaye M, and Estrada RL. 1970. Neurofibromatosis and hyperparathyroidism—a new syndrome? *Can Med Assoc J* 103:258–9.

Daniels SR, Loggie JMH, McEnery PT, and Towbin RB. 1987. Clinical spectrum of intrinsic renovascular hypertension in children. *Pediatrics* 80:698–704.

Dawson BV, Kazama R, and Paplanus SH. 1984. Association of carcinoid with neurofibromatosis. *South Med J* 77:511–3.

Dayal Y, Tallberg KA, Nunnemacher G, DeLellis RA, and Wolfe HJ. 1986. Duodenal carcinoids in patients with and without neurofibromatosis: a comparative study. *Am J Surg Pathol* 10:348–57.

Deal JE, Snell MF, Barratt TM, and Dillon MJ. 1992. Renovascular disease in childhood. *J Pediatr* 121:378–84.

Debure C, Fiessinger JN, Bruneval P, Vuong NP, Cormier JM, and Housset E. 1984. Lésions artèrielles multiples au cours de la maladie de von Recklinghausen: une observation. *Presse Med* 13:1776–8.

Devaney K, Kapur SP, Patterson K, and Chandra RS. 1991. Pediatric renal artery dysplasia: a morphologic study. *Pediatr Pathol* 11:609–21.

Donaldson MC, Ellison LH, and Ramsby GR. 1985. Hypertension from isolated thoracic coarctation associated with neurofibromatosis. *J Pediatr Surg* 20:169–71.

Douvier S, Goudet P, Giroud M, Mavel A, and Jahier J. 1987. Influence de la grossesse sur la maladie de Recklinghausen. *Presse Med* 16:916.

Dugoff L and Sujansky E. 1996. Neurofibromatosis type 1 and pregnancy. *Am J Med Genet* 66:7–10.

Edwards JNT, Fooks M, and Davey DA. 1983. Neurofibromatosis and severe hypertension in pregnancy. *Br J Obstet Gyencol* 90:528–31.

Elliott CM, Tajik AJ, Giuliani ER, and Gordon H. 1976. Idiopathic hypertrophic subaortic stenosis associated with cutaneous neurofibromatosis: report of a case. *Am Heart J* 92:368–72.

Etches PC and Pickering D. 1978. Apical systolic click and murmur associated with neurofibromatosis. *J Med Genet* 15:401–3.

Faggioli GL, Gargiulo M, Bertoni F, Tarantini S, and Stella A. 1992. Hypertension due to an aneurysm of the left renal artery in a patient with neurofibromatosis. *Ann Vasc Surg* 6:456–9.

Ferencz C, Rubin JD, McCarter RJ, Brenner JI, Neill CA, Perry LW, Hepner SI, and Downing JW. 1985. Congenital heart disease: prevalence at livebirth—The Baltimore-Washington Infant Study. *Am J Epidemiol* 121:31–6.

Ferner RE. 1994. Medical complications of neurofibromatosis 1. In: Huson SM and Hughes RAC, eds. *The Neurofibromatoses: A Pathogenic and Clinical Overview.* London: Chapman & Hall, pp. 316–30.

Feyrter F. 1949. Über die vasculäre Neurofibromatose, nach Utersuchungen am menschlichen Magen-Darmschlauch. *Virchows Arch* 317:221–65.

Finley JL and Dabbs DJ. 1988. Renal vascular smooth muscle proliferation in neurofibromatosis. *Hum Pathol* 19:107–10.

Fischberg C, Cotting J, Hack I, Laurini RN, and Payot M. 1996. Fatal double tracheoesophageal vascular compression and neurofibromatosis. *Arch Pediatr* 3:1253–7.

Fitzpatrick AP and Emanuel RW. 1988. Familial neurofibromatosis and hypertrophic cardiomyopathy. *Br Heart J* 60:247–51.

Fossali E, Minoja M, Intermite R, Spreafico C, Casalini E, and Sereni F. 1995. Percutaneous transluminal renal angioplasty in neurofibromatosis. *Pediatr Nephrol* 9:623–5.

Francis DMA and Mackie W. 1987. Life-threatening hemorrhage in patients with neurofibromatosis. *Aust NZ J Surg* 57:679–82.

Freimanis MG, Rodgers RW, and Samaan NA. 1984. Neurofibromatosis and primary hyperparathyroidism. *South Med J* 77:794–5.

Friedman JM and Birch PH. 1997. Type 1 neurofibromatosis: a descriptive analysis of the disorder in 1,728 patients. *Am J Med Genet* 70:138–43.

Friedman JM, Birch PH, and the NNFF International Database Participants. 1997. Cardiovascular malformations in neurofibromatosis type 1 (NF1). *Am J Hum Genet* 61:A98.

Geisler HE and Lloyd FP. 1963. Pregnancy complicated by invasive pheochromocytoma and neurofibromatosis. *Obstet Gynecol* 21:614–7.

Ginsburg DS, Hernandez E, and Johnson JWC. 1981. Sarcoma complicating von Recklinghausen disease in pregnancy. *Obstet Gynecol* 58:385–7.

Glenn F, Keefer EBC, Speer DS, and Dotter CT. 1952. Coarctation of the lower thoracic and abdominal aorta immediately proximal to celiac axis. *Surg Gynecol Obstet* 94:561–9.

Greene JF, Fitzwater JE, and Burgess J. 1974. Arterial lesions associated with neurofibromatosis. *Am J Clin Pathol* 62:481–7.

Griffiths ML and Theron EJ. 1978. Obstructed labour from pelvic neurofibroma. *S Afr Med J* 53:781.

Griffiths DFR, Williams GT, and Williams ED. 1983. Multiple endocrine neoplasia associated with von Recklinghausen's disease. *BMJ* 287:1341–3.

———. 1987. Duodenal carcinoid tumours, phaeochromocytoma and neurofibromatosis: islet cell tumour, phaeochromocytoma and the von Hippel-Lindau complex: two distinctive neuroendocrine syndromes. *Q J Med* 64:769–82.

Guthrie GP, Tibbs PA, McAllister RG, Stevens RK, and Clark DB. 1982. Hypertension and neurofibromatosis: case report. *Hypertension* 4:894–7.

Gutmann DH, Geist RT, Rose K, and Wright DE. 1995. Expression of two new isoforms of the neurofibromatosis type 1 gene product, neurofibromin, in muscle tissues. *Dev Dyn* 202:302–11.

Habiby R, Silverman B, Listernick R, and Charrow J. 1995. Precocious puberty in children with neurofibromatosis type 1. *J Pediatr* 126:364–7.

Hagymásy L, Tóth M, Szücs N, and Rigó J. 1998. Neurofibromatosis type 1 with pregnancy-associated renovascular hypertension and the syndrome of hemolysis, elevated liver enzymes, and low platelets. *Am J Obstet Gynecol* 179:272–4.

Halper J and Factor SM. 1984. Coronary lesions in neurofibromatosis associated with vasospasm and myocardial infarction. *Am Heart J* 108:420–2.

Halpern M and Currarino G. 1965. Vascular lesions causing hypertension in neurofibromatosis. *N Engl J Med* 273:248–52.

Hasegawa M, Tanaka H, Watanabe I, Uehara T, and Nasu M. 1984. Malignant schwannoma and follicular thyroid carcinoma associated with von Recklinghausen's disease. *J Laryngol Otol* 98:1057–61.

Hirayama K, Kobayashi M, Yamaguchi N, Iwabuchi S, Gotoh M, Inoue C, Yamada S, Ebata H, Ishida H, and Koyama A. 1996. A case of renovascular hypertension associated with neurofibromatosis. *Nephron* 72:699–704.

Holt JF. 1978. Neurofibromatosis in children. *AJR Am J Roentgenol* 130:615–39.

Holt JF and Wright EM. 1948. The radiologic features of neurofibromatosis. *Radiology* 51:647–64.

Hope DG and Mulvihill JJ. 1981. Malignancy in neurofibromatosis. *Adv Neurol* 29:33–56.

Horikawa M, Hirotaka S, Yamada S, and Ohtaki E. 1997. Case of von Recklinghausen disease associated with cerebral infarction. *J Child Neurol* 12:144–6.

Horyn G, Bourgeois-Dujols P, Palaric JC, and Giraud JR. 1988. Maladie de Recklinghausen et complications vasculaires au cours de la grossesse. *J Gynecol Obstet Biol Reprod (Paris)* 17:641–5.

Hosokawa T, Iwabuchi K, Ohe Y Sato H, Konno H, Haga S, and Sakakibara N. 1986. [General anesthesia for a patient with IHSS (idiopathic hypertrophic subaortic stenosis) and von Recklinghausen's disease]. *Masui* 35:450–4.

Hough DR, Chan A, and Davidson H. 1983. Von Recklinghausen's disease associated with gastrointestinal carcinoid tumors. *Cancer* 51:2206–8.

Huffman JL, Gahton V, Bowers VD, and Mills JL. 1996. Neurofibromatosis and arterial aneurysms. *Am Surg* 62:311–4.

Huson SM, Compston DAS, and Harper PS. 1989. A genetic study of von Recklinghausen neurofibromatosis in southeast Wales. II. Guidelines for genetic counselling. *J Med Genet* 26:712–21.

Huynh DP, Nechiporuk T, and Pulst SM. 1994. Differential expression and tissue distribution of type I and type II neurofibromins during mouse fetal development. *Dev Biol* 161:538–51.

Ing FF, Goldberg B, Siegel DH, Trachtman H, and Bierman FZ. 1995. Arterial stents in the manangement of neurofibromatosis and renovascular hypertension in a pediatric patient: case report of a new treatment modality. *Cardiovasc Intervent Radiol* 18:414–8.

Iraci G, Gerosa M, Scanarini M, Tomazzoli L, Fiore DL Pardatscher K, Rigobello L, and Secchi AG. 1980. Anterior optic gliomas with precocious or pseudoprecocious puberty. *Child Brain* 7:314–24.

Jansson S, Tisell L-E, Hansson G, and Stenström G. 1988. Multiple neuroectodermal abnormalities in pheochromocytoma patients. *World J Surg* 12:710–7.

Jarvis GJ and Crompton AC. 1978. Neurofibromatosis and pregnancy. *Br J Obstet Gynecol* 85:844–6.

Kapur BML, Sarin SK, Anand CS, and Varma K. 1983. Carcinoid tumour of ampulla of Vater associated with viscero-cutaneous neurofibromatosis. *Postgrad Med J* 59:734–5.

Kaufman RL, Hartmann AF, and McAlister WH. 1972. Family studies in congenital heart disease IV: congenital heart disease associated with neurofibromatosis. *Birth Defects Original Article Series,* vol. 8, no. 5. New York: Liss, pp. 92–5.

Kayes LM, Burke W, Riccardi VM, Bennett R, Ehrlich P, Rubenstein A, and Stephens K. 1994. Deletions spanning the neurofibromatosis 1 gene: identification and phenotype of five patients. *Am J Hum Genet* 54:424–36.

Keenan RA, Robinson DJ, and Briggs PC. 1982. Fatal spontaneous retroperitoneal hemorrhage caused by von Recklinghausen's neurofibromatosis. *J R Coll Surg Edinb* 27:310.

Kelly TE, Sproul GT, Huerta MG, and Rogol AD. 1998. Discordant puberty in monozygotic twin sisters with neurofibromatosis type 1 (NF1). *Clin Pediatr* 37:301–4.

Kurien A, John PR, and Milford DV. 1997. Hypertension secondary to progressive vascular neurofibromatosis. *Arch Dis Child* 76:454–5.

Larrieu AJ, Hashimoto SA, and Allen P. 1982. Spontaneous massive haemothorax in von Recklinghausen's neurofibromatosis. *Thorax* 37:151–2.

Latour H, Ferriére N, Baissus C, Renevier D, Martin O, Rebuffat G, and Chaptal PA. 1981. Sténose intimale isolée d'une artère rénale et hypertension artérielle curable dans la maladie de Recklinghuasen: association de sténoses hypoplastiques des troncs atortique et pulmonaire et de régurgitation sigmoïdienne aortique. *Arch Mal Coeur* 74:871–6.

Laue L, Comite F, Hench K, Loriaux DL, Cutler GB, and Prescovitz GH. 1985. Precocious puberty associated with neurofibromatosis and optic gliomas: treatment with lutenizing hormone releasing hormone analogue. *Am J Dis Child* 139:1097–1100.

Leão M and Ribeiro da Silva ML. 1995. Evidence of central nervous system involvement in Watson syndrome. *Pediatr Neurol* 12:252–4.

Le Douarin N. 1982. *The Neural Crest.* London: Cambridge University Press, pp. 91–107.

Lehrnbecher T, Gassel AM, Rauh V, Kirchner T, and Huppertz H-I. 1994. Neurofibromatosis presenting as a severe systemic vasculopathy. *Eur J Pediatr* 153:107–9.

Leier CV, DeWan CJ, and Anatasia LF. 1972. Fatal hemorrhage as a complication of neurofibromatosis. *Vasc Surg* 6:98–101.

Levisohn PM, Mikhael MA, and Rothman SM. 1978. Cerebrovascular changes in neurofibromatosis. *Dev Med Child Neurol* 20:789–93.

Lin AE and Garver KL. 1988. Cardiac abnormalities in neurofibromatosis. *Neurofibromatosis* 1:146–51.

Linnoila RI, Keister HR, Steinberg SM, and Lack EE. 1990. Histopathology of benign versus malignant sympathoadrenal paragangliomas: clinicopathologic study of 120 cases including unusual histologic features. *Hum Pathol* 21:1168–80.

Lipper S, Wilson CF, and Copeland KC. 1981. Pseudogynecomastia due to neurofibromatosis: a light microscopic and ultrastructural study. *Hum Pathol* 12:755–9.

Listernick R, Darling C, Greenwald M, Strauss L, and Charrow J. 1995. Optic pathway tumors in children: the effect of neurofibromatosis type 1 on clinical manifestations and natural history. *J Pediatr* 127:718–22.

Loh K-C, Shlossberg AH, Abbott EC, Salisbury SR, and Tan M-H. 1997. Phaeochromocytoma: a ten-year study. *Q J Med* 90:51–60.

Manger WM and Gifford RW. 1977. *Pheochromocytomas.* New York: Springer-Verlag.

Maron BJ. 1997. Hypertrophic cardiomyopathy. *Lancet* 350:127–33.

Maron BJ, Gardin JM, Flack JM, Gidding SS, Kurosaki TT, and Bild DE. 1995. Prevalence of hypertrophic cardiomyopathy in a general population of young adults: echocardiographic analysis of 4111 subjects in the CARDIA Study—coronary artery risk development in (young) adults. *Circulation* 92:785–9.

McAllister HA and Fenoglio JJ. 1978. Tumors of the cardiovascular system. *Atlas of Tumor Pathology,* 2nd series, fascicle 15. Washington, D.C.: Armed Forces Institute of Pathology, pp. 70–1.

Mendez HMM. 1985. The neurofibromatosis-Noonan syndrome. *Am J Med Genet* 21:471–6.

Meschede D, Froster UG, Gullotta F, and Nieschlag E. 1993. Reproductive failure in a patient with neurofibromatosis-Noonan syndrome. *Am J Med Genet* 47:346–51.

Meszaros WT, Guzzo F, and Schorsch H. 1966. Neurofibromatosis. *AJR Am J Roentgenol* 98:557–69.

Muhonen MG, Godersky JC, and VanGilder JC. 1991. Cerebral aneurysms associated with neurofibromatosis. *Surg Neurol* 36:470–5.

Mulvihill JJ. 1994. Malignancy: epidemiologically associated cancers. In: Huson SM and Hughes RAC, eds. *The Neurofibromatoses: A Pathogenic and Clinical Overview.* London: Chapman & Hall, pp. 305–15.

Nakamura H, Koga M, Sato B, Noma K, Morimoto Y, and Kishimoto S. 1986. von Recklinghausen's disease with pheochromocytoma and nonmedullary thyroid cancer. *Ann Intern Med* 105:796–7.

Neiman HL, Men E, Holt JF, Stern AM, and Perry BL. 1974. Neurofibromatosis and congenital heart disease. *AJR Am J Roentgenol* 122:146–9.

Nogami A, Hiroe M, and Marumo F. 1991. Regional sympathetic denervation in von Recklinghausen's disease with coronary spasm and myocarditis. *Int J Cardiol* 32:397–400.

Noonan J. 1994. Noonan syndrome: an update and review for the primary pediatrician. *Clin Pediatr (Phila)* 33:548–55.

North K. 1993. Neurofibromatosis type 1: review of the first 200 patients in an Australian clinic. *J Child Neurol* 8:395–402.

Norton KK, Xu J, and Gutmann DH. 1995. Expression of the neurofibromatosis I gene product, neurofibromin, in blood vessel endothelial cells and smooth muscle. *Neurobiol Dis* 2:13–21.

Noubani H, Poon E, Cooper RS, Kahn E, Kazadevich M, and Parnell VA. 1997. Neurofibromatosis with cardiac involvement. *Pediatr Cardiol* 18:156–8.

Ohtsuki Y, Sonobe H, Mizobuchi T, Takahashi K, Hayashi K, Iwata J, and Tahara E. 1989. Duodenal carcinoid (somatostatinoma) combined with von Recklinghausen's disease: a case report and review of the literature. *Acta Pathol Jpn* 39:141–6.

Okada E and Shozawa T. 1984. von Recklinghausen's disease (neurofibromatosis) associated with malignant pheochromocytoma. *Acta Pathol Jpn* 34:425–34.

Opitz JM and Weaver DD. 1985. The neurofibromatosis-Noonan syndrome. *Am J Med Genet* 21:477–90.

Pagès A, Marty C, Baldet P, and Péraldi R. 1970. Le syndrome neurfibromatose—carcinome médullaire thyroïdien—phéochromocytome. *Arch Anat Pathol* 18:137–42.

Pellock JM, Kleinman PK, McDonald BM, and Wixson D. 1980. Childhood hypertensive stroke with neurofibromatosis. *Neurology* 30:656–9.

Pentecost M, Stanley P, Takahashi M, and Isaacs H. 1981. Aneurysms of the aorta and subclavian and vertebral arteries in neurofibromatosis. *Am J Dis Child* 135:475–7.

Pernot C, Deschamps J-P, and Didier F. 1971. Stenose de l'artère pulmonaire taches cutanées pigmentaires et anomalies du squelette. *Arch Franc Pediatr* 28:593–603.

Pilmore HL, Na Nagara MP, and Walker RJ. 1997. Neurofibromatosis and renovascular hypertension presenting in early pregnancy. *Nephrol Dial Transplant* 12:187–9.

Planché C, Camilleri JP, El Abdel Hafez A, Zannier D, Mericer JN, and Artru B. 1983. Lésions de l'arche aortique dans la maladie de Recklinghausen. *Arch Mal Coeur* 76:607–13.

Pollard SG, Hornick P, Macfarlane R, and Calne RY. 1989. Renovascular hypertension in neurofibromatosis. *Postgrad Med J* 65:31–3.

Puls LE and Chandler PA. 1991. Malignant schwannoma in pregnancy. *Acta Obstet Gynecol Scand* 70:243–4.

Reubi F. 1944. Les vaisseaux et les glandes endocrines dans la neurofibromatose: le syndrome sympathiocontonique dans le maladie de Recklinghausen. *Schweiz Z Pathol Bacteriol* 7:168–236.

———. 1945. Neurofibromatose et lésions vasculaires. *Schweiz Med Wochenschr* 75: 463–5.

Riccardi VM. 1992. *Neurofibromatosis: Phenotype, Natural History, and Pathogenesis.* 2nd ed. Baltimore: Johns Hopkins University Press.

Riccardi VM, Boyd AE, and Garber AJ. 1985. Unpublished study cited in Riccardi VM. 1992. *Neurofibromatosis: Phenotype, Natural History, and Pathogenesis.* 2nd ed. Baltimore: Johns Hopkins University Press, pp. 186–7.

Rosenquist GC, Krovetz LJ, Haller JA, Simon AL, and Bannayan GA. 1970. Acquired right ventricular outflow obstruction in a child with neurofibromatosis. *Am Heart J* 79:103–8.

Rowen M, Dorsey TJ, Kegel SM, and Ostermiller WE. 1975. Thoracic coarctation associated with neurofibromatosis. *Am J Dis Child* 129:113–5.

Rubenstein AE, Mytilineou C, Yahr MD, Pearson J, and Goldstein M. 1981. Neurotransmitter analysis of dermal neurofibromas: implications for the pathogenesis and treatment of neurofibromatosis. *Neurology* 31:1184–8.

Ruppert RD, Buerger LF, and Chang WWL. 1966. Pheochromocytoma, neurofibromatosis and thyroid carcinoma. *Metabolism* 15:537–41.

Sachs RN, Buschauer-Bonnet C, Kemeny JL, Amouroux J, and Lanfranchi J. 1984. [Hypertrophic cardiomyopathy and von Recklinghausen's disease]. *Rev Med Interne* 5:154–6.

Salvadori A, Bigi R, Corradetti C, Occhi G, Partesana N, Zatta G, and Tarolo GL. 1986. [Recklinghausen disease and hypertrophic cardiomyopathy: Description of a case with regional hypertrophy]. *Minerva Cardioangiol* 34:771–3.

Salyer WR and Salyer DC. 1974. The vascular lesions of neurofibromatosis. *Angiology* 25:510–9.

Sasaki J, Miura S, Ohishi H, and Kikuchi K. 1995. [Neurofibromatosis associated with multiple intracranial vascular lesions: Stenosis of the internal carotid artery and peripheral aneurysm of Heubner's artery—report of a case]. *No Shinkei Geka* 23:813–7.

Saxena KM. 1970. Endocrine manifestations of neurofibromatosis in children. *Am J Dis Child* 120:265–71.

Schräder R, Kunkel B, Schneider M, and Kaltenbach M. 1986. Hypertrophische Kardiomyopathie bei einer Patientin Neurofibromatose von Recklinghausen. *Med Klin* 81:264–7.

Schürch W, Messerli FH, Genest J, Lefebvre R, Roy P, Cartier P, and Roho-Ortega JM. 1975. Arterial hypertension and neurofibromatosis: renal artery stenosis and coarctation of abdominal aorta. *Canad Med Assoc J* 113:879–85.

Scotto di Uccio V, Petrillo C, Chiosso M, and De Tommasis L. 1988. [Mitral valve prolapse and Recklinghausen's disease: description of a case]. *Minverva Cardioangiol* 36:331–3.

Scully RE, Mark EJ, McNeely WF, and McNeely BU. 1989. Case Records of the Massachusetts General Hospital: Case 15-1989. *N Engl J Med* 320:996–1004.

Senning Å and Johansson L. 1960. Coarctation of the abdominal aorta. *J Thoracic Cardiovasc Surg* 40:517–23.

Serleth HJ, Cogbill TH, and Gundersen SB. 1998. Ruptured pancreaticoduodenal artery aneurysms and pheochromocytoma in a pregnant patient with neurofibromatosis. *Surgery* 124:100–2.

Sharland M, Burch M, McKenna WM, and Paton MA. 1992. A clinical study of Noonan syndrome. *Arch Dis Child* 67:178–83.

Sharma JB, Gulati N, and Malik S. 1991. Maternal and perinatal complications in neurofibromatosis during pregnancy. *Int J Gynecol Obstet* 34:221–7.

Shelton NP. 1983. Fatal spontaneous retroperitoneal hemorrhage in a patient with von Recklinghausen's disease: a case report. *J Indiana State Med Assoc* 76:831.

Sherman SJ and Schwartz DB. 1992. Eclampsia complicating a pregnancy with neurofibromatosis: a case report. *J Reprod Med* 37:469–72.

Simmons TC, Henderson DR, Gletten F, Pascua L, and Greene C. 1987. The association of neurofibromatosis, psammomatous ampullary carcinoid tumor, and extrahepatic biliary obstruction. *J Clin Gastroenterol* 9:490–2.

Sobata E, Ohkuma H, and Suzuki S. 1988. Cerebrovascular disorders associated with von Recklinghausen's neurofibromatosis: a case report. *Neurosurgery* 22:544–9.

Solomon L, Kim YH, and Reiner L. 1976. Neurofibromatous pseudogynecomastia associated with prepubertal idiopathic gynecomastia. *NY State J Med* 76:932–5.

Stephens M, Williams GT, Jasani B, and Williams ED. 1987. Synchronous duodenal neuroendocrine tumours in von Recklinghausen's disease: a case report of co-existing gangliocytic paraganglioma and somatostatin-rich glandular carcinoid. *Histopathology* 11:1331–40.

Stern HJ, Saal HM, Lee JS, Fain PR, Goldgar DE, Rosenbaum KN, and Barker DF. 1992. Clinical variability of type 1 neurofibromatosis: is there a neurofibromatosis-Noonan syndrome? *J Med Genet* 29:184–7.

Stocker KM, Baizer L, Coston T, Sherman L, and Ciment G. 1995. Regulated expression of neurofibromin in migrating neural crest cells of avian embryos. *J Neurobiol* 27:535–52.

Stoll C, Alembik Y, and Dott B. 1995. Complex congenital heart disease, microcephaly, pheochromocytoma, and neurofibromatosis type I in a girl born from consanguineous parents. *Genet Couns* 6:217–20.

Suzuki H, Takahashi K, Yasumoto K, Fuse N, and Shibahara S. 1996. Differential tissue-specific expression of neurofibromin isoform mRNAs in rat. *J Biochem (Tokyo)* 120:1048–54.

Swapp GH and Main RA. 1973. Neurofibromatosis in pregnancy. *Br J Dermatol* 80:431–5.

Syme J. 1980. Neurofibromatosis as a cause of renovascular hypertension. *Australas Radiol* 24:62–6.

Taboada D, Alonso A, Moreno J, Muro D, and Mulas F. 1979. Occlusion of the cerebral arteries in Recklinghausen's diesease. *Neuroradiology* 18:281–4.

Tapp E and Hickling RS. 1969. Renal artery rupture in a pregnant woman with neurofibromatosis. *J Pathol* 97:398–402.

Tassabehji M, Strachan T, Sharland M, Colley A, Donnai D, Harris R, and Thakker N. 1993. Tandem duplication within a neurofibromatosis type I (NFI) gene exon in a family with features of Watson syndrome and Noonan syndrome. Am *J Hum Genet* 53:90–5.

Tenschert W, Holdener EE, Haertel MM, Senn H, and Vetter W. 1985. Secondary hypertension and neurofibromatosis: bilateral renal artery stenosis and coarctation of the abdominal aorta. *Klin Wochenschr* 63:593–6.

Tertsch D, Schön R, Ulrich FE, Alexander H, and Herter U. 1979. Pubertas praecox in neurofibromatosis of the optic chiasma. *Acta Neurochir* 28(Suppl):413–5.

Tomsick TA, Lukin RR, Chambers AA, and Benton C. 1976. Neurofibromatosis and intracranial arterial occlusive disease. *Neuroradiology* 11:229–34.

Vinik AA and Perry RR. 1997. Neoplasms of the gastroentereopancreatic endocrine system. In: Holland JF, Frei E, Bast RC, Kufe DW, Morton DL, and Weichselbaum RR, eds. *Cancer Medicine,* 4th ed. Baltimore: Williams & Wilkins, pp. 1605–39.

Virdis R, Balestrazzi P, Zampolli M, Donadio A, Street M, and Lorenzetti E. 1994. Hypertension in children with neurofibromatosis. *J Hum Hypertens* 8:395–7.

Wan A. 1988. Retro-peritoneal hemorrhage presenting as hip pain. *Arch Emerg Med* 5:246–7.

Watano K, Okamoto H, Takagi C, Matsuo H, Hirao N, and Kitabatake A. 1996. Neurofibromatosis complicated with XXX syndrome and renovascular hypertension. *J Intern Med* 239:531–5.

Watson DJ and Osofsky SG. 1981. Renovascular hypertension with a neural band across the renal artery in neurofibromatosis. *South Med J* 74:1145–6.

Watson GH. 1967. Pulmonary stenosis, café-au-lait spots, and dull intelligence. *Arch Dis Childh* 42:303–7.

Waxman BP, Buzzard AJ, Cox J, and Stephens MJ. 1986. Gastric and intestinal bleeding in multiple neurofibromatosis with cardiomyopathy. *Aust NZ Surg* 56:171–3.

Weissman A, Jakobi P, Zaidise I, and Drugan A. 1993. Neurofibromatosis and pregnancy: an update. *J Reprod Med* 38:890–6.

Welch TJ and McKusick MA. 1993. Cardiovascular case of the day: abdominal coarctation due to neurofibromatosis. *AJR Am J Roentgenol* 160:1313–4.

Wertelecki W, Superneau DW, Blackburn W, and Varakis JN. 1982. Neurofibromatosis, skin hemangiomas, and arterial disease. *Birth Defects Original Article Series, Vol. 18, no. 3B.* New York: Liss, pp. 29–41.

Westenend PH, Smedts F, de Jong MCJW, Lommers EJP, and Assmann KJM. 1994. A 4-year-old boy with neurofibromatosis and severe renovascular hypertension due to renal arterial dysplasia. *Am J Surg Pathol* 18:512–6.

Wheeler MH, Curley IR, and Williams ED. 1986. The association of neurofibromatosis, pheochromocytoma, and somatostatin-rich duodenal carcinoid tumor. *Surgery* 100:1163–9.

Wilcox CS. 1993. Use of angiotensin-converting enzyme inhibitors for diagnosing renovascular hypertension. *Kidney Int* 44:1379–90.

Wolkenstein P, Freche B, Zeller J, and Revuz J. 1996. Usefulness of screening investigations in neurofibromatosis type 1: a study of 152 patients. *Arch Dermatol* 132:1333–6.

Woody RC, Perrot LJ, and Beck SA. 1992. Neurofibromatosis cerebral vasculopathy in an infant: clinical, neuroradiographic, and neuropathologic studies. *Pediatr Pathol* 12:613–9.

Wu L-T, Chahinian AP, Baylin SB, Thompson NW, and Averbuch SD. 1997. Neoplasms of the neuroendocrine system. In: Holland JF, Frei E, Bast RC, Kufe DW, Morton DL, and Weichselbaum RR, eds. *Cancer Medicine,* 4th ed. Baltimore: Williams & Wilkins, pp. 1571–603.

Yoshida A, Hatanaka S, Ohi Y, Umekita Y, and Yoshida H. 1991. von Recklinghausen's disease associated with somatostatin-rich duodenal carcinoma (somatostatinoma), medullary thyroid carcinoma, and diffuse adrenal hyperplasia. *Acta Pathol Jpn* 41:847–56.

Zacharin M. 1997. Precocious puberty in two children with neurofibromatosis type I in the absence of optic chiasmal glioma. *J Pediatr* 130:155–7.

Zachos M, Parkin PC, Babyn PS, and Chait P. 1997. Neurofibromatosis type 1 vasculopathy associated with lower limb hypoplasia. *Pediatrics* 100:395–8.

Zochodne D. 1984. von Recklinghausen's vasculopathy. *Am J Med Sci* 287:64–5.

Zöller M, Rembeck B, Åkesson HO, and Angervall L. 1995. Life expectancy, mortality and prognostic factors in neurofibromatosis type 1. *Acta Derm Venereol (Stockh)* 75:136–40.

Zöller MET, Rembeck B, Odén A, Sameulsson M, and Angervall L. 1997. Malignant and benign tumors in patients with neurofibromatosis type 1 in a defined Swedish population. *Cancer* 79:2125–31.

II

Neurofibromatosis 2

13

Clinical Aspects

Mia MacCollin, M.D.

HISTORICAL PERSPECTIVE

In 1822 J. H. Wishart, then the president of the Royal College of Surgeons of Edinburgh, made a case report of an unfortunate 21-year-old man with a history of amblyopia and macrocephaly from childhood. From age 17 he had intermittent vomiting and from age 19, deafness. Seizures developed, and an attempt was made to resect a tumor protruding from his occiput. The surgical site became infected, and the patient died shortly afterward. At autopsy he was found to have multiple dural-based tumors, hydrocephalus, and multiple tumors at the skull base. Wishart's name has subsequently been associated with the "severe" form of NF2.

Seventy years after Wishart's observations, von Recklinghausen's famous monograph was published (English translation published in Crump, 1981) and the presence of skin and spinal cord tumors in both disorders became emphasized in the literature. In 1903, Henneberg and Koch observed that a clinically distinct form of NF existed, which lacked skin alterations typical of von Recklinghausen disease and included bilateral eighth cranial nerve tumors. They referred to this distinct disorder as "central" neurofibromatosis in contrast with the "peripheral" features of von Recklinghausen disease. Despite this observation, confusion regarding the differentiation between the two forms of NF persisted. For example, one of the first detailed cases of NF2 to be reported in the English language literature was that of Bassoe and Nuzum in 1915 (Fig. 13-1). They described a sporadically affected 15-year-old boy who had onset of intermittent left leg weakness associated with back pain at age 5. During his life he was also noted to have skin tumors and strabismus and immediately before his death a detailed neurologic evaluation revealed bilateral facial paresis and impaired left-sided hearing with evidence of spinal-cord dysfunction at multiple levels. At autopsy, multiple peripheral and central tumors were found, including bilateral cerebellopontine angle tumors "each the size of an English walnut." Although the authors made many astute observations regarding this and previous cases of NF, potential differentiation with "cutaneous" neurofibromatosis was made only

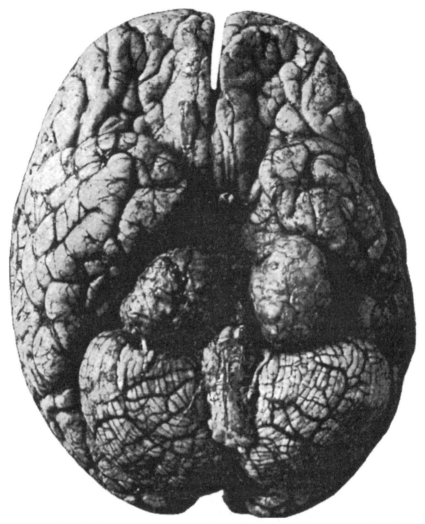

Figure 13-1. Typical autopsy appearance of large bilateral vestibular tumors deforming structures of the cerebellopontine angles at the skull base. *Source:* Bassoe and Nuzum 1915. Reprinted with permission.

in passing. Instead, the authors focused on the differentiation of neurofibromatosis (presumably both type 1 and type 2) from tuberous sclerosis primarily because of the presence of large glial cell "heaps" in the brains of their patient (subsequently known as glial hamartomas) and the hypothesis that the nerve sheath tumors of NF and the glial tumors of tuberous sclerosis shared a primary pathogenic mechanism, originating in "malformations in the primitive neurogenic tissues."

In 1929, Gardner and Frazier described a family with 38 affected members over five generations who had early onset of deafness and vestibular dysfunction, often with blindness and death at a young age. Transmission was autosomal dominant, with 50% of individuals at risk who reached adulthood manifesting the disorder and no evidence of incomplete penetrance or sex specificity. Interestingly, there was a marked increase in severity with generations in this kindred, manifested by both decreasing ages at deafness and death with passing generations. Two affected members were examined at autopsy and were found to have only bilateral cerebellopontine angle tumors, an early indication of intrafamilial homogeneity in NF2. Again these authors struggled with the classification of this disorder. Their review of the English and German literature noted that about 10% of all cases of eighth-nerve tumors in the literature were bilateral, and that 30 of these 37 bilateral cases were associated with other features of "neurofibromatosis." They argued that bilateral disease was further pathologically distinguished from unilateral disease because of the entrapment of nerve fibers in the former. Dr. Frazier concluded in his discussion that "some specific designation [should] be given to this syndrome other than von Recklinghausen's disease," but his remarks were most likely directed toward the subset of patients with NF2 who, like this kindred, do not have a tumor load outside of the cerebellopontine angle. With remarkable tenacity, Dr. Gardner provided follow-up on this family over the subsequent decades, culminating in a 1970 report detailing 97 members, most of whom could be considered to have the limited form of NF2 that bears his name (Young et al. 1970).

Several subsequent works have examined the form of NF characterized by bilateral cerebellopontine angle tumors, especially in its relationship to the more common or "peripheral" form of NF. In 1966 Rodgriguez and Berthrong reviewed 49 cases of "acoustic neurinomas" associated with meningioma and concluded that "the presence of multiple meningiomas and acoustic neurinomas in the same patient is almost certain evidence of the existence of Recklinghausen's neurofibromatosis, even if neurofibromas are not apparent to the observer." Half of their patients had gliomas and only 25% had a positive family history suggesting that this cohort consisted of especially severely affected individuals. Lee and Abbott (1969) described a large NF2 pedigree and noted that this particular type of "familial central nervous system neoplasia" was associated with ocular abnormalities, including congenital amblyopia and cataract. Kanter and colleagues (1980) examined the genetic and natural history of NF2, more closely documenting the high penetrance, clinical course, and marked differences between central and peripheral neurofibromatosis. These authors were the first to point out that malignant transformation, common in peripheral NF, was not seen in central NF. They also documented the unfortunate fact that patients with NF2 often face years of misdiagnosis before the underlying problem is recognized, citing a patient who saw 12 physicians in 17 years without being correctly diagnosed, despite the fact that her sister had bilateral vestibular schwannomas and her father had unexplained deafness.

CLINICAL CRITERIA

In 1987 and 1989, consensus development conferences were held at the National Institutes of Health to clarify the various clinical types of NF (Mulvihill et al. 1990). The conferees recommended the adoption of the term *neurofibromatosis 2 (NF2)* over central, bilateral vestibular, or bilateral acoustic neurofibromatosis. The importance of these efforts in terms of improved diagnostic specificity and pathophysiologic classification cannot be overstated. Formal diagnostic criteria (Table 13-1) for NF2, proposed at the 1987 conference, were the basis for genetic linkage studies and other work defining the nature of the NF2 genetic defect (Chapter 15). Modification of these criteria, based on rare cases said to lack bilateral vestibular tumors, have been proposed. Evans and colleagues (1992a) suggested that the presence of multiple meningioma or unilateral vestibular tumor with other NF2-related features is diagnostic. More recently, the Clinical Care Committee of the National Neurofibromatosis Foundation added a second category of "presumptive or probable NF2" (Table 13-2; Gutmann et al. 1997) for individuals meeting the Evans criteria but not NIH criteria. Diagnosis based on these revisions must be viewed with caution since many patients without bilateral vestibular schwannoma may in fact prove to have mosaic disease or other syndromes with different natural history and genetic risks than true NF2. Molecular analysis of the *NF2* gene may serve to further clarify these diagnostic categories in the near future (Chapter 15).

NATURAL HISTORY OF NF2

PRESENTATION

Most patients with NF2 are recognized when they present with symptoms referable to the eighth cranial nerve (Table 13-3). Although the tumors of NF2 originate on the vestibular branch of the nerve, auditory symptoms are usually noted first by the patient, including tinnitus and deafness. In the case of deafness, the

Table 13-1. NIH consensus criteria for NF2 from the NIH Consensus Development statement

---

The diagnostic criteria for NF2 are met if a person has either of the following:
1. Bilateral eighth nerve masses seen with appropriate imaging techniques (for example, CT or MRI)
2. A first-degree relative with neurofibromatosis 2 and either unilateral eighth nerve mass or two of the following:
   Neurofibroma
   Meningioma
   Glioma
   Schwannoma
   Juvenile posterior subcapsular
   Lenticular opacity

Source: Mulvihill et al. 1990.

Table 13-2. Proposed revisions to the NF2 clinical criteria

Definite NF2	Presumptive or Probable NF2
Bilateral vestibular schwannomas (VS) or Family history of NF2 (first-degree relative) plus 1. Unilateral VS < 30 years, or 2. Any two of the following: meningioma, glioma, schwannoma, juvenile posterior subcapsular lenticular opacities	Unilateral VS < 30 years plus at least one of the following: meningioma, glioma, schwannoma, juvenile posterior subcapsular lenticular opacities or Multiple meningiomas (two or more) plus unilateral VS < 30 years or one of the following: glioma, schwannoma, juvenile posterior subcapsular lenticular opacities

Source: Gutmann et al. 1997.

inability to use a phone with one ear is often an important clue, as it is the only test of unilateral hearing that occurs in everyday life. Deafness occasionally occurs suddenly, but more frequently presents insidiously with a lag in hearing abilities between the two ears. Some patients have a fluctuating course with episodes of sudden hearing loss, followed by complete or partial recovery. Other relatively common presentations include facial weakness, visual impairment, and painful peripheral-nerve tumors. Headache and seizure are distinctly uncommon modes of presentation. When questioned closely, often patients give a history of skin tumor that, in retrospect, is the first manifestation of their disorder.

The presentation of NF2 in children deserves special discussion (MacCollin and Mautner 1998; Mautner et al. 1993). Subtle skin tumors and posterior capsular cataract are often the first manifestations of NF2, but are unlikely to be recognized as such in the absence of an affected parent. Congenital amblyopia and peripheral-nerve tumors are other common clues to NF2 in children at risk. Completely asymptomatic children who are at risk may be diagnosed on the basis of radiographic surveillance protocols or molecular genetic testing as described below. Presence of café-au-lait macules alone in children at risk is not

Table 13-3. Presenting symptom of NF2 in two large clinical surveys

Symptom	Evans et al. 1992a*	Parry et al. 1994
Deafness and/or tinnitus	54%	41%
Balance dysfunction	8	3
Focal weakness or sensory change	18	19
Seizure	8	3
Skin tumor	*	13
Ocular	1	13
Genetic/radiographic diagnosis of asymptomatic family member	11	8

* Skin tumors and cataract excluded.

sufficiently specific to warrant concern. In a series of nine affected children, Mautner and colleagues (1993) found that, retrospectively, symptoms or signs of NF2 were present before age 5 in six patients, illustrating the need for vigilance in the pediatric population.

The average age of onset of symptoms in NF2 has been reported to be 18 to 22 years (Table 13-4). Uncommonly, NF2 will become symptomatic in a child younger than 10 or an adult over 35. When skin tumors and cataracts are more carefully considered as presenting problems, the average age of onset is less than 18 years (Mautner et al. 1996). Unfortunately, all major natural history studies have documented a pronounced lag between onset of symptoms and correct diagnosis, underscoring the great need for increased clinical recognition of this disorder.

CLINICAL COURSE

The clinical course of NF2 is extremely variable and dependent on tumor burden, surgical management, and complications. Most commonly, patients exhibit a progressive deterioration with loss of hearing, ambulation, and sight along with chronic pain due to their tumor burden. The rate of deterioration from age of diagnosis may vary from years to decades. Attempts have been made to subdivide NF2 into a severe or Wishart variant with an early presentation and fulminant course and milder or Gardner variant with a later age of onset and much less rapid course. The utility of this division in clinical practice is limited, since some patients may be fortuitously recognized and diagnosed early yet have a relatively benign course, while others subjected to aggressive surgical treatment may fare poorly even with a late age of onset. A small number of patients have only vestibular schwannoma with disability primarily related to the seventh and eighth cranial nerves if brain-stem compression is prevented. Despite the wide clinical variability among the NF2 population as a whole, there is intrafamilial homogeneity, which may be helpful in the counseling and treatment of patients with a positive family history. Genotype–phenotype relationships in this disorder may eventually aid in predicting the course of the disease in any one individual (see Chapter 15).

Earlier reports suggested that women with NF2 may be more severely affected than men, an interesting hypothesis in light of the presence of estrogen receptors on both sporadic schwannomas and meningiomas (Carroll et al. 1997;

Table 13-4. Clinical course of NF2 in two large clinical surveys

	Evans et al. 1992a	Parry et al. 1994
Average age at first symptom	21.6 years*	20.3 years
Average age of hearing loss	24 years	25.7 years
Average age at diagnosis of NF2	27.6 years	28.3 years

*Skin tumors and cataract excluded.

Martuza et al. 1988). This disparity has not been confirmed in large surveys of the disease, however, which find no difference between age of onset, deafness or other parameters of severity in men versus women (for example, Parry et al. 1994). Worsening of vestibular tumor symptoms and/or presentation of new symptoms during pregnancy has been documented in several cases (Allen et al. 1974; Evans et al. 1992a). Since NF2 tends to worsen during young adulthood exactly when pregnancy is most likely to occur, a cause-and-effect relationship will be difficult to prove. The study of Parry and colleagues (1994) documented a total of 25 pregnancies to 12 women with only a single case of significant worsening. Further study of pregnancy is needed in this disorder, and increased neurologic monitoring is probably warranted during pregnancy in women affected with NF2 until this issue is resolved.

The average age of death in the NF2 population has been reported to be 36 years; in the same study, actuarial survival from diagnosis was 15 years (Evans et al. 1992a). It is important to realize that several factors may have impact on this figure in the near future. Early recognition of the disease, both clinically and by presymptomatic diagnosis of offspring at risk, allows diagnosis of tumors at an earlier and presumably more surgically approachable stage. Improvements in imaging techniques have allowed detection of smaller tumors and better preoperative assessment of anatomy. Finally, advances in surgical techniques and the advent of rational medical and genetic therapies described below and in Chapter 14 will certainly improve outcome.

TUMOR TYPES ASSOCIATED WITH NF2

A detailed discussion of the tumors associated with NF2 is presented in Chapter 14. Briefly, these include schwannomas, meningiomas, ependymomas, and astrocytomas (Table 13-5). Although neurofibromas have been reported in NF2, caution must be used in interpreting specimens in which the entrapment of nerve fibers by NF2-associated schwannomas may falsely suggest that diagnosis. Schwannomas associated with NF2 clearly show sites of predilection with vestibular tumors being a nearly universal occurrence. One fourth of patients

Table 13-5. Percentage of NF2 patients found to have various tumor types*

Tumor Type	
Vestibular schwannoma	98%
Other cranial-nerve schwannoma	25
Meningioma	50
Spinal cord tumors	67
Astrocytoma/ependymoma	5
Skin tumor	68

*Diagnosis was frequently made on radiographic appearance, and some categories overlap (for example, spinal cord tumors may include astrocytomas, ependymomas and meningiomas). *Source:* Abstracted from Evans et al. 1992a, Parry et al. 1994, Mautner et al. 1996.

have other intracranial schwannomas, with the trigeminal nerve being the most frequently affected. Up to 80% of patients will have radiographic evidence of spinal schwannomas on careful examination; however, the vast majority of these will remain clinically silent. Peripheral-nerve tumors are much less common and less numerous than in patients with NF1 and are consequently less cosmetically burdensome. Almost all NF2-associated schwannomas are extremely slow growing and cause symptoms only after years of existence. Meningiomas appear in 50% of all patients with NF2, with the majority being intracranial. Unlike schwannomas, meningiomas have no common site of predilection. Glial tumors (ependymomas and astrocytomas) in NF2 are radiographically common but symptomatically rare.

OCULAR DYSFUNCTION

Visual impairment is a frustratingly common complication of NF2 and is a result of a variety of disparate processes (Table 13-6). Estimates of visual impairment in patients with NF2 vary from 33 to 75%, reflective of the population studied and the extent of the ophthalmologic examination reported (Bouzas et al. 1993; Mautner et al. 1996; Ragge et al. 1995). Direct involvement of ocular structures by NF2 includes both anterior and posterior elements. Juvenile posterior subcapsular lenticular opacity or cortical cataract are the most common ocular findings. These lesions may be an important clue to diagnosis in children, but become symptomatic in less than 20% of affected eyes. Retinal abnormalities, including hamartomas and epiretinal membranes are seen in up to one fourth of patients, primarily those most severely affected. Visual acuity may be affected when these malformations involve the macular region or lead to retinal detachment. About 10% of patients with NF2 have idiopathic strabismus and amblyopia as children. Further work is needed to define the exact etiology of this association.

Indirect impairment of visual function may be due to the tumor burden of NF2 itself or to iatrogenic injury. Chronically increased intracranial pressure leading to optic atrophy and blindness was frequently seen in patients with NF2 before routine surgical intervention (Gardner and Frazier 1929), but it is now rare. Orbital meningiomas and other tumors that directly affect the optic nerve

Table 13-6. Causes of visual impairment in patients with NF2

Cause*	
Cataract	70–80%
Retinal abnormality	22%
Juvenile amblyopia/strabismus	12%
Corneal opacification	11%
Orbital and optic nerve tumors	9%
Extraocular movement abnormality	9%

*Retinal abnormalities include retinal hamartoma and epiretinal membrane. Corneal opacification is most commonly due to damage to the fifth or seventh cranial nerve at surgery. *Source:* Abstracted from Bouzas et al. 1993 and Ragge et al. 1995.

and/or ocular motility are seen in 5 to 10% of patients (Bouzas et al. 1993; Ragge 1995). Optic nerve gliomas, common in patients with NF1, are not seen in the NF2 population. Finally, corneal injury is a common but often avoidable complication of surgical injury to the fifth and seventh cranial nerves (Seiff and Chang 1992; Rogers and Brand 1997). Incomplete lid closure, decreased corneal sensation and decreased tear production may all contribute to corneal damage. Patients should be closely monitored during the immediate postoperative period, when other medical and neurologic problems may eclipse the need for meticulous eye care, but when facial palsy is often at its most severe. Treatment including lubricating drops and ointments, gold weights and other prostheses, and temporary suturing of the eyelids should be pursued vigorously.

OTHER MANIFESTATIONS OF NF2

Unlike the many protean manifestations of NF1, patients with NF2 develop little pathology outside of their tumor burden. Occasional patients have been reported to have peripheral neuropathy or mononeuritis multiplex, the etiology of which is unclear (Evans et al. 1992a; Kilpatrick et al. 1992; Ohnishi and Nada 1972; Overweg-Plandsoen et al. 1996; Parry et al. 1994; Thomas et al. 1990). Many patients with NF2 have areflexia, which cannot be completely explained by tumor burden, leaving open the possibility that subclinical neuropathy is underrecognized. Careful dermatologic evaluation of patients with NF2 has revealed café-au-lait macules that are probably greater in size and number than in the general population but are not distinctive enough from the general population to be of use diagnostically (Evans et al. 1992a; Parry et al. 1994). Earlier references that emphasized café-au-lait macules in patients who clearly had NF2 may not have taken into account the prevalence of this finding in the genetically normal population. Specifically, NF2-affected adults do not reach the clinical criteria of six or more macules over 15 mm in greatest diameter that is nearly universally met in individuals affected with NF1. Other dermatologic features of NF1, such as generalized hyperpigmentation and freckling, are also not seen in NF2. Patients with NF2 do not have the associated cognitive problems, such as mental retardation and learning disability, that patients with NF1 have, although memory problems may become bothersome to those with large numbers of intracranial tumors late in the course of their disease. Certain pathologic features, discussed in more detail in Chapter 14, are nearly pathognomonic for NF2, but have no clinical significance during life.

ARE THERE CLINICAL SUBTYPES OF NF2?

The wide phenotypic spectrum of NF2 and its relatively homogenous appearance within kindreds has led to the proposal of subtypes within the disease (Table 13-7). The Wishart subtype, named for the Edinburgh physician who first reported an autopsy-proven case of NF2 in 1822, is applied to individuals with more than two intracranial tumors (in addition to bilateral vestibular tumors), spinal-cord ependymomas, and age at onset of less than 20 years. The Gardner subtype, named for the neurosurgeon who recognized the familial nature of this

Table 13-7. Criteria used to subtype NF2 individuals and families

Criterion	Gardner	Wishart	Lee/Abbott*
Vestibular schwannoma	Yes	Yes	Yes
Other intracranial tumors	< 2	≥ 2	NA
or			
Intramedullary spinal tumor	No	Yes	NA
Age at onset	≤ 20 years	< 20 years	NA
Retinal hamartoma	No	No	In index case or relative with NF2

*Individuals were allocated to the Lee/Abbott subtype if they or a blood relative with NF2 had a retinal hamartoma, regardless of other clinical findings. NA = not applicable. *Source:* Abstracted from Parry et al. 1994.

disorder in a relatively mildly affected kindred, is characterized by rare tumors outside of vestibular schwannomas and age of onset greater than 20 years. A third subset, characterized by prominent retinal pathology, has been designated "Lee/Abbott" in reference to the authors who first brought attention to the association of ocular abnormalities with genetic predisposition to vestibular tumors. Two statistical analyses of large cohorts of patients with NF2 have shown no evidence for a separate Lee/Abbott category of disease (Evans et al. 1992a; Parry et al. 1994). The same studies, however, showed that when individuals are assigned to one of the first two categories, affected family members are nearly always characterized as the same subtype, supporting the validity of this division. Furthermore, in these large cohorts of patients, significant differences were seen between subtypes in all measures of severity except for presence of cataract (Parry et al. 1994). Subtyping may be helpful in the counseling of sporadically affected individuals, but when other family members are affected, intrafamilial homogeneity may be more useful and specific in the prediction of clinical course. When counseling on the basis of subtypes, a clinician must also recognize that any one patient's course may be more dependent on age of recognition, aggressiveness of management, and iatrogenic complications than on the subtype. Finally, although genotype–phenotype studies have shown a strong correlation between truncating mutation and severe phenotype (see Chapter 15), no strict correspondence to the Gardner/Wishart categorization has been found.

CLINICAL GENETICS AND EPIDEMIOLOGY OF NF2

Unlike NF1, NF2 is a rare disorder, with most generalists unlikely to see more than one family in their practice. Because of its rarity, and frequent delayed or missed diagnosis, its incidence is difficult to estimate accurately. Evans et al. (1992c) estimated the incidence at birth to be approximately 1 in 40,000 in a population-based study, which would make NF2 approximately 10 times less frequent than NF1. Half of all affected individuals have no preceding family history of the disease, and in several cases de novo alteration in the *NF2* gene has been documented in the probands as compared with the unaffected parents (Mac-

Collin et al. 1994). The high rate of sporadic NF2 may reflect a relatively high mutation rate at the *NF2* locus and a low reproductive fitness, especially of severely affected patients.

Sporadic tumors of the types associated with NF2 are extremely common. For example, unilateral vestibular schwannoma has an incidence of about 1 per 100,000 per year (Eldridge and Parry 1992) and in two large autopsy series the incidence of occult vestibular schwannoma was even higher (0.82% to 0.87%) (Leonard and Talbot 1970; Stewart et al. 1975). It is estimated that less than 5% of individuals with vestibular schwannoma will have bilateral disease and NF2 (Eldridge and Parry 1992). Consistent with the high rate of sporadic disease, NF2 shows no racial, ethnic, or gender predilection.

NF2 shows autosomal dominant transmission with nearly full penetrance as measured by the radiographic presence of bilateral vestibular schwannoma by age 30. Rare cases of incomplete penetrance are reported in the literature (Kanter et al. 1980; Young et al. 1970) without complete radiographic investigation. A single obligate carrier from the family originally reported by Lee and Abbott (1969) has been found at autopsy at age 43 to have no vestibular tumor (Parry et al. 1994), although multiple other tumors were present. In two studies, a parent-of-origin effect on severity was observed, with the mean age in paternally inherited cases being 24 years and that of maternally inherited cases 18 years (Evans et al. 1992c; Kanter et al. 1980). Subsequent work has not confirmed this disparity (Parry et al. 1994), which may alternatively reflect a difference in the reproductive fitness of severely affected men versus severely affected women. Some workers have speculated that NF2 shows anticipation, with subsequent generations more severely affected than preceding ones. In two-generation kindreds, this may be due to a mitigating effect of mosaicism in the founders (Riccardi and Lewis 1988). This effect is particularly evident in the original five-generation family reported by Gardner (Young et al. 1970), but is difficult to reconcile with what we now know about the mutational basis of the disease (Chapter 15).

INITIAL DIAGNOSIS OF NF2

In nearly all individuals with NF2 bilateral vestibular schwannomas eventually develop, and this alone is enough to diagnose the disorder. In the presence of other cardinal features of NF2, especially multiple NF2-related tumors, a diagnosis of NF2 can be made using the revised criteria (see Table 13-2), but if there is no family history of the disease, this diagnosis should be viewed with skepticism until vestibular tumors can be shown. Conversely, vestibular tumors should be vigorously sought with annual high-quality imaging studies in any patient in whom NF2 is suspected because of the additional diagnostic certainty and the therapeutic choices that early definitive diagnosis affords. At present, molecular diagnostic tools are not helpful in the diagnosis or exclusion of NF2 in a proband because of the high incidence of "unfound" mutations in patients known to have NF2 (Chapter 15). When a diagnosis of NF2 is made or suspected, initial evaluation should also include a slit-lamp examination, a thorough skin and neurologic evaluation, and audiologic testing. Complete MRI of the spine may be considered if the diagnosis remains unclear or if unexplained neurologic deficits exist. Cervical MRI scan is important even in asymptomatic patients with NF2 before their first surgery because of the relatively high incidence of intramedullary cervical cord tumors.

Several protocols exist for the treatment of children who are at risk for NF2 because they have a parent with NF2 (Evans et al. 1992b; Harsh et al. 1995). Parents or guardians should be made aware as early as possible of the risk that NF2 may develop in their children, and couples should receive prenatal counseling by a genetics services provider whenever a pregnancy is contemplated. Prenatal diagnosis is available for most at-risk pregnancies based on mutation analysis of the affected parent or linkage analysis in families in which more than one individual is affected. In general, parents may be counseled that affected offspring will exhibit similar problems and time course as the affected parent, unless there is evidence of mosaicism in the parent, which may strongly mitigate the course and severity of the disease in the founding generation. Timing of testing of a child at risk will depend on many factors, including the course of NF2 in the parent and the attitude of the immediate family toward testing and presymptomatic intervention. Testing protocols may be discussed with the family in the pre-school age and school-age period, and testing should be strongly encouraged by the time a child reaches puberty. Before molecular testing, a thorough neurologic examination should be done on the individual at risk, and the risks and benefits of testing (including medical, social, and personal issues) should be discussed with the patient and his or her family by a qualified genetic services provider. When possible, molecular testing is preferable to clinical testing because of its greater accuracy. If molecular testing is not available for any reason, clinical testing may be substituted, but the program of surveillance must often be extended for many years in negative individuals (Evans et al. 1992b).

MANAGEMENT OF NF2

CLINICAL EVALUATION OF INDIVIDUALS KNOWN TO HAVE NF2

All patients in whom the diagnosis of NF2 is known or suspected should undergo comprehensive initial evaluation as noted above. Once a diagnosis is established, a strict monitoring program should be established. Immediately after diagnosis, more frequent examination and imaging may be required to determine the growth rate of the patient's tumors. Once this is established, however, most patients can be managed with a program of annual evaluation. At a minimum this should include a thorough review of any new neurologic symptoms and a complete neurologic examination along with the radiographic and audiologic procedures outlined below.

Imaging of vestibular schwannomas is best obtained by MRI scanning done at 3-mm slice thickness overlapping by 1.5 mm on both axial and coronal views of the internal auditory canals with and without the administration of contrast material (Fig. 13-2). CT evaluation, while useful for evaluating bony destruction

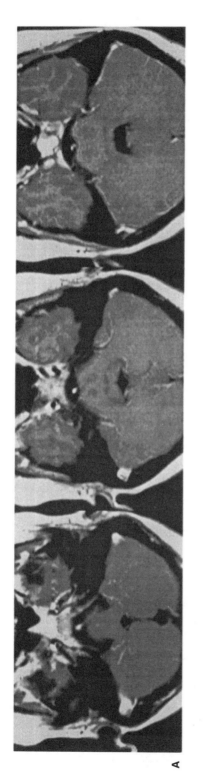

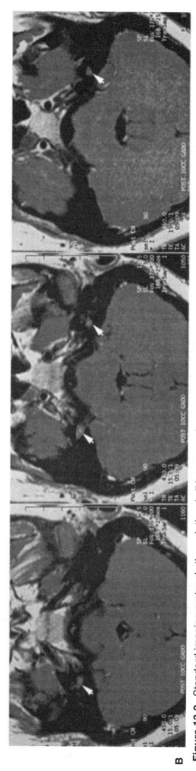

Figure 13-2. Standard imaging protocols through the skull base are often not adequate to detect small vestibular tumors. (A) Axial T$_1$-weighted, contrast-enhanced images at standard (5 mm) slice thickness in a 14-year-old at risk for NF2. This study was read as negative for vestibular tumors. (B) Similar study obtained 1 month later from the same patient at 3-mm slice thickness clearly demonstrates bilateral vestibular tumors (arrows).

caused by skull-based tumors, is filled with artifact in the region of the internal auditory canal and should never be substituted for annual MRI of vestibular tumors (Fig. 13-3). Annual spinal cord evaluation is reserved for those individuals with large or symptomatic spinal cord tumors and need not be repeated for individuals found to be free of tumor on initial evaluation. Other imaging methods that may reduce the cost and time of imaging (Shelton et al. 1996) are being developed, but are not yet validated in a large NF2 population.

Annual hearing evaluation is mandatory for patients with NF2 who have any functional hearing in either ear (Matthies and Samii 1997; Lawani et al. 1998). Audiologic evaluation provides a functional equivalent to the anatomic information provided by imaging studies, assists in evaluating the risks and benefits of surgical intervention, and is obviously important in the fitting of hearing aids for

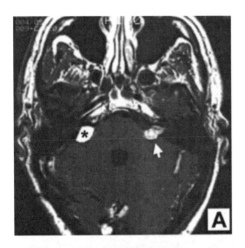

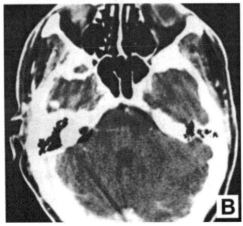

Figure 13-3. (A) T₁-weighted, contrast-enhanced MRI through the skull base in a 45-year-old man with NF2. A large left vestibular schwannoma with significant extracanalicular component is present (arrow). High signal due to fat packing at the site of resection of the contralateral tumor is seen in the right cerebellopontine angle (*). (B) Heat CT scan of the same patient at the same age. The anatomy of the skull base is nearly impossible to assess because of the artifact in the area.

patients with significant hearing impairment. Although audiology itself is not painful, many patients find hearing tests distressing, especially when they must confront unilateral hearing loss, which can be ignored in most everyday settings. Testing should be performed in a center with personnel experienced with vestibular tumors and should be reproducible and comparable to previous years' results. In most cases, hearing evaluation should be performed by a certified audiologist. Routine audiology includes both pure-tone measurements of sensitivity and speech intelligibility measurements of the quality of information that the patient receives. A number of special tests are available to further evaluate eighth-cranial-nerve function. The test most helpful for the patient with NF2 is auditory brain-stem response, an evoked potential recording that measures the acoustic impulse as it is transmitted from the periphery through the CNS. Auditory brain-stem response abnormalities are almost always present before functional hearing loss, and serial auditory brain-stem response is especially important in the presymptomatic patient who is contemplating surgical intervention (Matthies and Samii 1997). Despite its sensitivity, auditory brain-stem response should not be substituted for imaging studies for detection or follow-up of vestibular tumors (Zappia et al. 1997). Electronystagmography, which evaluates the integrity of the vestibular system, is uncomfortable for patients and is rarely necessary.

Genetic counseling is an important part of the annual examination of a patient with NF2 and should be tailored to the developmental or life stage of the patient. Depending on the family environment, even school age children may have questions about their future abilities to have children of their own. Sexually active teenagers and couples contemplating pregnancy should be counseled regarding the availability of prenatal and presymptomatic diagnosis as outlined above.

SURGICAL INTERVENTION

Surgical management of NF2-associated tumors is covered in detail in Chapter 14. Many surgical options exist for the management of vestibular schwannoma, ranging from translabyrinthine total removal to suboccipital debulking procedures. Because unilateral vestibular schwannoma is a relatively common otolaryngologic and neurosurgical problem, many centers have surgeons with great expertise in these procedures. Patients and families should be made aware, however, that vestibular schwannoma associated with NF2 may be a more difficult technical problem and may result in a worse surgical result than sporadic tumors. Although almost all families are aware of the risk of hearing loss in vestibular schwannoma surgery, many patients actually find that postoperative facial palsy and headache are more debilitating. Surgical management of other NF2-associated tumors is less bound by set protocols since the tumor location is less uniform. Unfortunately, the presence of a tumor alone is often taken to be indication for surgery. As is the case with NF1, poor timing of surgical intervention on a minimally active tumor may cause far more disability and disappointment than the tumor itself.

FACILITATING COMMUNICATION

All patients with NF2, regardless of their treatment, are at risk for deafness during their lifetime, and strategies for facilitating communication should be introduced from the initial clinic visit. Patients should receive their audiologic care in a center with personnel experienced in teaching lip-reading skills. Although many deaf adults are reluctant to learn sign language, acquisition of these skills is much easier while some hearing is preserved. Members of the patient's immediate family should be encouraged to attend sign classes with the patient. As deafness progresses, patients should be made aware of local private and public resources available for the hearing impaired. Amplification-type hearing aids may provide useful auditory function even in patients with fairly large tumors if they are fitted by an experienced center. Rarely, patients who are surgically deafened have vascular insult to the cochlea itself but preserved nerve function and may profit from a cochlear implant (Hoffman et al. 1992). Patients with more common proximal etiology of their deafness will, of course, get no benefit from a cochlear implant. Recently, the House Ear Institute, in conjunction with Cochlear Corporation, has modified the proximal electrode used in the cochlear implant to be placed into the lateral recess of the brainstem (Fig. 13-4). This auditory brain-stem implant (ABI) has produced spectacular results in a small number of deafened patients with NF2 (Otto et al. 1998), although implantation and follow-up of patients remains confined to a handful of specialized centers.

OTHER TREATMENT ISSUES

Anticipatory guidance is an important part of treatment of patients with NF2. Compassionately delivered information about the natural history of NF2 is important for families and individuals in planning both their personal and professional lives. Early in their course, patients may have balance dysfunction that is greater than they realize and are at high risk for accidental trauma. Hobbies or occupations that require ladders or working at heights should be especially discouraged. All patients should be counseled never to swim alone because of the risk of underwater disorientation and should probably not swim underwater, even with a companion. Chronic pain due to unresectable tumors or headache due to vestibular schwannoma surgery is a common symptom and should be managed by a pain clinic experienced in disability. Because NF2 is such a rare disorder, many patients and families feel extremely isolated and referral to support groups is an important part of treatment. A number of such organizations who offer face-to-face meetings, newsletters, and online resources are listed in the appendix.

Research in NF2 is now directed toward the development of rational medical therapies to prevent tumors from forming, inhibit the growth of existing tumors, or reduce the bulk of tumors that have already begun to cause symptoms. Hydroxyurea and antiestrogenic compounds are agents already in clinical trial for multiple meningiomas, with the former showing especially promising initial results (Lamberts et al. 1992; Schrell et al. 1997). Other therapies, such as

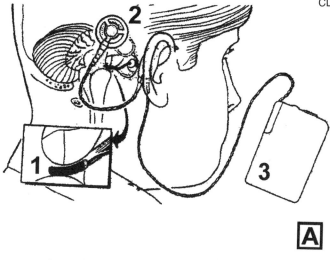

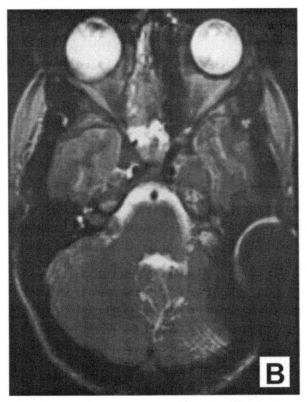

Figure 13-4. (A) Schematic representation of auditory brain-stem implant (ABI), showing placement of proximal implanted electrode array into the lateral recess (1), connection to subcutaneously placed transmitter (2), and external speech processor (3). (Courtesy of Cochlear Corporation, Englewood, Colo.) (B) T_2-weighted scan of skull base in a patient with ABI, showing artifact produced by the newer electrodes compatible with MR imaging (Heller et al. 1996).

antiangiogenesis agents, may be available in the near future (Takamiya et al. 1993), and contact with a research center specializing in NF is recommended for patients who wish to pursue such therapy.

PHENOTYPES RELATED TO NF2

PATIENTS WITH NF1 AND NF2

NF1 and NF2 are clinically and genetically distinct disorders that rarely present any diagnostic challenge to health care providers experienced in their diagnosis (Table 13-8). Infrequently, a young person with multiple skin tumors and spinal-cord involvement and a paucity of café-au-lait macules will provide an initial diagnostic dilemma. Most such cases can be resolved by careful examination with a Wood lamp, MRI scan through the internal auditory canal, and pathologic review of surgical specimens, recalling that neurofibroma pathology is seen in NF1 and schwannoma in NF2 (see Chapter 14).

Confusion between NF1 and NF2 is firmly embedded in the medical literature. A small number of cases meeting the clinical criteria for both NF1 and NF2 have been presented in the literature but most clearly describe patients with NF2 who only marginally meet NF criteria (Martuza and Ojemann 1982; Michaels et al. 1989). In a single case, a severely affected child with both NF1 and NF2 was born to a mother with NF2 and a father with NF1 (Sadeh et al. 1989). Much more commonly, persons who clearly have NF2 are described as having "NF" or "von Recklinghausen disease" (Argenyi et al. 1994; Lee and Abbott 1969; Rodriguez and Berthrong 1966). When interpreting the literature, it is important to view diagnostic categorization skeptically unless enough information is given to clearly categorize a patient. Patients reported before the advent of MRI scanning who have unexplained deafness present an especially difficult problem.

Table 13-8. Comparison of NF1 and NF2

	NF1	NF2
Incidence	1 in 3000	1 in 30,000
Typical age of onset	Infancy and early childhood	Adolescence and young adulthood
First manifestations	Café-au-lait macules, freckling	Hearing loss, balance dysfunction (cataract and skin schwannoma)
Typical tumor types	Neurofibromas, astrocytomas	Schwannomas, meningiomas
Optic nerve glioma?	Yes	No
Vestibular schwannoma?	No	Yes
Nontumorous manifestation	Many	Few
Increased risk of cancer?	Yes	No
Chromosomal location	Chromosome 17	Chromosome 22

MOSAIC NF2

Mosaic inactivation of the *NF2* gene is most likely an underrecognized condition. Mosaicism is obviously suggested in individuals with unilateral vestibular schwannoma and multiple other ipsilateral tumors (MacCollin et al. 1996; Fig. 13-5). However, individuals with bilateral vestibular schwannomas may also be mosaic (Evans et al. 1998; Kluwe and Mautner 1998). These individuals may have grossly asymmetric involvement of the eighth cranial nerves or a milder course than would otherwise be predicted from the nature of the causative mutation. Germline mosaicism of the *NF2* gene has been reported, resulting in affected siblings carrying identical *NF2* gene mutations with clinically normal parents (Parry et al. 1994). The causative mutation in this case could not be detected in lymphoblast DNA of either parent. It remains unclear what genetic risks persons with somatic mosaicism carry (i.e., to what extent somatic mosaicism may coexist with germline mosaicism). However, it would be expected that the non-mosaic affected offspring of a mosaic individual would have more severe disease than their mosaic parent.

Recognition of mosaic individuals may be problematic as they may not have bilateral vestibular schwannomas, and genetic analysis in peripheral tissues such as lymphocytes may not reveal the underlying mutation. Mosaicism should be considered in any individual with unilateral vestibular schwannoma and other NF2-related tumors, especially if the tumors are anatomically localized. Molecular genetic analysis of resected tumor material may be a viable alternative to analysis of peripheral tissues for definitive diagnosis of mosaicism. Germline mosaicism for *NF2* mutations appears to be sufficiently rare as to make screening of siblings of an affected individual with normal parents unnecessary.

SCHWANNOMATOSIS

Several literature reports have been made of individuals who had multiple pathologically proven schwannomas without vestibular schwannoma (Daras et al. 1993; Seppala et al. 1998; Shishiba et al. 1984; Wolkenstein et al. 1997). Strict diagnostic criteria have been proposed for this form of NF (Jacoby et al. 1997; Table 13-9). Although NF2 is an important diagnostic consideration in persons

Table 13-9. Diagnostic criteria for schwannomatosis

Definite Schwannomatosis	Presumptive or Probable Schwannomatosis
Two or more pathologically proven schwannomas *plus* Lack of radiographic evidence of vestibular nerve tumor at age > 18 years	Two or more pathologically proven schwannomas without symptoms of eighth-nerve dysfunction at age > 30 years Two or more pathologically proven schwannomas in an anatomically limited distribution (single limb or segment of spine) without symptoms of eighth-nerve dysfunction at any age.

Source: Adapted from Jacoby et al. 1997.

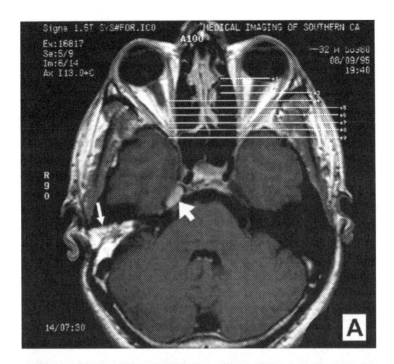

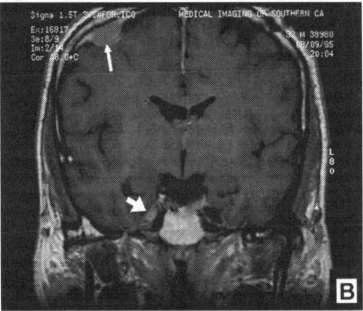

Figure 13-5. Typical radiographic appearance of mosaicism for the *NF2* gene in a 32-year-old man who had undergone resection of a unilateral vestibular schwannoma at age 29. (A) Axial scan through the skull base, showing residual fat packing at the site of tumor resection (small arrow) and appearance of a new tumor along the fifth cranial nerve (large arrow). No enhancement is seen in the contralateral internal auditory canal. (B) Coronal scan showing both the fifth-cranial-nerve tumor seen in panel A (large arrow) and a third tumor radiographically compatible with a meningioma (small arrow). Contrast-enhanced, T_1-weighted images.

with multiple schwannomas (Evans et al. 1997), there is a subgroup of patients who meet these criteria and do not go on to have NF2 and do not have offspring with NF2 (MacCollin et al. 1996). Patients with schwannomatosis primarily present with pain greater than neurologic disability, and chronic pain continues to be the defining issue of their clinical course. As a population, this clearly distinguishes them from the NF1 and NF2 populations, who may develop problems with chronic pain, but who primarily present with neurologic disability. This also makes patients with schwannomatosis prone to misdiagnosis or underdiagnosis, since long periods may pass before the underlying etiology of their pain is realized (Fig. 13-6). Surgical removal of schwannomas often cures pain, although recurrence is possible. For reasons not currently clear, schwannomatosis shows distinct genetics from both NF1 and NF2. Only rare patients will have a positive family history, and those who do show incomplete penetrance and widely variabile expressivity (Jacoby et al. 1997; MacCollin et al. 1996). Thus, it is prudent to examine a more extensive pedigree than is needed with NF1 or NF2. Schwannomatosis appears to be a genetically heterogeneous disorder, with familial cases showing linkage to chromosome 22 (Jacoby et al. 1997; Chapter 15).

OTHER SYNDROMES ASSOCIATED WITH SCHWANNOMAS

Carney complex is a rare, but well-documented syndrome of myxomas, spotty pigmentation, and endocrine overactivity, which exhibits autosomal dominant transmission (Carney 1995). Patients with Carney complex develop a variant of

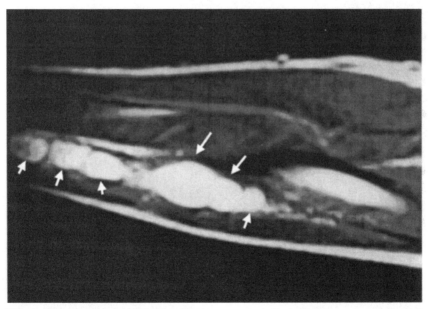

Figure 13-6. T_2-weighted MRI of the right forearm of a patient with schwannomatosis. Multiple masses appear along the course of the radial nerve (arrows). *Source:* MacCollin et al. 1996. Reprinted with permission.

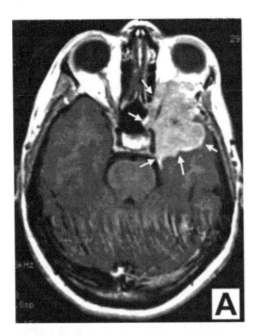

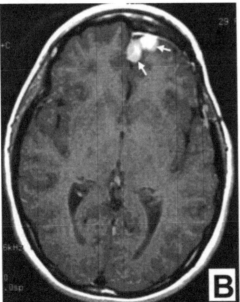

Figure 13-7. Multiple meningiomas in a 29-year-old woman without vestibular tumors. (A) Large multilobulated orbital tumor, outlined by arrows, that first caused proptosis at age 15. (B) Smaller dural-based masses in the left frontal lobe (arrows); at surgery at least four discrete tumors were noted.

schwannoma known as psammomatous melanotic schwannoma, which is uncommon in its sporadic form, and has not been reported in association with NF. Vestibular tumors and hearing impairment do not develop in patients with Carney complex. A single family has been described with multiple intradermal nevi, vaginal leiomyomas, and multiple schwannomas segregating in an autosomal dominant family (Gorlin and Koutlas 1998). Further study is needed to determine how common this association may be. Finally, granular-cell tumors, previously thought to be of myoblastic origin, have been classified as schwannian in derivation based on immunohistochemical data (Mazur et al. 1990). Granular-cell tumors may occur cutaneously, subcutaneously, or in deep structures. In about 10% of patients, tumors are multiple, and some patients with multiple tumors have had other stigmata of NF1 (Martin et al. 1990; Sahn et al. 1996). Granular-cell tumors (singular or multiple) have not been reported in association with NF2.

MULTIPLE MENINGIOMAS

In rare kindreds, multiple meningiomas may be transmitted as an autosomal dominant trait not linked to the *NF2* locus (Maxwell et al. 1998; Pulst et al. 1993). More frequently, an individual presents with two or more meningiomas and no family history of brain tumor (Fig. 13-7). Differential diagnosis of adults is a problem only when tumors arise in the cerebellopontine angle. Children with multiple meningiomas should be considered to have NF2 until proven otherwise. All persons with multiple meningiomas should have high-quality imaging of the internal auditory canals to rule out vestibular schwannoma since NF2 is much more common than familial multiple meningioma not linked to NF2. Sporadic patients with multiple meningiomas appear to be genetically heterogeneous (Chapter 15), an important point when counseling them on their genetic risks.

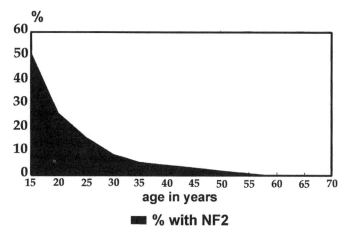

■ % with NF2

Figure 13-8. Age-specific risk of having NF2 on presenting with unilateral sporadic vestibular schwannoma. *Source:* Evans et al. 1993. Reprinted with permission.

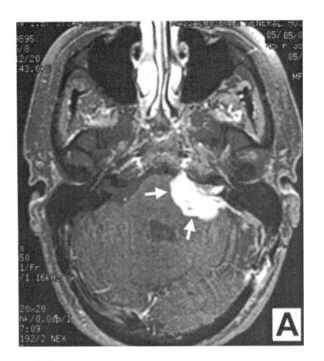

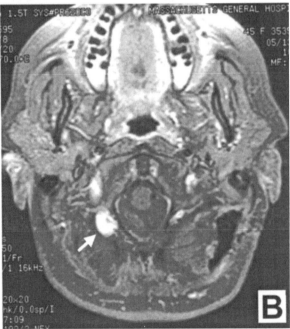

Figure 13-9. (A) Diagnostic dilemma presented by a 45-year-old woman with unilateral vestibular schwannoma (arrows). No contrast enhancement is seen in the opposite internal auditory canal. (B) Contralateral densely enhancing mass radiographically compatible with a second schwannoma in the deep tissues of the neck (arrow). Although she is unlikely to have true NF2, she may be mosaic for inactivating mutation, or may have two unrelated tumors.

YOUNG PATIENTS WITH SINGLE NF2-RELATED TUMORS

Tumors most commonly associated with NF2 such as vestibular schwannomas and meningiomas are rarely seen sporadically in the pediatric population, and their presence should always prompt a more through investigation for NF2. This issue is best studied for vestibular schwannoma, in which the risk of the development of bilateral tumors and NF2 is directly proportional to the age at which unilateral vestibular schwannoma develops (Fig. 13-8). Intracranial ependymomas and astrocytomas are more commonly seen in genetically normal children and probably do not warrant such a work-up.

DIAGNOSTIC DILEMMAS

As with NF1, diagnostic dilemmas are rare in NF2-related phenotypes when a patient is thorough investigations have been performed (Fig. 13-9). All patients suspected of having NF2 should undergo high-quality cranial MRI (defined above). If the diagnosis remains unclear, then neuroophthalmologic evaluation by a clinician familiar with NF2-related ocular findings, and pathologic review of previously resected surgical specimens, should be completed. All patients with evidence of bilateral vestibular schwannoma have NF2 by definition and need no further molecular confirmation. All patients with unilateral vestibular schwannoma and any other NF2-related feature should be carefully evaluated for mosaicism. The diagnosis of NF2 should be viewed with extreme suspicion in a patient with no bilateral vestibular schwannomas; the only exception to this rule is individuals with an NF2-related feature in whom a parent has bilateral vestibular schwannomas. Because NF2 is a fully penetrant disease, second-degree relatives of an individual affected with NF2 whose parents are not affected need not be evaluated for NF2.

REFERENCES

Allen J, Eldridge R, and Koerber T. 1974. Acoustic neuroma in the last months of pregnancy. *Am J Obstet Gynecol* 119:516–20.

Argenyi ZB, Thieberg M, Hayes C, and Whitaker D. 1994. Primary cutaneous meningioma associated with von Recklinghausen's disease. *J Cutan Pathol* 21:549–56.

Bassoe P and Nuzum F. 1915. Report of a case of central and peripheral neurofibromatosis. *J Nerv Ment Dis* 42:785–96.

Bouzas EA, Parry DM, Eldridge R, and Kaiser-Kupfer MI. 1993. Visual impairment in patients with neurofibromatosis 2. *Neurology* 43 (3 Pt1):622–3.

Carney JA. 1995. Carney Complex: the complex of myxomas, spotty pigmentation, endocrine overactivity, and schwannomas. *Semin Dermatol* 14:90–8.

Carroll RS, Zhang JP, and Black PM. 1997. Hormone receptors in vestibular schwannomas. *Acta Neurochir (Wien)* 139:188–92.

Crump T. 1981. Translation of case reports in Ueber die multiplen Fibrome der Haut und ihre Beziehung zu den multiplen Neuromen by F. v. Recklinghausen. *Adv Neurol* 29:259–75.

Daras M, Koppel B, Heise C, Mazzeo M, Poon T, and Duffy K. 1993. Multiple spinal intradural schwannomas in the absence of von Recklinghausen's disease. *Spine* 18:2556–9.

Eldridge R and Parry D. 1992. Vestibular schwannoma (acoustic neuroma). Consensus development conference. *Neurosurgery* 30:962–4.

Evans DGR, Huson SM, Donnai D, Neary W, Blair V, Newton V, Harris R. 1992a. A clinical study of type 2 neurofibromatosis. *Q J Med* 84:603–18.

Evans DGR, Huson S, Donnai D, Neary W, Blair V, Newton V, Strachan T, and Harris R. 1992b. A genetic study of type 2 neurofibromatosis in the United Kingdom. II. Guidelines for genetic counseling. *J Med Genet* 29:847–52.

Evans DGR, Huson SM, Donnai D, Neary W, Blair V, Teare D, Newton V, Strachan T, Ramsden R, and Harris R. 1992c. A genetic study of type 2 neurofibromatosis in the United Kingdom. I. Prevalence, mutation rate, fitness, and confirmation of maternal transmission effect on severity. *J Med Genet* 29:841–6.

Evans DGR, Ramsden R, Huson SM, Harris R, Lye R, and King TT. 1993. Type 2 neurofibromatosis: the need for supraregional care? *J Laryngol Otol* 107:401–6.

Evans DGR, Mason S, Huson S, Ponder M, Harding AE, and Strachan T. 1997. Spinal and cutaneous schwannomatosis is a variant form of type 2 neurofibromatosis: a clinical and molecular study. *J Neurol Neurosurg Psychiatry* 62:361–6.

Evans DGR, Wallace A, Wu, C, Trueman L, Ramsden R, Strachan T. 1998. Somatic mosaicism: a common cause of classic disease in tumor-prone syndromes? Lessons from type 2 neurofibromatosis. *Am J Hum Genet* 63:727–36.

Gardner WJ and Frazier CH. 1929. Bilateral acoustic neurofibromas. *Arch Neurol Psychol* 23:266–302.

Gorlin RJ and Koutlas IG. 1998. Multiple schwannomas, multiple nevi, and multiple vaginal leiomyomas: a new dominant syndrome. *Am J Med Genet* 78:76–81.

Gutmann DH, Aylsworth A, Carey JC, Korf B, Marks J, Pyeritz RE, Rubenstein A, and Viskochil D. 1997. The diagnostic evaluation and multidisciplinary management of neurofibromatosis 1 and neurofibromatosis 2. *JAMA* 278:51–7.

Harsh GR, MacCollin M, McKenna M, Nadol J, Ojemann R, and Short MP. 1995. Molecular genetic screening for chidren at risk of neurofibromatosis 2. *Arch Otol Head Neck Surg* 121:590–1.

Heller JW, Brackmann DE, Tucci DL, Nyenhuis JA, and Chou CK. 1996. Evaluation of MRI compatibility of the modified nucleus multichannel auditory brainstem and cochlear implants. *Am J Otolaryngol* 17:724–9.

Henneberg K and Koch M. 1903. Ueber "Centrale" Neurofibromatose und die Geschwulste des Klein-hirnbruckenwinkels (Acusticusneurome). *Arch Psy Nervenkr* (German) 36:251–304.

Hoffman RA, Kohan D, and Cohen NL. 1992. Cochlear implants in the management of bilateral acoustic neuromas. *Am J Otolaryngol* 13:525–8.

Jacoby LB, Jones D, Davis K, Kronn D, Short MP, Gusella J, and MacCollin M. 1997. Molecular analysis of the *NF2* tumor-suppressor gene in schwannomatosis. *Am J Hum Genet* 61:1293–1302.

Kanter WR, Eldridge R, Fabricant R, Allen JC, and Koerber T. 1980. Central neurofibromatosis with bilateral acoustic neuroma: genetic, clinical and biochemical distinctions from peripheral neurofibromatosis. *Neurology* 30:851–9.

Kilpatrick TJ, Hjorth RJ, and Gonzales MF. 1992. A case of neurofibromatosis 2 presenting with a mononeuritis multiplex. *J Neurol Neurosurg Psychiatry* 55:391–3.

Kluwe L and Mautner VF. 1998. Mosaicism in sporadic neurofibromatosis 2 patients. *Hum Mol Genet* 7:2051–5.

Lalwani AK, Abaza MM, Makariou EV, and Armstrong M. 1998. Audiologic presentation of vestibular schwannomas in neurofibromatosis type 2. *Am J Otolaryngol* 19:352–7.

Lamberts S, Tanghe H, Avezaat C, Braakman R, Wijngaarde R, Koper J, and de Jong H. 1992. Mifepristone (RU 486) treatment of meningiomas. *J Neurol Neurosurg Psychiatry* 55:486–90.

Lee DK and Abbott ML. 1969. Familial central nervous system neoplasia: Case report of a family with von Recklinghausen's neurofibromatosis. *Arch Neurol* 20:154–60.

Leonard JR and Talbot ML. 1970. Asymptomatic acoustic neurilemoma. *Arch Otolaryngol* 91:117–24.

MacCollin M and Mautner VF. 1998. The diagnosis and management of neurofibromatosis 2 in childhood. *Semin Pediatr Neurol* 5:243–52.

MacCollin M, Ramesh V, Jacoby LB, Louis D, Rubio MP, Pulaski K, Trofatter J, Short MP, Bove C, et al. 1994. Mutational analysis of patients with neurofibromatosis 2. *Am J Hum Genet* 55:314–20.

MacCollin M, Woodfin W, Kronn D, and Short MP. 1996. Schwannomatosis: a clinical and pathologic study. *Neurology* 46:1072–9.

Martin RW, Neldner KH, Boyd AS, and Coates PW. 1990. Multiple cutaneous granular cell tumors and neurofibromatosis in childhood: a case report and review of the literature. *Arch Dermatol* 126:1051–6.

Martuza R and Ojemann R. 1982. Bilateral acoustic neuromas: clinical aspects, pathogenesis and treatment. *Neurosurgery* 10:1–12.

Martuza RL, MacLaughlin DT, and Ojemann RG. 1988. Specific estradiol binding in schwannomas, meningiomas, and neurofibromas. *Neurosurgery* 9:665–71.

Matthies C and Samii M. 1997. Management of vestibular schwannomas (acoustic neuromas): the value of neurophysiology for evaluation and prediction of auditory function in 420 cases. *Neurosurgery* 40:919–29.

Mautner VF, Lindenau M, Baser M, Hazim W, Tatagiba M, Haase W, Samii M, Wais R, and Pulst SM. 1996. The neuroimaging and clinical spectrum of neurofibromatosis 2. *Neurosurgery* 38:880–6.

Mautner VF, Tatagiba M, Guthoff R, Samii M, and Pulst SM. 1993. Neurofibromatosis 2 in the pediatric age group. *Neurosurgery* 33:92–6.

Maxwell M, Shih S, Galanopoulos T, Hedley-Whyte E, and Cosgrove G. 1998. Familial meningioma: analysis of expression of neurofibromatosis 2 protein Merlin: report of two cases. *J Neurosurg* 88:562–9.

Mazur MT, Shultz JJ, and Myers JL. 1990. Granular cell tumor: immunohistochemical analysis of 21 benign tumors and one malignant tumor. *Arch Pathol Lab Med* 114:692–6.

Michaels V, Whisnant J, Garrity J, and Miller G. 1989. Neurofibromatosis type 1 with bilateral acoustic neuromas. *Neurofibromatosis* 2:213–7.

Mulvihill JJ, Parry DM, Sherman JL, Pikus A, Kaiser-Kupfer MI, and Eldridge R. 1990. NIH conference: neurofibromatosis 1 (Recklinghausen disease) and neurofibromatosis 2 (bilateral acoustic neurofibromatosis): an update. *Ann Intern Med* 113:39–52.

Ohnishi A and Nada O. 1972. Ultrastructure of the onion bulb-like lamellated structure observed in the sural nerve in a case of von Recklinghausen's disease. *Acta Neuropathol (Berl)* 20:258–63.

Otto SR, Shannon RV, Brackmann DE, Hitselberger WE, Staller S, and Menapace C. 1998. The multichannel auditory brainstem implant: performance in 20 patients. *Otolaryngol Head Neck Surg* 118 (3 Pt 1):291–303.

Overweg-Plandsoen WCG, Brouwer-Mladin R, Merel P, de Vries L, and Bijlsma EK. 1996. Neurofibromatosis type 2 in an adolescent boy with polyneuropathy and a mutation in the *NF2* gene. *J Neurol* 243:724–6.

Parry DM, Eldridge R, Kaiser-Kupfer MI, Bouzas EA, Pikus A, and Patronas N. 1994. Neurofibromatosis 2 (NF2): clinical characteristics of 63 affected individuals and clinical evidence for heterogeneity. *Am J Med Genet* 52:450–61.

Pulst SM, Rouleau G, Marineau C, Fain P, and Sieb J. 1993. Familial meningioma is not allelic to neurofibromatosis 2. *Neurology* 43:2096–8.

Ragge NK, Baser ME, Klein J, Nechiporuk A, Sainz J, Pulst SM, and Riccardi VM. 1995. Ocular abnormalities in neurofibromatosis 2. *Am J Ophthalmol* 120:634–41.

Riccardi V and Lewis R. 1988. Penetrance of von Recklinghausen neurofibromatosis: A distinction between predecessors and descendants. *Am J Hum Genet* 42:284–9.

Rodriguez HA and Berthrong M. 1966. Multiple primary intracranial tumors in von Recklinghausen's neurofibromatosis. *Arch Neurol* 14:467–75.

Rogers NK and Brand CS. 1997. Acoustic neuroma and the eye. *Br J Neurosurg* 11:292–7.

Sadeh M, Martinovits G, and Goldhammer V. 1989. Occurrence of both neurofibromatoses 1 and 2 in the same individual with a rapidly progressive course. *Neurology* 39:282–3.

Sahn EE, Dunlavey ES, and Parsons JL. 1996. Multiple cutaneous granular cell tumors in a child with possible neurofibromatosis. *J Am Acad Dermatol* 34:327–30.

Schrell UM, Rittig MG, Anders M, Koch UH, Marschalek R, Kiewewetter F, and Fahlbusch R. 1997. Hydroxyurea for treatment of unresectable and recurrent meningiomas. II. Decrease in the size of meningiomas in patients treated with hydroxyurea. *J Neurosurg* 86:840–84.

Seiff SR and Chang J. 1992. Management of ophthalmic complications of facial nerve palsy. *Otolaryngol Clin North Am* 25:669–90.

Seppala MT, Sainio MA, Haltia MJJ, Kinnunen JJ, Setala KH, and Jaaskelainen JE. 1998. Multiple schwannomas: schwannomatosis or neurofibromatosis type 2? *J Neurosurg* 89:36–41.

Shelton C, Harnsberger H, Allen R, and King B. 1996. Fast spin echo magnetic resonance imaging: clinical application in screening for acoustic neuroma. *Otolaryngol Head Neck Surg* 114:71–6.

Shishiba T, Niimura M, Ohtsuka F, and Tsuru N. 1984. Multiple cutaneous neurilemmomas as a skin manifestation of neurilemmomatosis. *J Am Acad Dermatol* 10:744–54.

Stewart TJ, Liland J, and Schuknecht HF. 1975. Occult schwannomas of the vestibular nerve. *Arch Otolaryngol* 101:91–5.

Takamiya V, Friedlander R, Brem H, Malick A, and Martuza R. 1993. Inhibition of angiogenesis and growth of human nerve-sheath tumors by AGM-1470. *J Neurosurg* 78:470–76.

Thomas PK, King RH, Chiang TR, Scaravilli F, Sharma AK, and Downie AW. 1990. Neurofibromatous neuropathy. *Muscle Nerve* 13:93–101.

Wishart JH. 1822. Case of tumours in the skull, dura mater, and brain. *Edinburgh Med Surg J* 18:393–7.

Wolkenstein P, Benchikhi H, Zeller J, Wechsler J, and Revuz J. 1997. Schwannomatosis: a clinical entity distinct from neurofibromatosis type 2. *Dermatology* 195:228–31.

Young DF, Eldridge R, and Gardner WJ. 1970. Bilateral acoustic neuroma in a large kindred. *JAMA* 214:347–53.

Zappia J, O'Connor C, Wiet R, and Dinces E. 1997. Rethinking the use of auditory brainstem response in acoustic neuroma screening. *Laryngoscope* 107:1388–92.

14

Associated Tumors

Mia MacCollin, M.D., and Anat Stemmer-Rachamimov, M.D.

SCHWANNOMAS

The most common tumor associated with NF2 is the schwannoma. Previous terminology for this tumor included both *neurinoma* and *neurilemoma* (or *neurilemmoma*). Macroscopically, schwannomas grow eccentric to the nerve and are well demarcated from surrounding tissue by a fibrous capsule. This is in contradistinction to neurofibromas, which grow within the nerve fiber and expand the nerve bundle as they grow. Schwannomas produce symptoms when nerve fibers or vascular structures are compromised by stretching over the increasing mass or by compression against adjacent bony structures. Microscopically, schwannomas are relatively homogeneous tumors, which reflects their origin from a single cell. Typical pathologic features make their distinction from other tumor types relatively easy in most cases (Fig. 14-1). Several pathologic features are more common in NF2-associated schwannomas relative to sporadic tumors; however, their presence or absence in any single tumor is not diagnostic of NF2 (Fig. 14-2; Hamada et al. 1997; Jaaskelainen et al. 1994; Sobel 1993). Schwannomas in NF2 show distinct sites of predilection, with the vestibular nerve uniformly affected and other sensory nerves affected more prominently than motor nerves (Martuza and Eldridge 1988).

VESTIBULAR SCHWANNOMA

The occurrence of eighth-nerve tumors is universal in patients with NF2, so much so that the diagnosis should be reconsidered in any adult who does not have bilateral eighth-nerve involvement. Although previously known as "acoustic neuromas," these tumors uniformly arise from the vestibular branch of the nerve leading to the currently accepted designation of "vestibular schwannoma" (Eldridge and Parry 1992). Despite their nerve of origin, most vestibular schwannomas present with auditory symptoms before patients become aware of vestibular dysfunction. A large body of literature exists on the growth rates of vestibular schwannoma, although relatively few patients in these studies have had bilateral tumors (Table 14-1). The majority of tumors grow slowly (less than

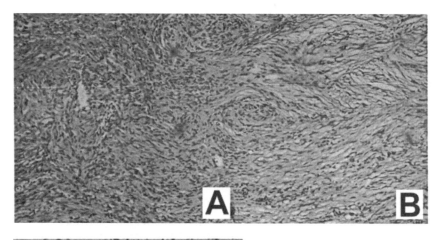

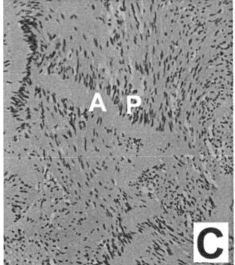

Figure 14-1. Typical histologic features seen in both sporadic and NF2-associated schwannomas. (A) Compact areas (Antoni A). (B) Loose areas (Antoni B). (C) Verocay bodies showing palisading of nuclei (P) around anuclear areas (A). (Original magnification, ×48.) *Source:* Photomicrograph courtesy of Dr. David Louis Neuropathology Department, Massachusetts General Hospital.

3 mm per year) and cause a slow decline in auditory function over a period of years. Less commonly, a patient will have sudden hearing loss or a fluctuating course with acute deterioration followed by recovery (Aslan et al. 1997; Selesnick and Jackler 1993). Left untreated, these tumors cause increasing balance dysfunction and other cranial-nerve impairments as they leave the internal auditory canal and enter the cerebellopontine angle. Eventually brain-stem compression and obstructive hydrocephalus result as the enlarging masses impinge on the pons (Fig. 14-3).

The diagnosis of vestibular schwannoma has become straightforward with the advent of MRI scanning. Previous use of skull x-ray examination and/or CT scanning made diagnosis possible only when tumors achieved a relatively large

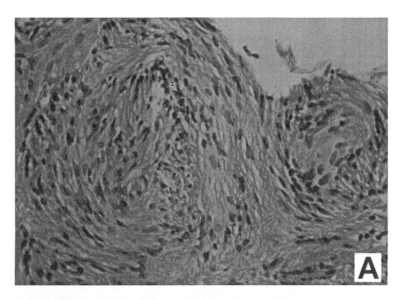

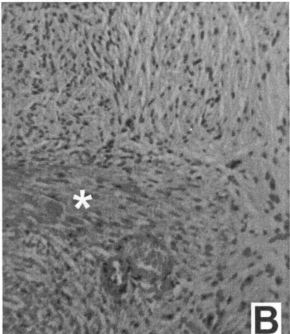

Figure 14-2. Histologic features more common in NF2-associated schwannomas than in their sporadic counterparts. (A) Lobularity, which can often be appreciated on both a gross and microscopic level. Lobularity is also seen in the histological drawing shown in Figure 14-4. (B) Entrapment of nerve (*). (Original magnification, ×80.)

Table 14-1. Studies examining growth rates of vestibular schwannomas

Study	N* (No. with NF2)	Average Growth Rate (Range)	Method of Determining Growth
Nedzelski et al. 1992	50 (0)	1.1 mm/year (–5.1–9.8)	Mean of AP and ML dimensions on CT images
Strasnick et al. 1994	51 (0)	1.1 mm/year(0–11)	Mean of AP and ML dimemsions, primarily on MR images
Charabi et al. 1995	123 (9)	3.2 mm/year (–3.2–30)	Mean of AP and ML dimensions, primarily on CT images
Wiet et al. 1995	53 (0)	1.6 mm/year (0–16.4)	AP or ML (whichever was greater), primarily on MR images
Abaza et al. 1996	22 (22)	0.3 cm³/year (0–4.9)	Volume change calculated as AP × ML × SI on MR images

AP = anteroposterior; ML = mediolaterial; SI = superior inferior.
*Except for the work of Abaza et al., these studies included only patients who met the criteria for "conservative management" or who self-selected against surgery.

size (see Fig. 13-3). Currently, tumors less than 3 mm can be routinely detected in children at risk (see Fig. 13-2). Tumors almost always originate inside the internal auditory canal at the point where the eighth nerve acquires a Schwann cell sheath. Auditory brain-stem response is less invasive and less costly than MRI and more specific and more sensitive than routine audiology or CT scanning in detecting vestibular tumors. Unfortunately, current auditory brain-stem response methods result in some detection failures for both large and small tumors (Wilson et al. 1997; Zappia et al. 1997), so it cannot be substituted for MRI.

The anatomy and pathology of vestibular schwannoma in patients with NF2 is somewhat distinct from that of sporadic vestibular schwannoma (Hamada et al. 1997; Jaaskelainen et al. 1994; Linthicum 1972; Sobel 1993). Often, on MRI scanning a multilobulated appearance is seen (Fig. 14-3C); this appearance is frequently also appreciated at surgery. The molecular basis of lobularity is not known since a multiclonal origin is unlikely given current molecular results (Chapter 15). Microscopically, lobularity and entrapment of nerve fibers are relatively common (see Fig. 14-2); in addition, collision tumors (intermingled meningiomas with vestibular schwannoma) are probably pathognomonic of some form of NF2 (Fig. 14-4).

Because sporadic vestibular schwannomas are relatively common tumors, accounting for 5 to 10% of all intracranial neoplasms in adults, a wide variety of treatment options are available. Nonsurgical treatments include watchful waiting (Charabi et al. 1995; Levo et al. 1997) and radiation therapy (Ito et al. 1997; Kondziolka et al. 1998; Linskey et al. 1992). Surgical approaches include total or partial tumor removal (Hecht et al. 1997; Nadol et al. 1992; Samii et al. 1997;

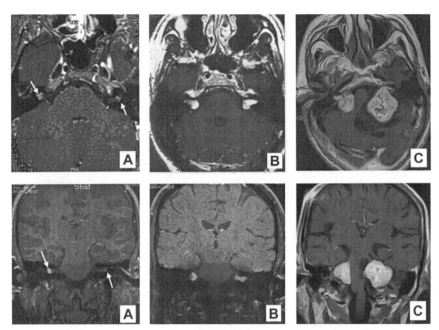

Figure 14-3. The natural history of vestibular schwannoma in NF2 in three affected members of the same kindred. (T₁-weighted, contrast-enhanced images.) (A) Axial (top) and coronal (bottom) images of a 16-year-old asymptomatic, at-risk adolescent. The diagnosis of NF2 is confirmed by the presence of bilateral enhancing masses in the internal auditory canals (arrows). (B) Similar studies of the 48-year-old affected parent of the patient shown in panel A. The tumors have now left the internal auditory canal and entered the cerebellopontine angle. At the time of this exam, the patient had progressive high-frequency hearing loss, but no other symptoms. (C) Images of the 75-year-old affected grandparent of the patient shown in panel A. The cystic and multilobulated nature of the tumors can now be appreciated. Progressive deformation of the pons has resulted in hydrocephalus, necessitating ventriculoperitoneal shunting.

Slattery et al. 1998), decompresive procedures, and auditory brain-stem or cochlear implantation (see Chapter 13). Tumor removal may be accomplished through a hearing-preservation procedure or a translabyrinthine approach, which allows greater exposure of the tumor bed, but results in deafness on the side operated on. Decompressive procedures, such as middle fossa craniotomy, may allow a large tumor to continue to grow without further damage to the seventh and eighth cranial nerve. Since the spectrum of therapeutic choices is much wider for patients with small asymptomatic tumors than for large or symptomatic ones, these options should be presented to the patient and family as early in the clinical course as possible.

In deciding on a treatment strategy for vestibular tumors associated with NF2, patients and care providers must consider both the risks and the benefits of the various approaches and the chance of future hearing loss on the contralateral

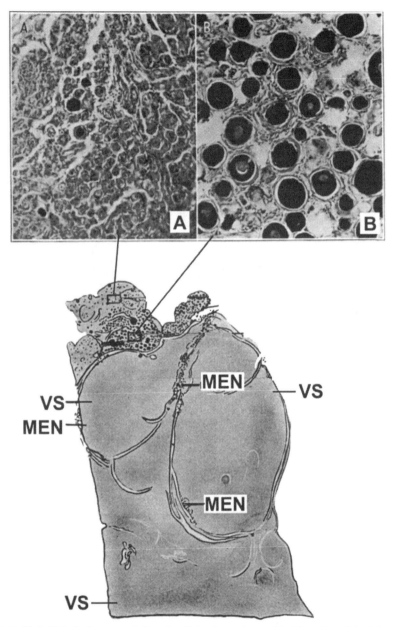

Figure 14-4. Historical representation of collision tumor in a patient from the original Gardner kindred. Overlying transitional meningioma has areas where whorl formation predominates (A) and others with numerous psammoma bodies (B) (original magnification, approximately ×85). The drawing of the vestibular tumor (VS) reveals that it is multilobulated with meningioma (MEN) "investing the nodules." *Source:* Adapted with permission from the Archives of Neurology and Psychiatry, 1940, volume 44, page 85, copyright 1940, American Medical Association.

side. In patients with preserved hearing on both sides and small intracanalicular tumors (less than 15 mm), total tumor removal of the larger side may be attempted. Most experienced centers report success rates (as measured by retained hearing postoperatively) of 60 to 70% for patients in this category (Samii et al. 1997; Slattery et al. 1998), but the issues of long-term tumor recurrence or hearing function remain open (McKenna et al. 1992). In patients with larger tumors, tumors that extend into the cerebellopontine angle (CPA), or tumors with a lobulated appearance, the chance of hearing preservation declines markedly.

In addition to deafness, intervention carries a number of other risks. Postprocedure facial palsy, either transient or permanent, may be more distressing to patients than hearing loss and may result in ocular damage due to corneal exposure (Rogers and Brand 1997). Other significant risks of surgery include bulbar palsy due to lower-cranial-nerve damage and headache, especially with the suboccipital approach. Risks of radiation therapy include lack of long-term tumor control, difficulty in subsequent surgical intervention (Slattery and Brackmann 1995) and potential malignant transformation (Baser et al. 1996). In patients with larger tumors or significant hearing loss on one side, watchful waiting is often the most prudent strategy. Intervention should be considered in these patients when hearing loss accelerates, or when brain-stem compression produces other symptoms. All patients with bilateral vestibular schwannoma should also receive counseling on facilitating communication as outlined in Chapter 13.

OTHER CRANIAL-NERVE SCHWANNOMAS

Schwannomas will develop on other cranial nerves in over 25% of all patients with NF2 (Fig. 14-5; Evans et al. 1992; Parry et al. 1994). The fifth cranial nerve is the most prominently affected, with tumors frequently extending forward into the cavernous sinus. Third-cranial-nerve tumors may cause diplopia and functional amblyopia. Their relationship to congenital strabismus is an interesting and unexplored area. Jugular fossa involvement by lower-cranial-nerve tumors may lead to unrecognized swallowing dysfunction and aspiration and warrants presymptomatic functional studies. The growth rate and natural history of other cranial-nerve schwannomas have not been studied in patients with NF2 or in patients with sporadic tumors. Without these data, there is little rationale for presymptomatic treatment of other cranial nerve tumors, and intervention is best reserved for those directly caused symptoms or imminent brain-stem compression. When treatment is considered for cranial-nerve schwannomas, it remains primarily surgical at this point. Tumors that are surgically inaccessible (such as those involving cavernous sinus) or symptomatic tumors in patients late in their disease may be arrested with radiation therapy.

SPINAL SCHWANNOMAS

Spinal schwannomas develop in up to 80% of all patients with NF2, although most are small asymptomatic tumors overlooked in life (Mautner et al. 1995). In the cervical and thoracic spine, these tumors nearly always begin on the dorsal root in the intravertebral foramen and progress to form a dumbbell configuration

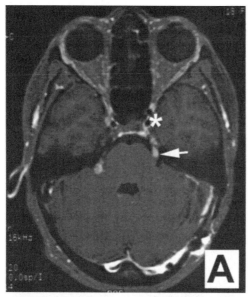

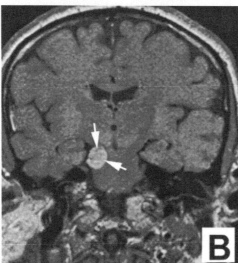

Figure 14-5. Cranial-nerve schwannomas in patients with NF2. (Contrast-enhanced, T_1-weighted images.) (A) Fifth-cranial-nerve tumor (arrow) growing forward into the cavernous sinus (*). (B) Fourth-cranial-nerve tumor (arrows).

(Fig. 14-6), indistinguishable from that of neurofibromas in patients with NF1. The cauda equina may become riddled with small tumor masses, suggestive of metastatic disease, but despite this radiographic appearance, these tumors infrequently cause significant symptoms. Because intervention is rarely, if ever, warranted on an asymptomatic patient, and because tumors grow slowly and cause symptoms over a long period of time, screening studies of the thoracic and lumbar spinal cord are probably not warranted in an asymptomatic patient. For similar reasons, patients known to have small dumbbell tumors or cauda equina

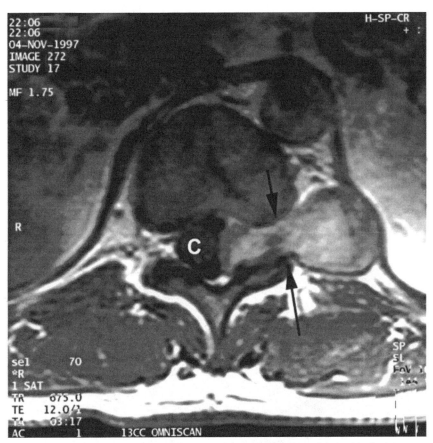

Figure 14-6. Spinal-cord schwannoma in a patient with NF2 that originated in the intravertebral foramen (arrows) and grew both medially and laterally in a dumbbell configuration. Medial growth is significantly displacing the spinal cord (C), and the patient presented with progressive difficulties in ambulation. (Contrast-enhanced, T_1-weighted images.)

masses probably do not need to have imaging performed on an annual basis unless symptoms are increasing. Treatment for spinal schwannomas remains surgical, including both complete resection and debulking, and should be reserved for patients with severe and/or progressive symptoms as significant neurologic impairment may result from surgery itself.

PERIPHERAL SCHWANNOMAS

Schwannomas may arise on any nerve distal to the spinal cord. Tumors arising on major deep nerves of the extremities are most likely to become symptomatic, causing pain or progressive weakness (Fig. 14-7). Mononeuritis multiplex causing weakness and atrophy of a single limb may mimic peripheral nerve tumor, but remains a diagnosis of exclusion after appropriate radiographic evaluation.

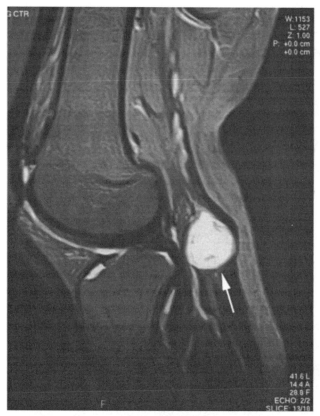

Figure 14-7. Schwannoma of the tibial nerve arising in the popliteal fossa (arrow). In addition to bilateral vestibular tumors, this patient had multiple nodular tumors of the arms, some of which caused intense pain on minimal trauma. (Contrast-enhanced, T_1-weighted image.)

Hard, nodular, subcutaneous tumors, primarily of the limbs or trunk, that may be painful with minor trauma develop in about half of patients (Mautner et al. 1997). Surgical resection of peripheral schwannoma may often be accomplished without significant nerve damage as they arise eccentric to the nerve with a distinct capsule.

Cutaneous schwannomas are seen in up to half of all patients with NF2 (Evans et al. 1992; Mautner et al. 1996; Parry et al. 1994). Unlike the numerous cutaneous neurofibromas seen in a typical patient with NF1, cutaneous tumors associated with NF2 may be quite subtle and are often appreciated only after a detailed inspection of the skin (Fig. 14-8). Typical NF2-associated cutaneous tumors are well circumscribed and only slightly raised from the surrounding skin. Often the affected skin surface is roughened and the hair arising from the area is darker, thicker, and coarser than in adjacent areas. Cutaneous tumors in patients

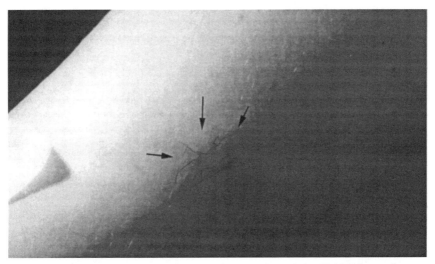

Figure 14-8. Cutaneous schwannoma on the forearm of a patient with NF2 (arrows). *Source:* Photograph courtesy of Dr. Victor Mautner, Department of Neurology, Klinikum North.

with NF2 are usually present in young children and do not become significantly larger or more numerous with age. Because skin tumors appear at a young age, they are a valuable diagnostic marker in a child at risk. In children with no family history, cutaneous tumors may cause diagnostic confusion with NF1, and biopsy may be necessary to clarify the underlying process.

NEUROFIBROMAS

Although neurofibroma was one of the original NIH diagnostic criteria for NF2 (Mulvihill et al. 1990), subsequent revisions (Gutmann et al. 1997) have omitted it because of the recognition that most nerve sheath tumors associated with NF2 have the pathology of a schwannoma and not of a neurofibroma (Halliday et al. 1991; Mautner et al. 1997). Some reports of NF2-related pathology describe tumors as "neurofibromas" because of features such as embedded nerve fibers (Smith et al. 1993), however, entrapment of nerve fibers can be seen in schwannomas from patients with NF2 and should not alone prompt a diagnosis of neurofibroma (Table 14-2). In addition, cutaneous schwannomas with a plexiform pathology may resemble plexiform neurofibromas, especially at low magnification (Fig. 14-9). Further work is needed to determine if neurofibromas do occur with any significant frequency in NF2, but the finding of a pathologically verified neurofibroma should raise some suspicion regarding the diagnosis, especially in an atypical patient.

Table 14.2. Comparison of schwannoma and neurofibroma

Characteristic	Schwannoma	Neurofibroma
Relationship to nerve	Eccentric and well demarcated from axons	Intrinsic with entrapment of axons
Encapsulation	Yes	No
Composition	Homogeneous (Schwann cells)	Heterogeneous (Schwann cells, fibroblasts, perineurial cells, mast cells, axons, mucinous matrix)
Cell density	Biphasic with hypercellular (Antoni A) and hypocellular (Antoni B) areas	Low to moderate without abrupt changes in cellularity
Association with NF	NF2 and schwannomatosis	NF1
Malignant transformation	No	Occasional with plexiform tumors

MENINGIOMAS

Meningioma develops in approximately half of individuals with NF2 (Evans et al. 1992; Parry et al. 1994). Unlike schwannoma, there is no overwhelming site of predilection of intracranial meningioma, although as noted above, meningioma intermingled or adjacent to vestibular schwannoma is nearly pathognomonic for NF2 or mosaic NF2 (see Fig. 14-4). Meningioma of the orbit deserves special vigilance, since these tumors may compress the optic nerve and cause visual loss (Fig. 14-10). Orbital meningioma presenting in childhood may be confused with optic nerve gliomas, but the latter occur only in patients with NF1. Meningioma at the skull base causing brainstem compression is an important late cause of mortality in patients with NF2. Meningioma may also affect the spine (Fig. 14-11) and may rarely arise in distal sites such as the lung and skin (Argenyi et al. 1994). A subset of patients with NF2 appear to be especially predisposed to development of intracranial tumors, with plaquelike involvement of nearly every meningeal surface late in the disease. Few tumors develop in other kindreds (Gardner and Frazier 1929).

Diagnosis of meningioma in patients with NF2 is usually straightforward, since the radiographic appearance of most tumors is quite distinct. Confusion may arise when meningioma occurs in the CPA. Vestibular schwannomas almost always have a prominent intercanalicular component, while CPA meningiomas may indent the internal auditory meatus, but do not usually progress down into the internal auditory canal. Cavernous sinus involvement by meningioma may be difficult to differentiate from fifth cranial nerve schwannoma. In general, cavernous sinus meningiomas encase the carotid and nervous elements of the sinus, making their surgical removal much more complex than that of schwannomas, which tend to displace these structures. Pathologically, meningiomas from patients with NF2 have been reported to be predominantly fibroblastic, although one report revealed equal numbers of fibroblastic and meningothelial tumors (Louis et al. 1995).

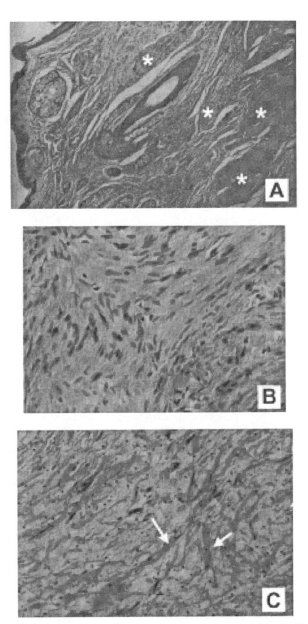

Figure 14-9. Cutaneous plexiform schwannomas may easily be confused with plexiform neurofibromas, especially at low magnification. (A) Low magnification of a skin tumor from a patient with NF2, showing plexiform schwannoma seen as multiple nodules in small nerve twigs (*). (Original magnification, ×48.) (B) Higher magnification of the tumor seen in panel A reveals that the tumor nodules are composed of homogeneous aggregates of Schwann cells. (Original magnification, ×320.) (C) In contrast, a plexiform neurofibroma (not from a patient with NF2) shows a heterogeneous mixture of proliferating cells in a myxoid matrix with numerous splayed nerve fibers (arrows). (Original magnification, ×48.)

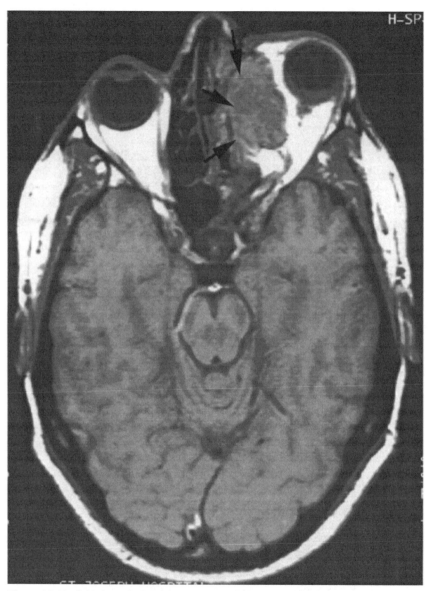

Figure 14-10. Orbital meningioma (arrows) in a patient with NF2 first noted to cause proptosis at age 10. Despite considerable lateral and downward displacement of the globe, this 31-year-old man had binocular vision with 20/20 acuity in the affected eye.

The course of meningioma in NF2 is often very indolent with tumors being present for years to decades before symptoms appear. Aggressive presymptomatic treatment is probably not warranted. Indications for consideration of surgical treatment include worsening neurologic symptoms, rapid growth rate of tumors, especially at the skull base, and development of edema surrounding a

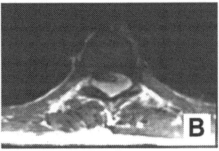
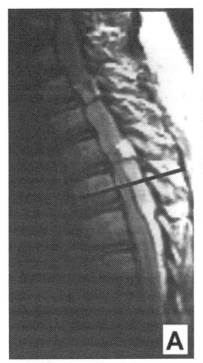

Figure 14-11. Spinal-cord meningioma in a 14-year-old with NF2 who presented with an acute sensory level at T4. (T_1-weighted, contrast-enhanced images.) (A) Sagittal view shows enhancing lesion extending over several spinal segments. (B) Axial view of the level of the line in A shows tumor surrounding but not invading the spinal cord.

tumor (Fig. 14-12). Radiation may be considered in meningiomas that are not surgically accessible, especially those of the cavernous sinus and skull base. Medical therapy of meningioma may be a possibility in the near future (Matsuda et al. 1994; Schrell et al. 1997; Yazaki et al. 1995) and will be an important adjuvant for patients with NF2 in whom large tumor burdens develop late in the course of their disease.

EPENDYMOMAS AND ASTROCYTOMAS

Estimates of the percentage of patients with NF2 who have glial-cell tumors vary widely, from 6% (Evans et al. 1992; Parry et al. 1994) to 33% (Mautner et al. 1995). The latter probably represents a better estimate of the true incidence in a population that has undergone comprehensive radiographic evaluation, while the former represents an upper estimate of the incidence of patients with symptoms. Ependymomas in NF2 patients are especially likely to occur in the cervical cord and cervical medullary junction but rarely grow to a size that causes symptoms (Fig. 14-13; Jones and MacCollin 1997). Biopsy to confirm diagnosis is not war-

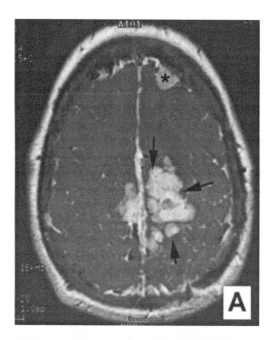

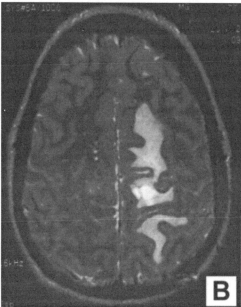

Figure 14-12. (A) Contrast-enhanced, T_1-weighted image, showing multiple dural-based tumors consistent with meningiomas in a patient with NF2, including a small frontal mass (*) and a larger multilobulated mass posteriorly (arrows). (B) T_2-weighted images of the same region, showing considerable edema around the posterior mass, but not the frontal tumor. The patient presented with a worsening of right focal motor seizures, which resolved after resection of the posterior tumors.

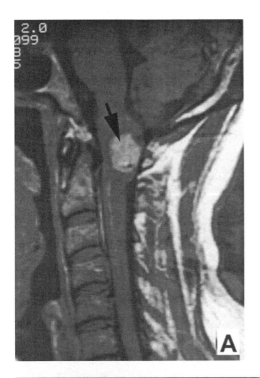

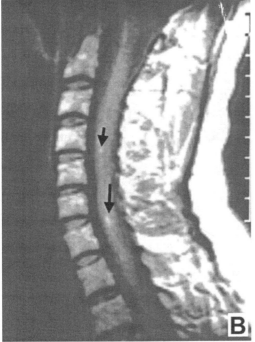

Figure 14-13. Ependymoma in patients with NF2. (T_1-weighted, contrast-enhanced images.) (A) Large cystic mass enlarging the cervical medullary junction (arrow) and causing progressive spasticity. (B) More-typical appearance of small dots of enhancement (arrows), which are consistent with either ependymoma or astrocytoma and are asymptomatic.

ranted in a patient with NF2, unless very rapid unexplained growth occurs. Pathologically, no distinctions are known between NF2-associated glial tumors and sporadically occurring ones (Fig. 14-14); however, this area has not been studied in detail. Treatment of sporadic ependymomas is aggressive, with attempted total resection and adjunctive radiation and/or chemotherapy for residual disease (McCormick et al. 1990). In light of the relatively indolent course of NF2-associated tumors and the additional tumor burden, it is unlikely that such aggressive treatment is warranted, even in a patient with symptoms.

MALFORMATIVE AND HAMARTOMATOUS LESIONS

In addition to the tumors described above, there are a variety of malformative lesions frequently encountered in patients with NF2. These lesions arise from Schwann cells (schwannosis, Schwann cell tumorlets), meningeal cells (meningioangiomatosis), and glial cells (glial microhamartomas) and may reflect the susceptibility of these cells to abnormal proliferation (Louis et al. 1995). While meningioangiomatosis and schwannosis may be encountered in patients who do not have NF2, microhamartomas have been described only in patients with NF2. The relationship between these malformative lesions and the frank neoplastic lesions seen in NF2 is unclear.

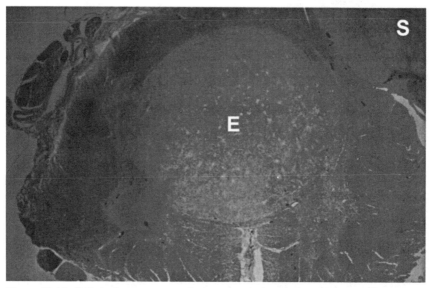

Figure 14-14. Pathologic appearance of a large cervical ependymoma (E), which has nearly replaced the spinal-cord substance. A schwannoma originating from the dorsal root at the same level can also be seen (S). (Original magnification, ×48.) *Source:* Photomicrograph courtesy of Dr. David Louis, Neuropathology Department, Massachusetts General Hospital.

MENINGIOANGIOMATOSIS

Meningioangiomatosis was first described in 1915 by Bassoe and Nuzum and named by Worster-Drought et al. in 1937. It appears as a nodular intracortical mass that may extend to overlying leptomeninges with the formation of a gritty meningeal plaquelike lesion (Fig. 14-15). Histologically, meningioangiomatosis

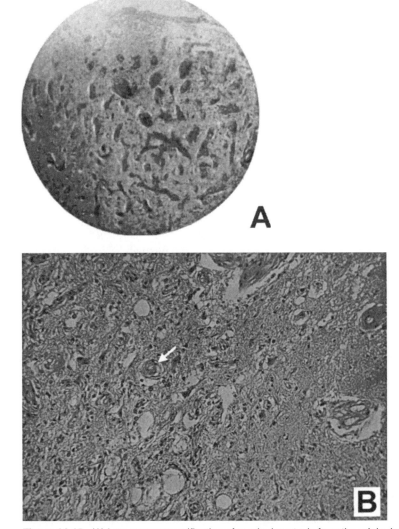

Figure 14-15. (A) Low-power magnification of meningiomatosis from the original autopsy report of Bassoe and Nuzum (1915) (original magnification not given). (*Source:* Bassoe and Nuzum 1915. Reprinted with permission.) (B) High-power magnification of meningioangiomatosis, showing proliferating small vessels (arrow) surrounded by spindled cells. (Original magnification, ×80.)

is characterized by proliferating small vessels and perivascular aggregates of spindle cells, thought to be of meningothelial lineage. The degree of spindle-cell proliferation is variable; some lesions are very cellular, and the spindle cells predominate, while in other lesions the vessels are more prominent, with few perivascular cells. Associated histologic features that may be encountered are degenerative changes of the vascular component, such as hyalinization of vessel walls, calcification, and bone formation.

Meningioangiomatosis also occurs in patients who do not have NF2 (sporadic meningioangiomatosis). In these cases it is often a single lesion in children or young adults with seizures. On the other hand, in patients with NF2 the lesions are often multiple and asymptomatic, detected only at autopsy (Bassoe and Nuzum 1915; Halper et al. 1986; Rubinstein 1986; Worster-Drought et al. 1937). Although meningioangiomatosis may rarely be associated with a frank meningioma, it has very low proliferative activity (Prayson 1995; Stemmer-Rachamimov et al. 1997), supporting the clinical impression of a static or very slowly growing lesion.

GLIAL MICROHAMARTOMAS

Glial microhamartomas are a frequent and typical lesion of NF2; autopsy estimates of their prevalence in patients with NF2 vary from 100% (Wiestler et al. 1989) to 45% (Rubinstein 1986). These glial nodules are small clusters of polymorphic cells with atypical nuclei and eosinophilic cytoplasm (Fig. 14-16). A detailed microscopic examination of the brain showed distribution in the cerebral cortex, thalamus, and basal ganglia (Wiestler et al. 1989), but other studies have found them more widespread, including in the cerebellum and spinal cord (Louis et al. 1995). The hamartomas stain for S100 protein but not for neuronal pro-

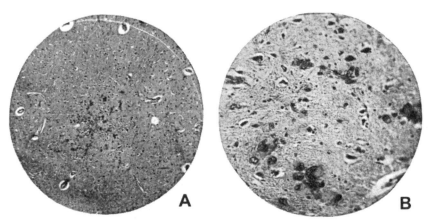

Figure 14-16. Microglial hamartomas, known as "heaps" in the original autopsy report of Bassoe and Nuzum (1915). (A) Low-power magnification, showing a cortical nodule in the center of the field. (B) Higher-power magnification, showing a classic small aggregate of dysplastic glial cells. (Original magnifications not given.) (*Source*: Bassoe and Nuzem 1915. Reprinted with permission.)

teins, and are therefore thought to be of astrocytic lineage. The glial hamartomas of NF2 are not associated clinically with mental retardation or epilepsy. It is unlikely that they provide a substrate for neoplastic transformation because their distribution is different from that of gliomas and they lack proliferative activity (Wiestler et al. 1989).

SCHWANNOSIS AND TUMORLETS

Schwannosis and tumorlets are small nodular proliferations of Schwann cells. Two forms of schwannosis have been defined: intramedullary schwannosis, at the junction of the dorsal nerve root with the dorsal gray horn, and perivascular schwannosis, in the perivascular spaces of the central spinal cord (Rubenstein 1986). Schwannosis is not specific for NF2 and is often encountered in association with chronic lesions of the spinal cord such as compression or following trauma. It is therefore thought to represent a reactive process. In patients with NF2, however, these lesions are more exuberant and numerous.

In addition to the development of frank schwannomas, the peripheral nerves, especially the cauda equina of patients with NF2, may be riddled with numerous small Schwann cell nodules that histologically have the appearance of schwannomas. Molecular study of these "tumorlets" in a single autopsy case showed loss of NF2 protein expression, consistent with early tumorigenesis (Stemmer-Rachamimov et al. 1998).

MALIGNANCY IN NF2

Unlike NF1, NF2 confers a minimal increased risk of malignancy over that of the general population. Increased risk of de novo malignancy (such as pheochromocytoma or leukemia in patients with NF1) probably does not occur. Rarely, aggressive tumors of meningeal or Schwann cell origin occur (Higami et al. 1998), and in several cases this has followed treatment with therapeutic radiation (Baser et al. 1996). The exact risks for malignancy in NF2 and the additional risk conferred by radiation therapy are areas for future study.

REFERENCES

Abaza MM, Makariou E, Armstrong M, and Lalwani AK. 1996. Growth rate characteristics of acoustic neuromas associated with neurofibromatosis type 2. *Laryngoscope* 106:694–9.

Argenyi Z, Thieberg M, Hayes C, and Whitaker D. 1994. Primary cutaneous meningioma associated with von Recklinghausen's disease. *J Cut Pathol* 21:549–56.

Aslan A, De Donato G, Balyan FR, Falcioni M, Russo A, Taibah A, and Sanna M. 1997. Clinical observations on coexistence of sudden hearing loss and vestibular schwannoma. *Otolaryngol Head Neck Surg* 117:580–2.

Baser M, MacCollin M, Sujansky E, Evans DGR, and Rubenstein A. 1996. Malignant nervous system tumors in patients with neurofibromatosis 2. Paper presented at FASEB summer research conference on neurofibromatosis, Snowmass, Colorado, June 30, 1996.

Bassoe P and Nuzum F. 1915. Report of a case of central and peripheral neurofibromatosis. *J Nerv Ment Dis* 42:785–96.

Charabi S, Thomsen J, Mantoni M, Charabi B, Jorgensen B, Borgesen SE, Gyldensted C, and Tos M. 1995. Acoustic neuroma (vestibular schwannoma): growth and surgical and nonsurgical consequences of the wait-and-see policy. *Otolaryngol Head Neck Surg* 113:5–14.

Eldridge R and Parry D. 1992. Vestibular schwannoma (acoustic neuroma). Consensus development conference. *Neurosurgery* 30:962–4.

Evans DGR, Huson SM, Donnai D, Neary W, Blair V, Newton V, and Harris R. 1992. A clinical study of type 2 neurofibromatosis. *Q J Med* 84:603–18.

Gardner W and Frazier C. 1929. Bilateral acoustic neurofibromas. *Arch Neurol Psychiatry* 23:266–302.

Gardner WJ and Turner O. 1940. Bilateral acoustic neurofibromas: further clinical and pathologic data on hereditary deafness and Recklinghausen's disease. *Arch Neurol Psychiatry* 44:76–99.

Gutmann D, Aylsworth A, Carey J, Korf B, Marks J, Pyeritz R, Rubenstein A, and Viskochil D. 1997. The diagnostic evaluation and multidisciplinary management of neurofibromatosis 1 and neurofibromatosis 2. *JAMA* 278:51–7.

Halliday AL, Sobel RA, and Martuza RL. 1991. Benign spinal nerve sheath tumors: their occurrence sporadically and in neurofibromatosis types 1 and 2. *J Neurosurg* 74:248–53.

Halper J, Scheithauer B, Okazaki H, and Laws ERJ. 1986. Meningio-angiomatosis: a report of six cases with special reference to the occurrence of neurofibrillary tangles. *J Neuropath Exp Neurol* 45:426–46.

Hamada Y, Iwaki T, Fukui M, and Tateishi J. 1997. A comparative study of embedded nerve tissue in six NF2-associated schwannomas and 17 nonassociated NF2 schwannomas. *Surg Neurol* 48:395–400.

Hecht CS, Honrubia VF, Wiet RJ, and Sims HS. 1997. Hearing preservation after acoustic neuroma resection with tumor size used as a clinical prognosticator. *Laryngoscope* 107:1122–6.

Higami Y, Shimokawa I, Kishikawa M, Okimoto T, Ohtani H, Tomita M, Tsujino A, and Ikeda T. 1998. Malignant peripheral nerve sheath tumors developing multifocally in the central nervous system in a patient with neurofibromatosis type 2. *Clin Neuropatho* 17:115–20.

Ito K, Durita H, Sugasawa K, Mizuno M, and Sasaki T. 1997. Analyses of neuro-otological complications after radiosurgery for acoustic neurinomas. *Int J Radiat Oncol Biol Phys* 39:983–8.

Jaaskelainen J, Paetau A, Pyykko I, Blomstedt G, Palva T, and Troupp H. 1994. Interface between the facial nerve and large acoustic neurinomas. Immunohistochemical study of the cleavage plane in NF2 and non-NF2 cases. *J Neurosurg* 80:541–7.

Jones R and MacCollin M. 1997. The natural history of ependymoma in patients with neurofibromatosis 2. *Neurology* 48:A35.

Kondziolka D, Lunsford LD, McLaughlin MR, and Flickinger JC. 1998. Long-term outcomes after radiosurgery for acoustic neuromas. *New Engl J Med* 339:1426–33.

Levo H, Pyykko I, and Blomstedt G. 1997. Non-surgical treatment of vestibular schwannoma patients. *Acta Otolaryngol Suppl (Stockh)* 529:56–8.

Linskey ME, Lunsford LD, and Flickinger JC. 1992. Tumor control after sterotactic radiosurgery in neurofibromatosis pateints with bilateral acoustic tumors. *Neurosurgery* 31:829–38.

Linthicum FH. 1972. Unusual audiometric and histologic findings in bilateral acoustic neurinomas. *Ann Oto Rhinol Laryngol* 81:433–7.

Louis DN, Ramesh V, and Gusella J. 1995. Neuropathology and molecular genetics of neurofibromatosis 2 and related tumors. *Brain Pathol* 5:163–72.

McCormick P, Torres R, Post K, and Stein B. 1990. Intramedulallary ependymoma of the spinal cord. *J Neurosurg* 72:523–32.

McKenna M, Halpin C, Ojemann R, Nadol J, Montgomery W, Levine R, Carlisle E, and Martuza R. 1992. Long-term hearing results in patients after surgical removal of acoustic tumors with hearing preservation. *Am J Otolaryngol* 13:134–6.

Martuza RL and Eldridge R. 1988. Neurofibromatosis 2 (bilateral acoustic neurofibromatosis). *N Engl J Med* 318:684–8.

Matsuda Y, Kawamoto K, Kiya K, Kurisu K, Sugiyama K, and Uozumi T. 1994. Antitumor effects of antiprogesterones on human meningiomas cells in vitro and in vivo. *J Neurosurg* 80:527–34.

Mautner VF, Lindenau M, Baser M, Hazim W, Tatagiba M, Haase W, Samii M, Wais R, and Pulst SM. 1996. The neuroimaging and clinical spectrum of neurofibromatosis 2. *Neurosurgery* 38:880–6.

Mautner VF, Lindenau M, Baser M, Kluwe L, and Gottschalk J. 1997. Skin abnormalities in neurofibromatosis 2. *Arch Dermatol* 133:1539–43.

Mautner VF, Tatagiba M, Lindenau M, Funsterer C, Pulst SM, Kluwe L, and Zanella F. 1995. Spinal tumors in patients with neurofibromatosis type 2: MR imaging study of frequency, multiplicity, and variety. *AJR Am J Roentgenol* 165:951–5.

Mulvihill JJ, Parry DM, Sherman J, Pikus A, Kaiser-Kupfer M, and Eldridge R. 1990. NIH conference: neurofibromatosis 1 (Recklinghausen disease) and neurofibromatosis 2 (bilateral acoustic neurofibromatosis): an update. *Ann Intern Med* 113:39–52.

Nadol JB, Chiong CM, Ojemann RG, McKenna M, Martuza R, Montgomery W, Levine R, Ronner S, and Glynn R. 1992. Preservation of hearing and facial nerve function in resection of acoustic neuroma. *Laryngoscope* 102:1153–8.

Nedzelski J, Schessel D, Pfleiderer A, Kassel E, and Rowed D. 1992. Conservative management of acoustic neuromas. *Otolaryngol Clin North Am* 25:691–705.

Parry DM, Eldridge R, Kaiser-Kupfer M, Bouzas E, Pikus A, and Patronas N. 1994. Neurofibromatosis 2 (NF2): clinical characteristics of 63 affected individuals and clinical evidence for heterogeneity. *Am J Med Genet* 52:450–61.

Prayson R. 1995. Meningioangiomatosis: a clinicopathologic study including MIB1 immunoreactivity. *Arch Pathol Lab Med* 119:1061–4.

Rogers N and Brand C. 1997. Acoustic neuroma and the eye. *Br J Neurosurg* 11:292–7.

Rubinstein L. 1986. The malformative central nervous system lesions in the central and peripheral forms of neurofibromatosis: a neuropathological study of 22 cases. *Ann NY Acad Sci* 486:14–29.

Samii M, Matthies C, and Tatagiba M. 1997. Management of vestibular schwannomas (acoustic neuromas): auditory and facial nerve function after resection of 120 vestibular schwannomas in patients with neurofibromatosis 2. *Neurosurgery* 40:696–706.

Schrell U, Rittig M, Anders M, Koch U, Marschalek R, Kiewewetter F, and Fahlbusch R. 1997. Hydroxyurea for treatment of unresectable and recurrent meningiomas. II. Decrease in the size of meningiomas in patients treated with hydroxyurea. *J Neurosurg* 86:840–4.

Selesnick SH and Jackler RK. 1993. Atypical hearing loss in acoustic neuroma patients. *Laryngoscope* 103 (4 Pt 1):437–41.

Slattery W and Brackmann D. 1995. Results of surgery following sterotactic irradiation for acoustic neuromas. *Am J Otolaryngol* 16:315–9.

Slattery W, Brackmann D, and Hitselberger W. 1998. Hearing preservation in neurofibromatosis type 2. *Am J Otolaryngol* 19:638–43.

Smith P, Bigelow D, Kletzker G, Leoneti J, Pugh B, and Mishler E. 1993. Hearing preservation following a transtemporal resection of an acoustic schwannoma: a case report. *Am J Otolaryngol* 14:434–6.

Sobel RA. 1993. Vestibular (acoustic) schwannomas: Histologic features in neurofibromatosis 2 and in unilateral cases. *J Neuropathol Exp Neurol* 52:106–13.

Stemmer-Rachamimov A, Horgan M, Taratuto A, Munoz D, Smith T, Frosch M, and Louis D. 1997. Meningioangiomatosis is associated with neurofibromatosis 2 but not with somatic alterations of the NF2 gene. *J Neuropathol Exp Neurol* 56:485–9.

Stemmer-Rachamimov A, Yasushi I, Lim ZY, Jacoby LB, MacCollin M, Gusella J, Ramesh V, and Louis D. 1998. Loss of the NF2 gene and merlin occur by the tumorlet stage of schwannoma development in neurofibromatosis 2. *J Neuropathol Exp Neurol* 57:1164–7.

Strasnick B, Glasscock M, Haynes D, McMenomey S, and Minor L. 1994. The natural history of untreated acoustic neuromas. *Laryngoscope* 104:1115–9.

Wiestler OD, von Siebenthal K, Schmitt HP, Feiden W, and Kleihues P. 1989. Distribution and immunoreactivity of cerebral micro-hamartomas in bilateral acoustic neurofibromatosis (neurofibromatosis 2). *Acta Neuropathol (Berl)* 79:137–43.

Wiet R, Zappia J, Hecht C, and O'Connor C. 1995. Conservative management of patients with small acoustic tumors. *Laryngoscope* 105 (8 Pt 1):795–800.

Wilson DF, Talbot JM, and Mills L. 1997. A critical appraisal of the role of auditory brain stem response and magnetic resonance imaging in acoustic neuroma diagnosis. *Am J Otolaryngol* 18:673–81.

Worster-Drought C, Dickson WE, and McMenemey WH. 1937. Multiple meningeal and perineural tumours with analogous changes in the glia and ependyma (neurofibroblastosis). *Brain* 60:85–117.

Yazaki T, Takamiya Y, Costello PC, Mineta T, Menon AG, Rabkin SD, and Martuza RL. 1995. Inhibition of angiogenesis and growth of human non malignant and malignant meningiomas by TNP-470. *J Neurooncol* 23:23–9.

Zappia J, O'Connor C, Wiet R, and Dinces E. 1997. Rethinking the use of auditory brainstem response in acoustic neuroma screening. *Laryngoscope* 107:1388–92.

15

Molecular Biology

Mia MacCollin, M.D., and James F. Gusella, Ph.D.

CLONING OF THE *NF2* GENE

Initial work in the localization of the *NF2* gene used linkage analysis in a small number of families affected with NF2 (Rouleau et al. 1987) and loss-of-heterozygosity studies in NF2-related tumors (Seizinger et al. 1987). Both approaches converged on the long arm of human chromosome 22. In 1993, an affected patient and her daughter were found to have an aberration consistent with a deletion in this region on Southern blot analysis (Trofatter et al. 1993). Using the method of exon trapping, expressed sequences within this region were isolated and a message with alterations in two other NF2-related tumors was identified (Trofatter et al. 1993). The putative protein product was named "merlin" (moesin, ezrin, radizin like protein) for its unexpected relationship with several cytoskeletal elements. At the same time, a second group isolated this transcript and named the protein product "schwannomin" in recognition of its role in preventing the formation of schwannomas (Rouleau et al. 1993).

The *NF2* gene spans 110 kb and comprises 16 constitutive exons and one alternatively spliced exon. Despite its relatively restricted phenotype, *NF2* is widely expressed. On Northern blot, *NF2* messenger RNA can be detected in three different size ranges (7, 4.4, and 2.6 kb) most likely due to variable length of 3′ untranslated material. Because exon 16 is both alternatively spliced and contains an in-frame stop codon, two different isoforms of the NF2 protein can be made. Isoform 1 is a protein of 595 amino acids produced from exons 1 through 15 and exon 17, and is the dominant form in most tissues. Presence of the alternatively spliced exon 16 substantially changes the C terminus of the protein, replacing 16 amino acids with 11 novel residues in isoform 2.

The *NF2* gene is remarkably conserved through evolution. The mouse isoform, isolated by two groups shortly after cloning of the human gene (Haase et al. 1994; Hara et al. 1994), maps to mouse chromosome 11 in a region of synteny with human 22q. It is similarly alternatively spliced in the 3′ end and is 98% identical to human NF2 at the amino acid level. Interestingly, however, mice heterozygous for an *NF2* mutation develop a phenotype of malignant tumors quite distinct from that of human NF2 (McClatchey et al. 1998).

EXPRESSION AND FUNCTION OF NF2

The NF2 protein can be detected as a 65- to 69-kD protein in many different cell types (den Bakker et al. 1995; Gonzalez-Agosti et al. 1996; Scherer and Gutmann 1996). Endogenous NF2 is localized to the plasma membrane of Schwann and other cell types and to motile regions in human fibroblast and meningioma cells. In the normal central nervous system, NF2 is widely expressed in coarse cytoplasmic granules in both glia and neurons, with less exuberant expression in other cells (Stemmer-Rachamimmov et al. 1997b). NF2 protein cannot be detected, even in a truncated form, in most NF2-related tumors (Gutmann et al. 1997; Stemmer-Rachamimmov et al. 1997a).

On the basis of sequence similarity, the NF2 protein was determined to be a member of the protein 4.1 family of cytoskeleton-associated proteins (Tsukita et al. 1997; Table 15-1). This was an unexpected finding, since no other family members are associated with tumor formation and only one, protein 4.1 itself, is associated with human genetic disease (hereditary elliptocytosis). The ERM proteins (ezrin, moesin, radixin), to which the NF2 protein is most closely related, share 70 to 75% amino acid identity and a common structure (Fig. 15-1). These proteins localize to motile regions of the cell, including microvilli, cellular protrusions, and leading and ruffling edges. ERM proteins interact with the Rho family of GTPases in a signaling cascade, which controls the organization of the spectrin–actin cytoskeleton and cell adhesion. Although less is currently known about NF2 protein physiology and function than about other ERM family members, similar interactions with the cytoskeleton are beginning to be identified (Deguen et al. 1998; Pelton et al. 1998; Xu and Gutmann 1998).

MUTATIONS IN PATIENTS WITH NF2

The mutational analysis of patients with NF2 has proceeded at a much more rapid pace than that of patients with NF1 because of the much smaller size of the gene and transcript. In at least two studies, exon scanning methods have detected germline mutations in two thirds of all individuals studied with typical bilateral

Table 15-1. Other band 4.1 family members

	Function
Protein 4.1	Maintains membrane stability and cell shape by connecting membrane proteins with the cytoskeleton
Talin	Found at focal adhesions at cell–cell or cell–substrate contacts
Moesin	Found at or near membrane in filopodia or other cell-surface protrusions
Exrin	Co-localized with actin in cell-surface structures
Radixin	Found in adherens junction, where it is proposed to cap actin filaments

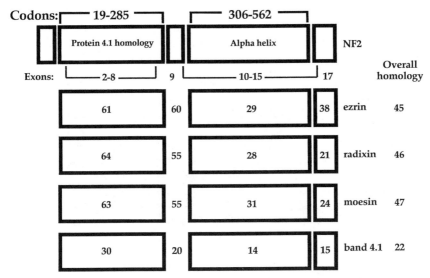

Figure 15-1. The NF2 protein is a member of the band 4.1 family of cytoskeleton-associated proteins. This schematic diagram depicts the domains of the NF2 protein, which include a region of homology in the amino terminal half that defines membership in the protein 4.1 family, an α-helical domain and a terminus affected by alternative splicing. The percentage amino acid identity with the three most closely related family members ezrin, radixin, and moesin and with band 4.1 itself is shown within each region. The C terminus of the ERM proteins contains an actin-binding region not found in the NF2 protein.

vestibular schwannoma (MacCollin et al. 1994; Parry et al. 1996). A wide variety of mutations have been identified in all *NF2* exons, except for exons 16 and 17 (Fig. 15-2). The vast majority of the alterations are predicted to truncate the protein product, due to introduction of a stop codon, a frameshift with premature termination or a splicing alteration, supporting the view that loss of the protein's normal function is crucial to the development of tumors. C to T transitions in CGA codons causing nonsense mutation are an especially frequent occurrence. Less than 10% of detected germline mutations involve in-frame deletions and missense mutations, although the identification of these events is crucial in determining the essential tumor-suppressor regions of this protein. Small numbers of patients have been reported to have gene deletions detected by Southern blot or flanking microsatellite analysis (Evans et al. 1998; Trofatter et al. 1993; Watson et al. 1993). No frequent polymorphisms, even in codon wobble positions, have been reported in the *NF2* gene.

SOMATIC MUTATIONS

The finding of acquired, somatic mutations or "second hits" in *NF2*-related tumor material is crucial to the confirmation of its role as a tumor-suppressor gene. Study of sporadic and *NF2*-derived schwannomas has shown grossly trun-

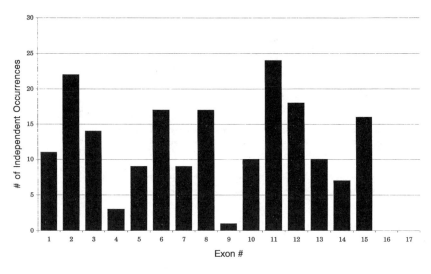

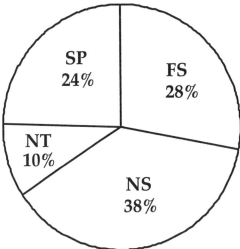

Figure 15-2. A wide variety of mutations have been identified throughout the *NF2* gene. (A) The number of independent occurrences of germline mutation in 189 unrelated patients with NF2. Relatively low rates of change are seen in exon 9, no causative mutations have yet been identified in the alternative spliced exons 16 and 17, and "warm spots" of mutation in exons 2, 6, 8, and 11 all correspond to CpG islands. (B) Sequence analysis in these studies demonstrates that germline *NF2* mutations are overwhelmingly truncating in nature. SP = splice-site mutations; FS = frameshifting insertions, deletions, and complex rearrangements; NS = nonsense mutations; NT = nontruncating insertions and deletions and missense mutations. *Source:* Data from Bourn et al. 1994, 1995; Evans et al. 1998; Kluwe et al. 1996, 1998; MacCollin et al. 1994, 1996; Merel et al. 1995; Parry et al. 1996; Rouleau et al. 1993; Ruttledge et al. 1996; Sainz et al. 1995; Scoles et al. 1996; Trofatter et al. 1993.

cating mutation in the vast majority, with out-of-frame deletion an especially common mechanism of mutation (e.g., Jacoby et al. 1996; Lekanne-Deprez et al. 1994; Welling et al. 1996). As has been seen with germline changes, there is no "hotspot" of mutation and all exons are relatively equally affected, with the exception of exons 16 and 17. Many schwannomas also show loss of polymorphic markers on chromosome 22, indicating large deletions or loss of the entire homologous chromosome. As would be expected, when the tumor is derived from an individual with NF2, the markers lost are always those on the chromosome carrying the normal copy of the gene. No differences have been reported between mutations detected in vestibular versus nonvestibular tumors nor between tumors derived from patients with NF2 versus patients with sporadic tumors, although this is an area that deserves further study.

Analysis of meningiomas, the second most common tumor type in NF2, has revealed slightly different results. For example, in a comprehensive analysis of 70 sporadic meningiomas, 43 mutations were detected in 41 tumors (Wellenreuther et al. 1995). Similar to the results in schwannoma, only 1 of the 43 involved a nontruncating event. Mutational events were much more frequent in tumors that had lost heterozygosity for chromosome 22 markers, supporting the hypothesis that *NF2* is the meningioma suppressor locus on chromosome 22. These authors found that *NF2* mutations occurred much more frequently in fibroblastic and transitional meningiomas (Stangl et al. 1997; Wellenreuther et al. 1995); however, pathologic study shows that meningiomas from patients with NF2 may be heterogeneous (Louis et al. 1995). These and other studies (e.g., Lekanne-Deprez et al. 1994; Ruttledge et al. 1994) suggest that *NF2* is a tumor suppressor for meningioma but that another gene or genes not on chromosome 22 may also fill this role.

Analysis of sporadic ependymomas has shown conflicting results. Rubio and colleagues (1994) were able to show *NF2* mutation in only one tumor from eight examined. A second study using slightly different methodologies found *NF2* mutation in five of seven spinal cord ependymomas studied (Birch et al. 1996). Since the distribution of *NF2*-associated ependymomas is mostly if not exclusively spinal (see Chapter 14), these differences may lie in the anatomic location of the tumors examined. *NF2* mutations in astrocytomas are notably absent (e.g., Rubio et al. 1994; Watkins et al. 1996), despite the clinically reported association of astrocytoma with NF2 (see Chapter 14). Molecular genetic study of glial tumors resected from patients with NF2 has not been reported.

Loss of heterozygosity has been observed for chromosome 22q markers in many different types of tumors not characteristic of NF2. Screening for mutations that affect the *NF2* gene in such tumors has yielded mixed results. Only a handful of putative mutations of the *NF2* gene have been found in malignant melanoma, breast adenocarcinoma, and colon cancer, and none has been seen in ovarian carcinoma or hepatocellular carcinoma (Arakawa et al. 1994; Bianchi et al. 1994; Englefield et al. 1994; Kanai et al. 1995). Two reports demonstrate a high rate of *NF2* mutation in malignant mesothelioma (Bianchi et al. 1995; Sekido et al. 1995). The significance of these results for patients with NF2 is unclear.

GENOTYPE–PHENOTYPE RELATIONSHIPS IN NF2

A strong effect of the genotype on the resulting phenotype in NF2 is suggested by the clinical observations outlined in Chapter 13 that intrafamilial homogeneity is marked in NF2. This is especially pronounced when NF2 is compared with NF1, which shows striking heterogeneity amongst affected family members. Several studies have supported the hypothesis that the underlying *NF2* gene mutation is predictive of the resulting phenotype when the gross variables of mild versus severe disease are examined (Bourn et al. 1994, 1995; Evans et al. 1998; Kluwe et al. 1996, 1998; MacCollin et al. 1994, 1996; Merel et al. 1995; Parry et al. 1996; Rouleau et al. 1993; Ruttledge et al. 1996; Sainz et al. 1995; Scoles et al. 1996; Trofatter et al. 1993). In these studies, a total of 110 independently occurring nonsense and frameshift mutations have produced severe disease in 95 cases studied (86%), while splice-site mutation has produced severe disease in only 49% of cases and rare nontruncating changes have produced severe disease in only 33% of cases. Despite studies in other tumor-suppressor genes that have linked position within the gene to specific manifestations, no effect of the position of the mutation has been determined in NF2.

Several of these studies have also presented a more detailed analysis of the effects of genotype on phenotype (Evans et al. 1998; Kluwe et al. 1996; Parry et al. 1996; Ruttledge et al. 1996; Table 15-2). Overall, patients with nonsense or frameshift mutations have earlier ages at onset and diagnosis and greater numbers of tumors than any other group of patients. At the other end of the spectrum, families in whom mutations cannot be identified by exon scanning have late ages of onset and diagnosis and a low frequency of nonvestibular tumors (Parry et al. 1996). Such families may have larger deletions or insertions not identified by the methods used in these studies (Watson et al. 1993), mutations in introns and untranslated regulatory elements, or mosaicism not detectable in the tissue analyzed (Bijlsma et al. 1997; MacCollin et al. 1997a). Also of importance to the clinician is that families with splice-site mutation display far more intrafamilial

Table 15-2. Relationship of phenotypic variables to underlying mutation type*

	Total	Nonsense/ Frameshift	Splice-Site	Missense	Unfound
Mean age of hearing loss (years)	26	22	30	36	24
Meningioma (%)	51	74	35	28	24
Spinal tumor (%)	56	76	40	28	46
Skin tumor (%)	65	90	37	20	71
Families (N)	81	51	13	6	11
Individuals (N)	128	62	31	18	17

*Mean ages of onset and diagnosis were defined differently in the two studies, but tended to parallel the ages of hearing loss within each cohort. Similar results were reported by Kluwe et al. (1998) and Ruttledge et al. (1996). Source: Adapted from Parry et al. (1996) and Evans et al. (1998).

variability than other families (Kluwe et al. 1998), so caution should be exercised when giving anticipatory guidance to these families. Further work is needed to define the exact parameters that may reliably be used to predict clinical course using the underlying genotype. These studies also point out an irony in current *NF2* screening protocols, since patients with mild phenotypes may be more likely to seek molecular diagnostic services than those with severe manifestations and are the least likely to have identifiable *NF2* gene changes using current techniques.

MOLECULAR BIOLOGY OF RELATED PHENOTYPES

MOSAIC NF2

As noted in Chapter 13, mosaic inactivation of the *NF2* gene is most likely an underrecognized condition. Molecular confirmation of mosaicism has been reported in patients with typical bilateral vestibular schwannomas (Bourn et al. 1994; Bijlsma et al. 1997; Evans et al. 1998), unilateral vestibular schwannoma with other *NF2*-related tumors (MacCollin et al. 1997a), and schwannomatosis (MacCollin et al. 1997b). As would be expected, when patients with similar mutations are compared, mosaicism has a mitigating effect on the phenotype. The relatively high incidence of mosaicism in a diverse array of phenotypes may make mutational analysis in tumor specimens preferable to that in an unaffected tissue such as lymphocytes. Mosaicism should also be considered whenever applying linkage testing in the offspring of founders (Bijlsma et al. 1997).

MULTIPLE MENINGIOMAS

As noted above, mutational analysis of sporadic meningiomas suggest that *NF2* may act as a tumor suppressor for this tumor type but that other elements may also play such a role. Molecular analysis of patients with multiple meningioma has shown similar heterogeneity. In a study of 12 such patients, 4 had tumors that were molecularly shown to be independently occurring events (Stangl et al. 1997). All 4 were female with only two tumors and fell into the age range in which sporadic meningioma is common. In 6 patients, separate tumors were found to contain identical mutations and loss of heterozygosity of the second allele. Because the mutations could not be detected in paired blood samples from these patients, noncontiguous spread of a single tumor was postulated. It was noted that no pathologic bridges of tumor tissue existed between the tumors, supporting the radiographic and clinical impression that they were indeed separate tumors. More detailed analysis of these patients is needed to ensure that they do not represent mosaicism for the *NF2* gene. Finally, in 2 patients, no mutations could be detected in the *NF2* gene. Although family studies were not presented, it is likely that this third group represents mutation in a second genomic locus, a hypothesis that is also supported by limited linkage data (Pulst et al. 1993).

SCHWANNOMATOSIS

Molecular analysis of patients with schwannomatosis has shown that, like patients with multiple meningioma, the phenotype may result from a variety of genetic mechanisms (Jacoby et al. 1997). Some patients with schwannomatosis are mosaic for *NF2* mutation, and these patients do not necessarily show anatomically limited distribution of their tumors (MacCollin et al. 1997b). A second group appear not to have alteration at the *NF2* locus, although an analysis of large numbers of these patients has not yet been done to confirm that impression. In the final group of patients, which thus far includes all familial cases, there is a remarkable tendency for somatic instability at the *NF2* locus. Like patients with NF2, these patients share a common chromosome 22 allele in familial cases, and tumors from these patients exhibit loss of heterozygosity of the *trans* allele to that shared in the family. Also like patients with NF2, multiple pathologically homogeneous tumors with *NF2* gene mutations develop in these patients. Unlike patients with NF2, however, the mutations in each separate tumor are distinct, in both type and location within the gene. The mechanism for the instability of the *NF2* locus remains unclear at the current time.

USE OF MUTATION ANALYSIS IN CLINICAL CARE

The success of mutational analysis in germline specimens has led to the availability of presymptomatic and prenatal diagnosis for the offspring of a majority of classically affected patients with NF2. Presymptomatic diagnosis may reduce the financial and emotional burdens on these families and assist in the early detection of NF2 in children, but such testing should be done only by persons who are experienced in the provision of genetic services and who are aware of the many ramifications that such testing may have on the patient and his or her family. Proband testing, molecular confirmation of the diagnosis of NF2 in a person known to have bilateral vestibular schwannoma, is currently of no clinical utility, since the diagnosis of NF2 remains a clinical one.

With further understanding of genotype–phenotype relationships, targeted anticipatory guidance may be offered to persons known to be affected with classic NF2, reducing the cost of caring for this population while improving medical and surgical management. Early experimental results suggest that subpopulations of patients at high risk for spinal-cord tumors or ocular manifestations may be identifiable, leading to increased surveillance in persons most at risk and reducing the burden of repeated tests on those at lesser risk. For most patients with related phenotypes and for children with NF2-related single tumors, molecular analysis probably best begins in tumor material. As outlined above, many of these individuals harbor somatically acquired changes that will not be detected in blood specimens. Furthermore, unlike NF2, outlying phenotypes and genetic predisposition to tumor formation can be ruled out in a small number of patients who can be definitely shown to have acquired mutations only. Clearly, further work is needed in this area to define the full utility of molecular testing.

GENE THERAPY

The prospects for gene or protein product replacement to halt or reverse the growth of NF2-related tumors are perhaps slightly better than those for NF1-related tumors, because of the smaller size of the transcript and protein product. Current research focuses on the development of model systems (McClatchey et al. 1998) and effective delivery systems (Ikeda et al. 1999).

REFERENCES

Arakawa H, Hayashi N, Nagase H, Ogawa M, and Nakamura Y. 1994. Alternative splicing of the NF2 gene and its mutation analysis of breast and colorectal cancers. *Hum Mol Genet* 3:565–8.

Bianchi AB, Hara T, Ramesh V, Gao J, Klein-Szanto AJ, Morin F, Menon AG, Trofatter JA, Gusella JF, Seizinger BR, et al. 1994. Mutations in transcript isoforms of the neurofibromatosis 2 gene in multiple human tumour types. *Nat Genet* 6:185–92.

Bianchi AB, Mitsunaga SI, Cheng JQ, Klein WM, Jhanwar SC, Seizinger B, Kley N, Klein-Szanto AJ, and Testa JR. 1995. High frequency of inactivating mutations in the neurofibromatosis type 2 gene (NF2) in primary malignant mesotheliomas [see comments]. *Proc Natl Acad Sci USA* 92:10854–8.

Bijlsma EK, Wallace AJ, and Evans DG. 1997. Misleading linkage results in an NF2 presymptomatic test owing to mosaicism. *J Med Genet* 34:934–6.

Birch B, Johnson F, Parsa A, Desai R, Yoon J, Lycette C, Li YM, and Bruce J. 1996. Frequent type 2 neurofibromatosis gene transcript mutations in sporadic intramedullary spinal cord ependymomas. *Neurosurgery* 39:135–40.

Bourn D, Carter SA, Evans DG, Goodship J, Coakham H, and Strachan T. 1994. A mutation in the neurofibromatosis type 2 tumor-suppressor gene, giving rise to widely different clinical phenotypes in two unrelated individuals. *Am J Hum Genet* 55:69–73.

Bourn D, Evans G, Mason S, Tekes S, Trueman L, and Strachan T. 1995. Eleven novel mutations in the NF2 tumour suppressor gene. *Hum Genet* 95:572–4.

Deguen B, Merel P, Goutebroze L, Giovannini M, Reggio H, Arpin M, Thomas G. 1998. Impaired interaction of naturally occurring mutant NF2 protein with actin-based cytoskeleton and membrane. *Hum Mol Genet* 7:217–26.

den Bakker M, Riegman P, Hekman A, Boersma W, Janssen P, van der Kwast T, and Zwarthoff E. 1995. The product of the NF2 tumour suppresssor gene localizes near the plasma membrane and is highly expressed in muscle cells. *Oncogene* 10:757–63.

Englefield P, Foulkes WD, and Campbell IG. 1994. Loss of heterozygosity on chromosome 22 in ovarian carcinoma is distal to and is not accompanied by mutations in NF2 at 22q12. *Br J Cancer* 70:905–7.

Evans DG, Trueman L, Wallace A, Collins S, and Strachan T. 1998. Genotype/phenotype correlations in type 2 neurofibromatosis (NF2): evidence for more severe disease associated with truncating mutations. *J Med Genet* 35:450–5.

Gonzalez-Agosti C, Xu L, Pinney D, Beauchamp R, Hobbs W, Gusella J, and Ramesh V. 1996. The merlin tumor suppressor localizes preferntially in membrane ruffles. *Oncogene* 13:1239–47.

Gutmann D, Giordano M, Fishback A, and Guha A. 1997. Loss of merlin expression in sporadic meningiomas, ependymomas and schwannomas. *Neurology* 49:267–70.

Haase VH, Trofatter JA, MacCollin M, Tarttelin E, Gusella JF, and Ramesh V. 1994. The murine NF2 homologue encodes a highly conserved merlin protein with alternative forms. *Hum Mol Genet* 3:407–11.

Hara T, Bianchi AB, Seizinger BR, and Kley N. 1994. Molecular cloning and characterization of alternatively spliced transcripts of the mouse neurofibromatosis 2 gene. *Cancer Res* 54:330–5.

Ikeda K, Saeki Y, Gonzalez-Agosti C, Ramesh V, Chiocca EA. 1999. Overexpression of merlin by vector-mediated gene transfer inhibits the proliferation of primary human meningioma cells. In press, *J Neurosurg.*

Jacoby LB, Jones D, Davis K, Kronn D, Short MP, Gusella J, and MacCollin M. 1997. Molecular analysis of the NF2 tumor-suppressor gene in schwannomatosis. *Am J Hum Genet* 61:1293–302.

Jacoby L, MacCollin M, Barone R, Ramesh V, and Gusella J. 1996. Frequency and distribution of NF2 mutations in schwannomas. *Genes Chromosomes Cancer* 17:45–55.

Kanai Y, Tsuda H, Oda T, Sakamoto M, and Hirohashi S. 1995. Analysis of the neurofibromatosis 2 gene in human breast and hepatocellular carcinomas. *Jpn J Clin Oncol* 25:1–4.

Kluwe L, Bayer S, Baser M, Hazim W, Wolfgang H, Funsterer C, and Mautner VF. 1996. Identification of NF2 germ-line mutations and comparison with neurofibromatosis 2 phenotypes. *Hum Genet* 98:534–8.

Kluwe L, MacCollin M, Tatagiba M, Thomas S, Hazim W, Haase W, and Mautner VF. 1998. Phenotypic variability associated with 14 splice-site mutations in the NF2 gene. *Am J Med Genet* 18:228–33.

Lekanne-Deprez RH, Bianchi AB, Groen NA, Seizinger BR, Hagemeijer A, van Drunen E, Bootsma D, Koper JW, Avezaat CJ, Kley N, et al. 1994. Frequent NF2 gene transcript mutations in sporadic meningiomas and vestibular schwannomas. *Am J Hum Genet* 54:1022–9.

Louis DN, Ramesh V, and Gusella JF. 1995. Neuropathology and molecular genetics of neurofibromatosis 2 and related tumors. *Brain Pathol* 5:163–72.

MacCollin M, Braverman N, Viskochil D, Ruttledge M, Davis K, Ojemann R, Gusella J, and Parry D. 1996. A point mutation associated with a severe phenotype of neurofibromatosis 2. *Ann Neurol* 40:440–5.

MacCollin M, Jacoby L, Jones D, Ojemann R, Feit H, and Gusella J. 1997a. Somatic mosaicism of the neurofibromatosis 2 tumor suppressor gene. *Neurology* 48:A429.

MacCollin M, Kronn D, Davis K, Jones D, and Jacoby L. 1997b. Schwannomatosis resulting from somatic mosaicism of the NF2 gene. *Ann Neurol* 42:513.

MacCollin M, Ramesh V, Jacoby LB, Louis DN, Rubio MP, Pulaski K, Trofatter JA, Short MP, Bove C, Eldridge R, et al. 1994. Mutational analysis of patients with neurofibromatosis 2. *Am J Hum Genet* 55:314–20.

McClatchey AI, Saotome I, Mercer K, Crowley D, Gusella JF, Bronson RT, and Jacks T. 1998. Mice heterozygous for a mutation at the NF2 tumor suppressor locus develop a range of highly metastatic tumors. *Genes Dev* 12:1121–33.

Merel P, Khe HX, Sanson M, Bijlsma E, Rouleau G, Laurent-Puig P, Pulst S, Baser M, Lenoir G, Sterkers JM, et al. 1995b. Screening for germ-line mutations in the NF2 gene. *Genes Chromosomes Cancer* 12:117–27.

Parry D, MacCollin M, Kaiser-Kupfer M, Pulaski K, Nicholson HS, Bolesta M, Eldridge R, and Gusella J. 1996. Germline mutations in the neurofibromatosis 2 (NF2) gene: Correlations with disease severity and retinal abnormalities. *Am J Hum Genet* 59:529.

Pelton P, Sherman L, Rizvi T, Marchionni M, Wood P, Friedman R, Ratner N. 1998. Ruffling membrane, stress fiber, cell spreading and proliferation abnormalities in human Schwannoma cells. *Oncogene* 17:2195–209.

Pulst SM, Rouleau GA, Marineau C, Fain P, and Sieb JP. 1993. Familial meningioma is not allelic to neurofibromatosis 2. *Neurology* 43:2096–8.

Rouleau GA, Merel P, Lutchman M, Sanson M, Zucman J, Marineau C, Hoang-Xuan K, Demczuk S, Desmaze C, Plougastel B, et al. 1993. Alteration in a new gene encoding a putative membrane-organizing protein causes neurofibromatosis type 2. *Nature* 363:515–21.

Rouleau GA, Wertelecki W, Haines JL, Hobbs WJ, Trofatter JA, Seizinger BR, Martuza RL, Superneau DW, Conneally PM, and Gusella JF. 1987. Genetic linkage of bilateral acoustic neurofibromatosis to a DNA marker on chromosome 22. *Nature* 329:246–8.

Rubio MP, Correa KM, Ramesh V, MacCollin MM, Jacoby LB, von Deimling A, Gusella JF, and Louis DN. 1994. Analysis of the neurofibromatosis 2 gene in human ependymomas and astrocytomas. *Cancer Res* 54:45–7.

Ruttledge MH, Sarrazin J, Rangaratnam S, Phelan CM, Twist E, Merel P, Delattre O, Thomas G, Nordenskjold M, Collins VP, et al. 1994. Evidence for the complete inactivation of the NF2 gene in the majority of sporadic meningiomas. *Nat Genet* 6:180–4.

Ruttledge M, Andermann A, Phelan C, Claudio J, Han F, Chretien N, Rangaratnam S, MacCollin M, Short MP, Parry D, Michels V, Riccardi V, Weksberg R, Kitamura K, Bradburn J, Hall B, Propping P, and Rouleau G. 1996. Type of mutation in the neurofibromatosis type 2 gene (NF2) frequently determines severity of disease. *Am J Hum Genet* 59:331–42.

Sainz J, Figueroa K, Baser ME, Mautner VF, and Pulst SM. 1995. High frequency of nonsense mutations in the NF2 gene caused by C to T transitions in five CGA codons. *Hum Mol Genet* 4:137–9.

Scherer SS and Gutmann D. 1996. Expression of the neurofibromatosis 2 tumor suppressor gene product, merlin, in Schwann cells. *J Neurosci Res* 46:595–605.

Scoles DR, Baser ME, and Pulst SM. 1996. A missense mutation in the neurofibromatosis 2 gene occurs in patients with mild and severe phenotypes. *Neurology* 47:544–6.

Seizinger BR, Rouleau G, Ozelius LJ, Lane AH, St George-Hyslop P, Huson S, Gusella JF, and Martuza RL. 1987. Common pathogenetic mechanism for three tumor types in bilateral acoustic neurofibromatosis. *Science* 236:317–9.

Sekido Y, Pass HI, Bader S, Mew DJ, Christman MF, Gazdar AF, and Minna JD. 1995. Neurofibromatosis type 2 (NF2) gene is somatically mutated in mesothelioma but not in lung cancer. *Cancer Res* 55:1227–31.

Stangl A, Wellenreuther R, Lenartz D, Kraus J, Menon A, Schramm J, Wiestler O, and von Deimling A. 1997. Clonality of multiple meningiomas. *J Neurosurg* 86:853–8.

Stemmer-Rachamimmov AO, Xu L, Gonzalez-Agosti C, Burwick J, Pinney D, Beauchamp R, Jacoby L, Gusella J, Ramesh V, and Louis D. 1997a. Universal absence of merlin, but not other ERM family members, in schwannomas. *Am J Pathol* 151:1649–54.

Stemmer-Rachamimmov AO, Gonzalez-Agosti C, Xu L, Burwick JA, Beauchamp R, Pinney D, Louis DN, and Ramesh V. 1997b. Expression of NF2 encoded Merlin and related ERM family proteins in the human central nervous system. *J Neuropathol Exp Neurol* 56:735–42.

Trofatter JA, MacCollin MM, Rutter JL, Murrell JR, Duyao MP, Parry DM, Eldridge R, Kley N, Menon AG, Pulaski K, et al. 1993. A novel moesin-, ezrin-, radixin-like gene is a candidate for the neurofibromatosis 2 tumor suppressor. *Cell* 72:791–800. [Published erratum appears in *Cell* 1993 75(4):826.]

Tsukita S, Yonemura S, and Tsukita S. 1997. ERM (ezrin/radixin/moesin) family: from cytoskeleton to signal transduction. *Curr Opin in Cell Biol* 9:70–5.

Watkins D, Ruttledge MH, Sarrazin J, Rangaratnam S, Poisson M, Delattre JY, and Rouleau GA. 1996. Loss of heterozygosity on chromsome 22 in human gliomas does not inactivate the neurofibromatosis type 2 gene. *Cancer Genet Cytogenet* 92:73–8.

Watson CJ, Gaunt L, Evans G, Patel K, Harris R, and Strachan T. 1993. A disease-associated germline deletion maps the type 2 neurofibromatosis (NF2) gene between the Ewing sarcoma region and the leukaemia inhibitory factor locus. *Hum Mol Genet* 2:701–4.

Wellenreuther R, Kraus JA, Lenartz D, Menon AG, Schramm J, Louis DN, Ramesh V, Gusella JF, Wiestler OD, and von Deimling A. 1995. Analysis of the neurofibromatosis 2 gene reveals molecular variants of meningioma. *Am J Pathol* 146:827–32.

Wellenreuther R, Waha A, Vogel Y, Lenartz D, Schramm J, Wiestler OD, and von Deimling A. 1997. Quantitative analysis of neurofibromatosis type 2 gene transcripts in meningiomas supports the concept of distinct molecular variants. *Lab Invest* 77:601–6.

Welling DB, Guida M, Goll F, Pearl DK, Glasscock ME, Pappas DG, Linthicum FH, Rogers D, and Prior T. 1996. Mutational spectrum in the neurofibromatosis type 2 gene in sporadic and familial schwannomas. *Hum Genet* 98:189–93.

Xu H and Gutmann D. 1998. Merlin differentially associates with the microtubule and actin cytoskeleton. *J Neurosci Res* 51:403–15.

Appendix

Resources for Patients and Their Families

SUPPORT GROUPS

Many patients and families with neurofibromatosis benefit from referral to a lay support group (Albon 1996; Benjamin et al. 1993; Huson and Upadhyaya 1994). Affected families may feel isolated, especially if their regular physician is not familiar with neurofibromatosis. Support groups provide an opportunity for individuals and families with neurofibromatosis to share experiences, concerns, and solutions to problems related to the disease. Support groups also serve as advocates for patients with neurofibromatosis and can help them obtain necessary services. One of the most important functions of support groups is promoting an understanding of neurofibromatosis in society as a whole. In addition, support groups enable affected families to participate in fund-raising and research related to neurofibromatosis.

Table A-1 lists some national neurofibromatosis support organizations. The table also includes telephone numbers and World Wide Web addresses for these organizations. The contact information may change, but Web sites maintained by these organizations often include current links to the others. Many of the larger national support organizations have chapters or affiliates throughout the country. Contact information for local affiliates can be obtained from the appropriate national office. The International Neurofibromatosis Association serves as an umbrella organization for the various national neurofibromatosis support groups. Information on the International Neurofibromatosis Association can be obtained from the National Neurofibromatosis Foundation in the United States.

PATIENT EDUCATION MATERIALS

Educational materials are available for patients with neurofibromatosis and their families from many of the NF support groups and, in the United States, from the March of Dimes. In addition, many national neurofibromatosis organizations and their local affiliates publish informative newsletters. The Internet has a great deal of information on neurofibromatosis. The quality of the available material varies from anecdotal to authoritative. Some of the information is incorrect or out of date. The Web sites maintained by the National Neurofibromatosis Foundation (www.nf.org) and Massachusetts General Hospital (neurosurgery.mgh.harvard. edu/NFR) are especially useful. The Internet also provides access to many bulletin boards and other resources designed to put affected families in contact with each other.

Table A–1. Some national neurofibromatosis support groups

Country	Organization	Telephone	World Wide Web and/or e-mail Address
Australia	Neuro-fibroma-tosis Association of Australia, Inc.	02 9628 5044	R.Pynor@echs.usyd.edu.au
Belgium	Association Belge pour personnes atteintes de la neurofibromatose	32.3.766.13.41	
Denmark	Dansk Forening for Neurfibromatosis Recklinghausen	45 3167 0367	
Germany	Von Recklinghausen Gesellschaft e. V.	040/52 71-2822	VRGes@aol.com
Italy	Assocazione Neurofibromatosi	0521.771457	
	Lottiamo Insieme per la NeuroFibromatosi Associazione	049/8213528	
Switzerland	Goupe d'entraide romand—NF	022-794 56 23	
United Kingdom	The Neurofibromatosis Foundation	0181-547-1636	www.nfa.zetnet.co.uk e-mail: nfa@zetnet.co.uk
United States	The National Neurofibromatosis Foundation, Inc.	800-323-7938 or 212-344-6633	www.nf.org e-mail:NNFF@nf.org
	Neurofibromatosis, Inc.	800-942-6825 or 301-577-8984	www.nfinc.org e-mail: NFInc1@aol.com
	The Acoustic Neuroma Assoication	404-237-8023	www.anausa.org e-mail ANAusa@aol.com

REFERENCES

Albon J. 1996. Gender response to neurofibromatosis 1. *Soc Sci Med* 42:99–109.

Benjamin CM, Colley A, Donnai D, Kingston H, Harris R, and Kerzin-Storrar L. 1993. Neurofibromatosis type 1 (NF1): knowledge, experience, and reproductive decision of affected patients and families. *J Med Genet* 30:567–74.

Huson SM and Upadhyaya M. 1994. Neurofibromatosis 1: clinical management and genetic counselling. In: Huson SM and Hughes RAC, eds *The Neurofibromatoses: A Pathogenic and Clinical Overview*. London: Chapman & Hall, pp. 355–81.

Index

Page numbers in *italics* denote figures; those followed by "t" denote tables.